Ovarian Cancer

UICC Monograph Series · Volume 11

Ovarian Cancer

Edited by

F. Gentil · A. C. Junqueira

With 126 figures

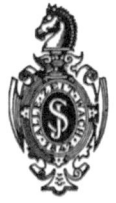

Springer-Verlag Berlin Heidelberg New York 1968

Dr. F. Gentil and Dr. A. C. Junqueira
Cancer Institute, Hospital A. C. Camargo, São Paulo/Brasil

ISBN 978-3-642-87757-5   ISBN 978-3-642-87755-1 (eBook)
DOI 10.1007/978-3-642-87755-1

Title-No. 7522

Foreword

The incidence of ovarian cancer has progressively increased during the past decade, and its mortality rate has followed a similar course. Conversely, in cancer of the uterine cervix, the mortality rate has diminished. Detection and early diagnosis have been the two responsible factors in achieving the decrease in the number of deaths occurring in cancer of the cervix. The reverse is true in cancer of the ovary: diagnosis as a rule is only established late, when dissemination has already occurred, thus making the control of the disease much more difficult.

Clinical staging thus far has not been in use at many centers, and it therefore becomes very difficult to compare results of treatment since we do not know the exact anatomical extent of the disease.

Histopathological classification in cancer of the ovary is still a very controversial subject and a uniform terminology is urgently required.

Management of patients with cancer of the ovary varies widely from one institution to another. There is no agreement as to how to treat an ovarian neoplasm; by surgery alone, or, by using radiation and chemotherapy as a complement to the operative treatment.

In an effort to shed more light on these items, the Patient Care Committee of the UICC held this symposium, which was unique in the broadness of its scope pertaining to every phase of ovarian cancer.

The M.D. Anderson Hospital was chosen as the site of the symposium for two very important reasons: 1. because Dr. R. Lee Clark, its director, is a member of the Patient Care Committee, and 2. because of the important contributions this institution has made in the field of modern cancerology.

We would like to take this opportunity on behalf of the UICC to express our deep gratitude to the M. D. Anderson Hospital for the facilities and the hospitality extended to us, and our sincere appreciation to all the participants.

Fernando Gentil
Antonio C. Junqueira

Table of Contents

U.I.C.C. Patient Care Committee Members

1962—1966

Dr. FERNANDO GENTIL (Chairman), São Paulo, Brasil

Dr. ANTONIO CARLOS JUNQUEIRA (Secretary), São Paulo, Brasil

Dr. GEORGE T. PACK, New York, U.S.A.

Dr. H. L. KOTTMEIER, Stockholm, Sweden

Dr. MASSARU KURU, Tokyo, Japan

Dr. R. LEE CLARK, jr., Texas, U.S.A.

Dr. MARTIN MIQUEO NARANCIO, Montevideo, Uruguay

Dr. ELPIDIO VALENCIA, Manila, Philippines

Dr. MARIO MARGOTTINI, Rome, Italy

Dr. V. I. YANISHEVSKY (Professor), Moscow, U.S.S.R.

Participants

F. GENTIL, M.D., Chairman, Chief of Surgical Service, Cancer Institute, Hospital A. C. Camargo, São Paulo, Brasil

A. C. JUNQUEIRA, M.D., Secretary, Chief of Service, Clinical Research on Radiotherapy and Chemotherapy, Cancer Institute, Hospital A. C. Camargo, Assistant. Department of Pharmacology. São Paulo Medical School, São Paulo, Brasil

G. BRULÉ, M.D., Chief of Solid Tumor Chemotherapy Service, Institut Gustave-Roussy (Villejuif), Paris, France

A. BRUNSCHWIG, M.D., Chief of Gynecology, Memorial, James Ewing Hospitals, New York City, U.S.A.

B. BURNS, jr., M.D., Associate Gynecologist — Section of Gynecology — Department of Surgery, The University of Texas M.D. Anderson Hospital and Tumor Institute, Houston, Texas, U.S.A.

I. DAVIDSOHN, M.D., Professor and Chairman, Department of Pathology, Chicago Medical School Director, Department of Experimental Pathology, Mount Sinai Hospital Medical Center, Chicago, Illinois, U.S.A.

L. DELCLOS, M.D., Associate Radiotherapist and Associate Professor of Radiology, The University of Texas M.D. Anderson Hospital and Tumor Institute Houston, Texas, U.S.A.

G. FLETCHER, M.D., Chief Radiotherapist and Professor of Radiology, The University of Texas M.D. Anderson Hospital and Tumor Institute, Houston, Texas, U.S.A.

J. GRAHAM, M.D., Head, Department of Gynecology, Roswell Park Memorial Institute, Buffalo, New York, U.S.A.

R. GRAHAM, D.Sc., Associate Gynecologist and Cytologist, Roswell Park Memorial Institute, Buffalo, New York, U.S.A.

G. GRICOUROFF, M.D., Head of the Pathological Department, Foundation Curie, Paris, France

H. L. KOTTMEIER, M.D., Professor of Gynecology, Radiumhemmet, Stockholm, Sweden

M. LENZ, M.D., Professor Emeritus of Clinical Radiology, Columbia University, Consultant Radiotherapist — Presbyterian and Montefiore Hospitals, New York City, U.S.A.

A. Luisi, M.D., Pathologist, Cancer Institute, Hospital A. C. Camargo — São Paulo, Brasil

J. H. Muller, M.D., Chief of the Departments of Radiology and Pathology, Universitäts-Frauenklinik, Zürich, Switzerland

* Prof. L. A. Novikova, Head, Department of Gynecology, Institut Experimentalnoy i Klinicheskoy Onkologii, Academia Meditsinkikh Nauk, Moscow, U.S.S.R.

S. S. Roberts, M.D., Attending Surgeon and Acting Head of Department, Illinois Research & Educational Hospitals, Associate Professor of Surgery and Acting Head of Department, University of Illinois, College of Medicine, Chicago, Illinois, U.S.A.

F. Rutledge, M.D., Chief, Section of Gynecology — Department of Surgery, The University of Texas M.D. Anderson Hospital and Tumor Institute, Houston, Texas, U.S.A.

* Prof. L. Santesson, M.D., Director, Department of Pathology, Radiumhemmet, Stockholm, Sweden

R. E. Scully, M.D., Pathologist, Massachusetts General Hospital, Associate Clinical Professor of Pathology, Harvard Medical School, Boston, Massachusetts, U.S.A.

Prof. G. Teilum, M.D., Director, University Institute of Pathological Anatomy, Copenhagen, Denmark

    * Contributed paper but did not attend.

General Classification of Ovarian Tumours

L. SANTESSON, M. D.

Director, Department of Pathology, Radiumhemmet, Stockholm, Sweden

H. L. KOTTMEIER, M. D.

Professor of Gynecology, Department of Pathology, Radiumhemmet, Stockholm, Sweden

Introduction

Ovarian cancer is not an entity but a group of diseases. Studies of the results of treatment must be based on homogenous groups of tumours and not on mixtures of histologically and biologically different tumour types. Furthermore, there still exists a considerable degree of confusion as to which tumours should be considered as true carcinomas. It is the lack of generally accepted definitions of the various histological forms that has resulted in the extreme differences in long-term results given by various authors. The importance of establishing a standardized, internationally accepted classification of ovarian tumours, so that the results of different clinics may be accurately compared, is obvious.

Since WALDEYER, in 1870, presented a classification partly based on histogenesis, many classifications of ovarian neoplasms, emphasizing different features of these tumours, have been given. As our knowledge of the complex ovarian structures has increased, the different systems of classification have been changed and the fundamental tumour types been more and more clearly defined.

Classification

Among the ovarian neoplasms, those related to the Müllerian epithelium constitute the vast majority of real ovarian tumours.

They consist of the serous and the mucinous cystomas and the endometrioid tumour types. It is obvious that the classification of these, the most common, primary epithelial tumours of the ovary, must be as concise and clearly delineated as possible, both as to the division among the three types and to the borderline between benign and malignant tumours in each tumour type. Experience has shown that *between obviously benign and obviously malignant neoplasms there exists a group of tumours that, in their clinical behaviour, resemble true carcinomas in as much as they give rise to implantation-metastases and ascites — but have quite a different course.* The general epithelial structures are maintained as in benign tumours but the epithelial cells show signs of proliferative activity, nuclear abnormalities and pathological mitosis. However, there is no visible evidence of infiltrative destructive growth in the connective tissue of the growth. The outcome in these cases is quite different from that of true carcinomas, which is why it is essential to separate tumours of proliferating cystadenomas without stromal invasion from the ovarian cancers (Figs. 1 and 2).

Fig. 3 gives the survival rate in cases of seropapillary cystoma of low potential malignancy compared with the rate in serous carcinomas. Unfortunately many

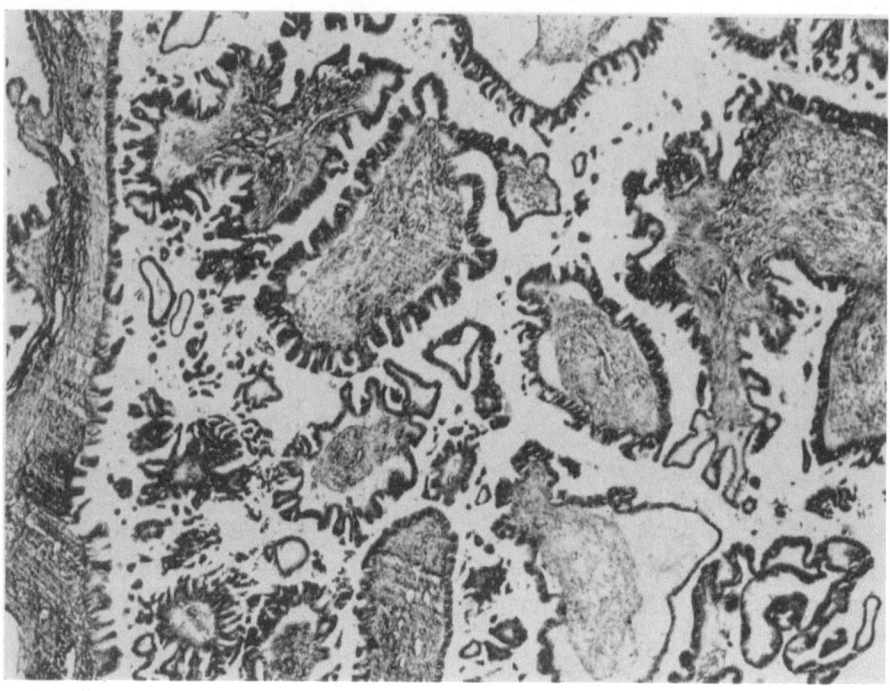

Fig. 1. Patient H. R., age 26. Ovarian tumour. Proliferating serous papillary cystadenoma, "possibly malignant", (Ib). Primary tumour. Photo-micrograph ×90

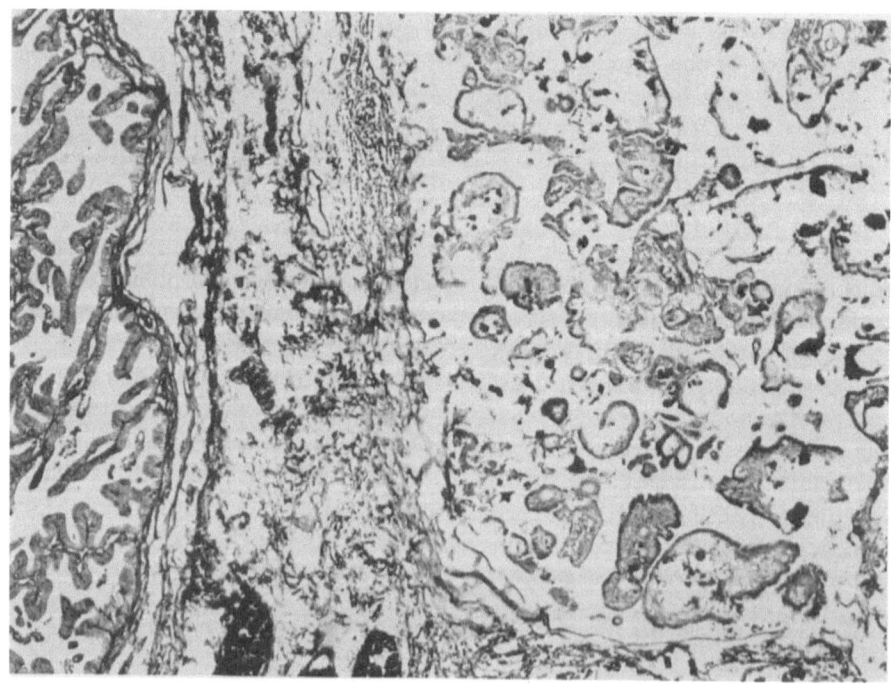

Fig. 2. Same as Fig. 1. Implantation in the tube × 90

clinicians do not separate cases of so-called questionable cancer from true. carcinomas; for this reasons an estimate of the results attained is impossible.

It is true that patients with a possibly malignant cystadenoma may occasion-ally succumb to the disease without the neoplasm having developed into an in-filtrative destructive growth. Further studies are required to establish in detail the cellular structures of these tumours (Figs. 4 and 5). It is also possible that

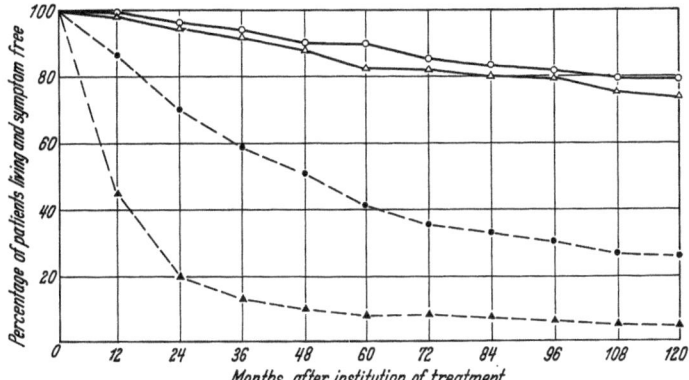

Fig. 3. Survival rate of cystomas 10year (375 cases)

——○—— Low potential malignancy: surgically completely removed (54 cases).   ——▵—— Low potential malignancy: surgically not completely removed (75 cases).   ⋯⋯•⋯⋯ Carcinomas: surgically completely removed (96 cases).   ⋯⋯▴⋯⋯ Carcinomas: surgically not completely removed (150 cases)

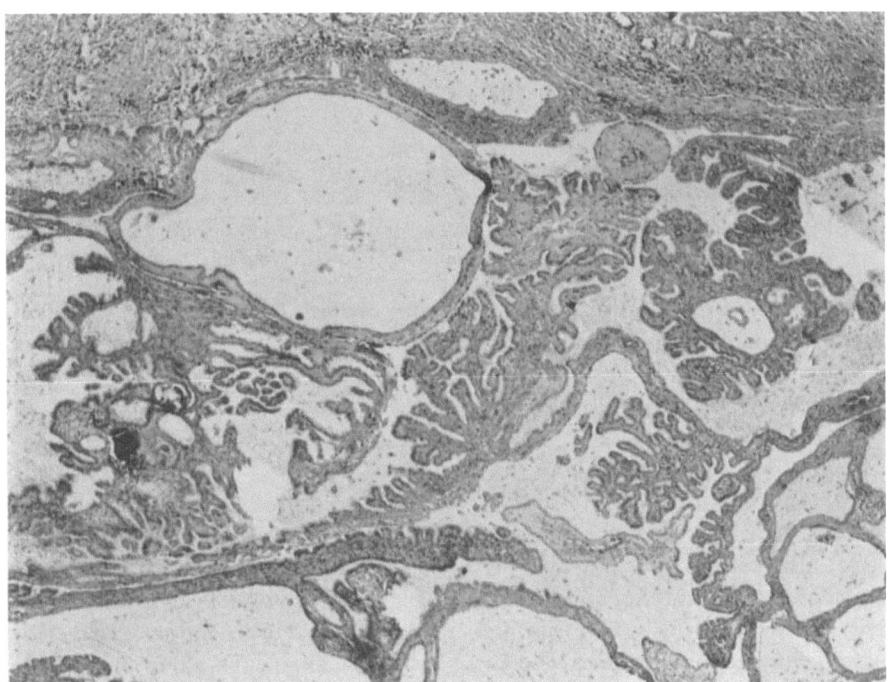

Fig. 4. Patient E. J., age 45. Ovarian tumour. Proliferating serous papillary cystadenoma, "possibly malignant", (Ib). Primary tumour. Photo-micrograph ×50

1*

in some cases the implantation metastases may regress, while in others the
tumour may spread and kill the patient.

Clinical and histological malignancy
does not always correspond in mucinous
tumours. Occasionally a benign muci-

these tumours have been designated as
endometrioid in order to point out that
endometrioid carcinoma structurally resembles adenocarcinoma of the endometrium.

Endometrioid carcinoma occurred in
as much as 30.3 per cent of 911 *true*

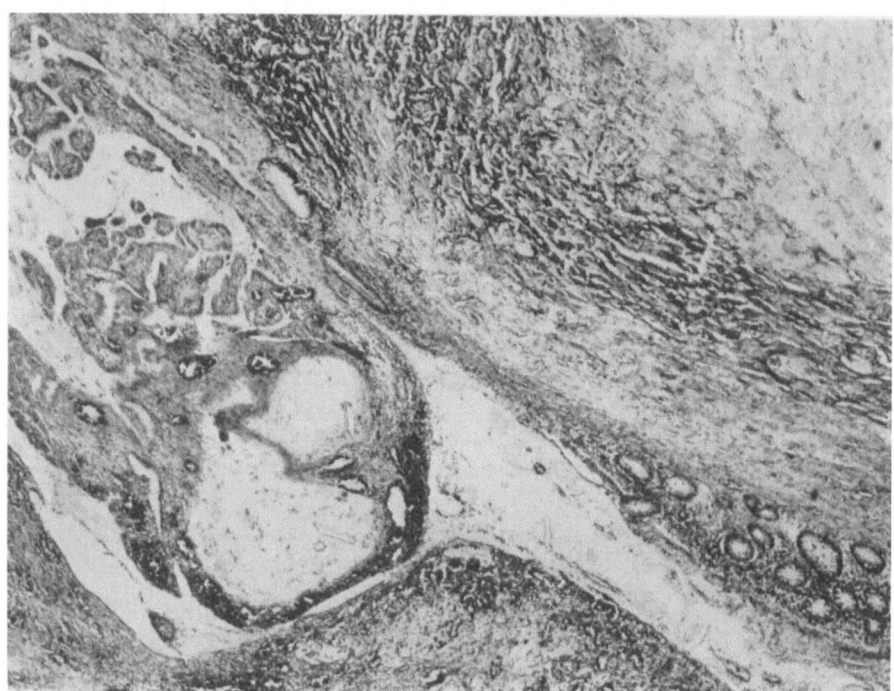

Fig. 5. Same as Fig. 4. Malignant growth through the colon wall. Note sero-papillary tumour in the
intestinal lumen adjacent to normal mucosa. Photo-micrograph × 50

nous growth may rupture and give rise
to pseudomyxoma peritonei, which will
kill the patient. Nevertheless, it is *important to subdivide the tumours with regard
to the histopathological pattern.*

During a study to determine the
relative prognostic significance of different types of ovarian carcinoma, it was
noted that neoplasms resembling adenocarcinoma of the endometrium appeared
to have a better prognosis than serous
and undifferentiated carcinomas (Figs.
6, 7). In the histopathological classification of epithelial ovarian tumours proposed by the International Federation of
Gynecology and Obstetrics (Table I),

ovarian carcinomas treated at the Radiumhemmet in 23 years. The figure is
remarkably high. Long and Taylor
give a figure of 16.7 per cent in
120 cases examined. Endometrioid carcinomas do not produce symptoms
pathognomonic of this tumour. In contrast to serous carcinomas, the tumour
remains for a long time in the true pelvis
and grows slowly. Distant metastases
appear rather late in endometrioid neoplasms. This explains partly the higher
survival rate for endometrioid carcinomas. Fig. 8b gives the 10-year survival
rate in 216 cases of serous, 38 of mucinous, 201 of endometrioid and 47 cases

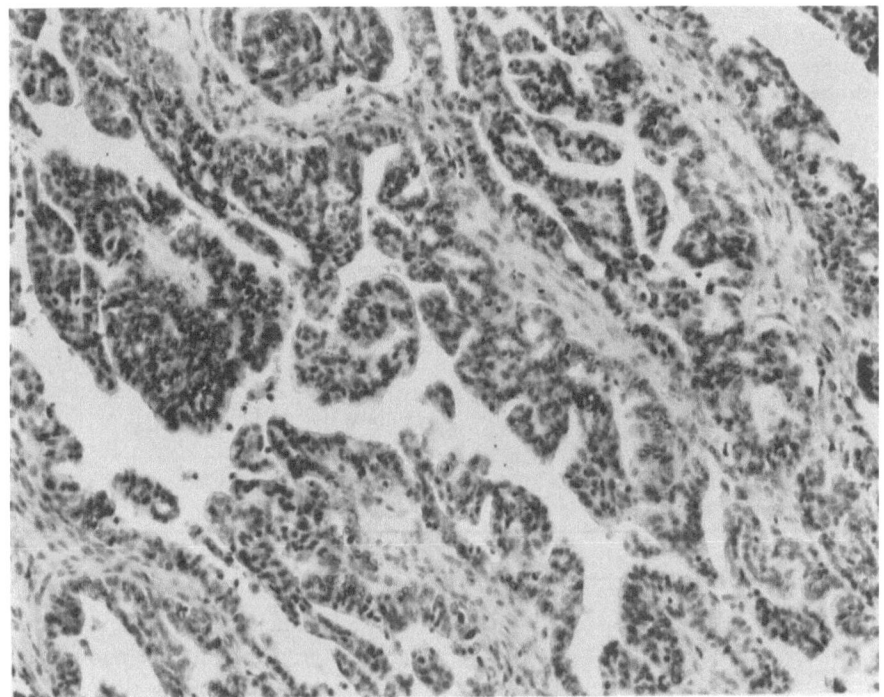

Fig. 6. Patient J. O., age 57. Ovarian tumour. Endometrioid carcinoma (IIIc). Highly differentiated with adenomatous structures similar to endometrial carcinoma. Photo-micrograph × 225

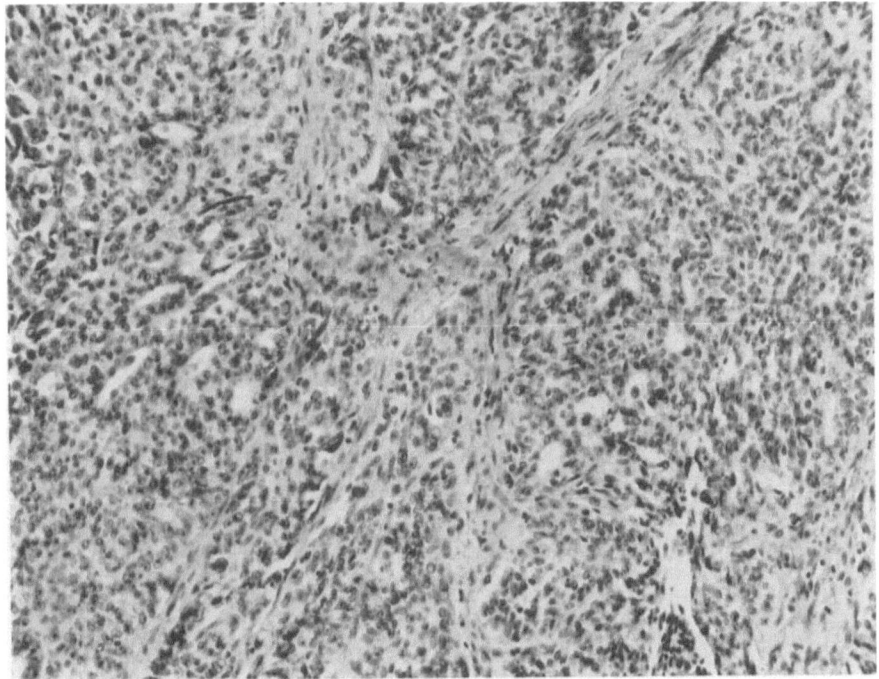

Fig. 7. Same as Fig. 6. Area with moderate differentiation. Predominantly solid structures. Photo-micrograph × 225

I. *Serous cystomas*

a) Serous benign cystadenomas

b) Serous cystadenomas with proliferating activity of the epithelial cells and nuclear abnormalities but with no infiltrative destructive growth (low potential malignancy)

c) Serous cystadenocarcinomas

II. *Mucinous cystomas*

a) Mucinous benign cystadenomas

b) Mucinous cystadenomas with proliferating activity of the epithelial cells and nuclear abnormalities but with no infiltrative destructive growth (low potential malignancy)

c) Mucinous cystadenocarcinomas

III. *Endometrioid tumours* (similar to adenocarcinomas in the endometrium)

a) Endometrioid benign cysts

b) Endometrioid tumours with proliferating activity of the epithelial cells and nuclear abnormalities but with no infiltrative destructive growth (low potential malignancy)

c) Endometrioid adenocarcinomas

IV. *Concomitant carcinomas, unclassified carcinomas* (tumours which cannot be allotted to any of the groups I, II, or III).

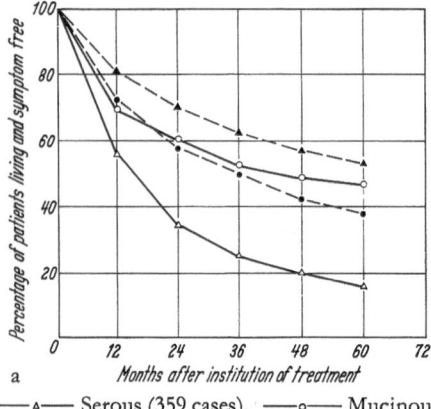

a

Months after institution of treatment

——▲—— Serous (359 cases). ——○—— Mucinous (66 cases). ······▲······ Endometrioid (276 cases). ······●······ Mesonephroid (66 cases)

of mesonephroid carcinoma treated at the Radiumhemmet. The remarkable differences in survival rate show the importance of separating the cases with regard to the histopathological pattern.

SANTESSON was the first to indicate the relatively high incidence of endometrioid carcinoma. Since the first publication by HERXHEIMER (1907) only a small number of similar tumours, presumably deriving from endometriosis, have been reported by many authors. In 1954 DOCKERTY applied the term endometrial-like carcinoma to a group of

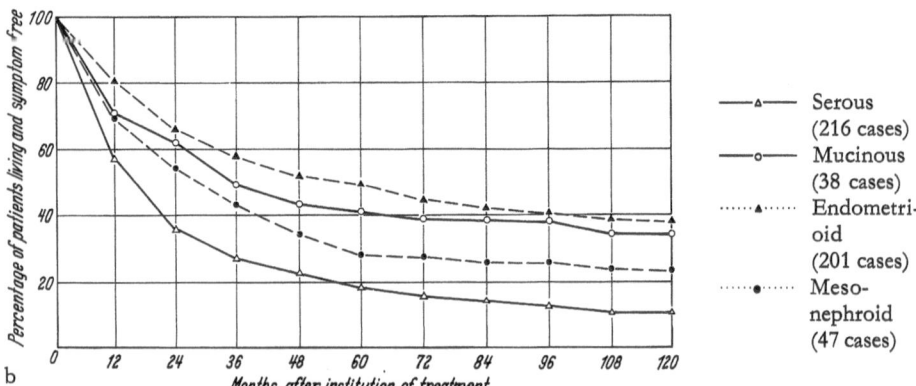

b

Months after institution of treatment

——▲—— Serous (216 cases)

——○—— Mucinous (38 cases)

······▲······ Endometrioid (201 cases)

······●······ Mesonephroid (47 cases)

Fig. 8a and b. a) 5-year survival rates of ovarian carcinoma (767 cases). b) 10-year survival rates of ovarian carcinoma (502 cases) ovarian neoplasms. It seems probable that endometrioid carcinomas derive from ovarian endometriosis although only occasionally can this source be proved. However, benign endometriosis was seen in about 30 per cent of 276 patients with endometrioid carcinoma treated at the Radiumhemmet.

As to the endometrioid carcinomas, cases of endometrioid "carcinomas" of low potential malignancy are rare compared with the number of corresponding serous and mucinous tumours in the Radiumhemmet series.

In Table II are reported cases of semimalignant and malignant ovarian

Table II. *Ovarian neoplasms treated at Radiumhemmet in the years 1921 through 1940, 1953, 1954, 1958 and 1959*

	No. of cases	Per cent of all cases
Germ cell tumour	78	5.7
Granulosa and theca cell tumour	109	8.0
Serous "carcinoma" low potential malignancy.	174	12.8 ⎱ 39.2
Serous true carcinoma	359	26.4 ⎰
Mucinous "carcinoma" low potential malignancy	71	5.2 ⎱ 10.0
Mucinous true carcinoma	66	4.8 ⎰
Endometrioid "carcinoma" low potential malignancy	12	0.9 ⎱ 21.0
Endometrioid true carcinoma	276	20.1 ⎰
Mesonephroid "carcinoma" low potential malignancy	6	0.4 ⎱ 5.2
Mesonephroid true carcinoma	66	4.8 ⎰
Undifferentiated carcinoma	57	4.2
Metastatic carcinoma	87	6.4
Total number of cases	1361	

The coexistence of ovarian and uterine carcinoma is not at all infrequent and is seen especially in cases of endometrioid ovarian carcinoma. In the individual patient, it may be impossible to decide which organ was the primary site of the cancer. Previously such cases were reported as carcinoma uteri and ovary. Sometimes the carcinoma may be of multicentric origin as indicated especially by HUBER. We have considered it wise to regard the ovarian neoplasm as the primary growth when symptoms and clinical findings indicate an ovarian disease. In 89 of 276 cases of endometrioid carcinoma, microscopic examination of the endometrium revealed an adenocarcinoma. The survival rate in these cases is remarkably enough, similar to that in pure endometrioid carcinomas.

tumours treated at the Radiumhemmet in the years 1921 through 1940, 1953, 1954, 1958 and 1959. Only neoplasms histologically proved are included in the series. All slides have been reviewed.

We have emphasized the significance of keeping endometrioid neoplasms separated from serous and mucinous tumours. Serous tumours amount to 39.2 per cent, endometrioid to 21 per cent and mucinous to 10 per cent of 1,361 neoplasms treated at the Radiumhemmet.

Seventy-two cases have been considered to be of mesonephric type. This neoplasm is characterized by large, clear cuboidal cells and resembles in other respects an adenocarcinoma. The clinical course of a mesonephric carcinoma corresponds to that of an endometrioid growth. It is essential to separate mesonephric carcinomas from the so-called mesonephromas of Schiller, which are of germ cell origin and are the subject of presentation by TEILUM in this book.

Even though a careful examination is made of the ovarian growth, there will remain a group of carcinomas which cannot be classified as being of serous, mucinous, endometrioid or mesonephric type. A neoplasm of this type that cannot be allotted to any of the four types mentioned should be reported as an unclassified carcinoma. The Radiumhemmet series includes 57 such tumours, i.e. 4.2 per cent.

From a histopathological and clinical point of view it is essential to separate metastatic carcinomas, sarcomas, teratomas, germ cell tumours and functioning tumours from the neoplasms related to the Müllerian epithelium. Occasionally it is difficult to decide whether the carcinoma is primary in the ovary or metastatic.

Granulosa cell tumour is the most common of functioning ovarian neoplasms. Unfortunately these tumours are often designated as granulosa cell carcinomas and are included in therapeutic statistics on ovarian carcinoma. Granulosa cell tumours grow slowly but may metastasize. There does not seem to exist a correlation between clinical course and histological type. However, the incidence of recurrences is much greater in sarcomatoid than in folliculoid and cylindromatous tumours. This is why a division of the cases with regard to the histological structures is desirable from a prognostic and therapeutic point of view. An important clinical observation is that, usually, recurrences do not appear until many years after the primary tumour was removed. Occasionally it is difficult to distinguish a sarcomatoid granulosa cell tumour from a Krukenberg carcinoma. The differential diagnosis between a cellular thecoma and a

sarcomatoid granulosa cell tumour may require special staining of the fibrils. The correct diagnosis is important as in general the thecoma is a benign growth, while recurrences have occurred in 70 per cent of sarcomatoid granulosa cell tumours treated at Radiumhemmet.

In our survey of ovarian neoplasms, attention has not been paid to such tumours as dermoids, benign ovarian cysts, fibromas, Brenner tumours, etc. All these growths should be separated from other ovarian neoplasms in statistics. Brenner tumour is, in our experience, a benign growth although, sometimes, it is seen in connection with especially mucinous carcinomas.

Finally, we refer to the various types of non-neoplastic cysts of the ovary. We do not intend to discuss the classification of these benign lesions but we would like to emphasize that the differential diagnosis between a non-neoplastic cyst and an incipient malignant tumour may be difficult. A needle biopsy through the vagina or the rectum may help to clarify the diagnosis.

Summary

The need for a standardized, internationally accepted histologic classification of ovarian tumours is emphasized. The variation in long-term results reported by different authors is the result of a lack of uniform definition of the many histological types of tumours found in this site. Criteria for classification of the most common primary epithelial tumours, the serous and mucinous cystomas and the endometrioid tumour type, as well as the so-called borderline neoplasms, should be carefully delineated because of the difference in prognosis. Statistics from the Radiumhemmet are presented to show the difference in results obtained for patients with the different types of tumours.

Malignant Ovarian Tumours of Mullerian Origin: Some Aspects

Antonio Luisi, M. D.

Titular de Patologia, Instituto Central Hospital A.C. Camargo, São Paulo, Brasil

Introduction

The fundamentals of nomenclature and the classification of tumours are based on histopathology; the identification of these tumours is established by comparison between their microscopic structure and the standard features of the corresponding normal tissues. The more the structure of a given tumour varies from the normal, the more difficult the recognition of the primary tissue and, consequently, the proper classification and identification of the neoplasm becomes. This is the explanation for a number of neoplasms not specifically diagnosed, for, since histopathologic identification is based solely on morphological grounds, to recognize tumours without these identifying features would be impossible.

The study of the ovarian tumours is particularly difficult, since the morphological relations of the tumour with the normal components of the gonad are not as yet established or have not been recognized; this fact leads to different interpretations of the same microscopic picture.

In view of this lack of morphological correlation, we may study the microscopic features of neoplasms, comparing them with the evolutionary phases of embryonic development. This method is important and its fundamentals are based on the theory that neoplasms are tissular proliferations that repeat, in those arising in the ovary, the various phases of the urogenital ridge development (Bassis, 1960).

Histopathological examination of some ovarian tumours has disclosed features similar to those of the tubal, endometrial and endocervical epithelia. When this resemblance and the derivation of the Fallopian tube and the uterus from the Müllerian ducts are considered, the logical conclusion is that those ovarian tumours reproducing these structures are of Müllerian origin.

The histogenetic explanation is based either on the presence of embryonic residues of the Müllerian ducts in the ovaries or, what is more widely accepted, on the fact that the superficial epithelium and the subjacent stroma, having the same origin as the Müllerian ducts, have the potentiality of reproducing the same structures. This potentiality is exemplified in Fig. 1, 2 and 3.

The epithelial tumours of the ovary that resemble the tubal epithelium are the serous tumours. There is practically unanimity among the authors that these tumours are of Müllerian origin. The likeness is such that Barzillai (1949) proposed the designation of *Endosalpingioma* for one kind of these serous tumours and adopted as a subtitle the expression *Benign seropapillary tumour of the ovary of Müllerian tubal type.*

The ovarian tumours reproducing endometrial features are generally designed as *endometrioid tumours*. The interpretation of their origin is variable, depending upon several concepts of the origin of the endometrial elements detected in the ovary. Two concepts are that the source can be (1) *local*, because of the potentiality of the superficial epithelium and of the ovarian stroma, or else the Müllerian embryonal residues; (2) *distant*, by transtubal implantation

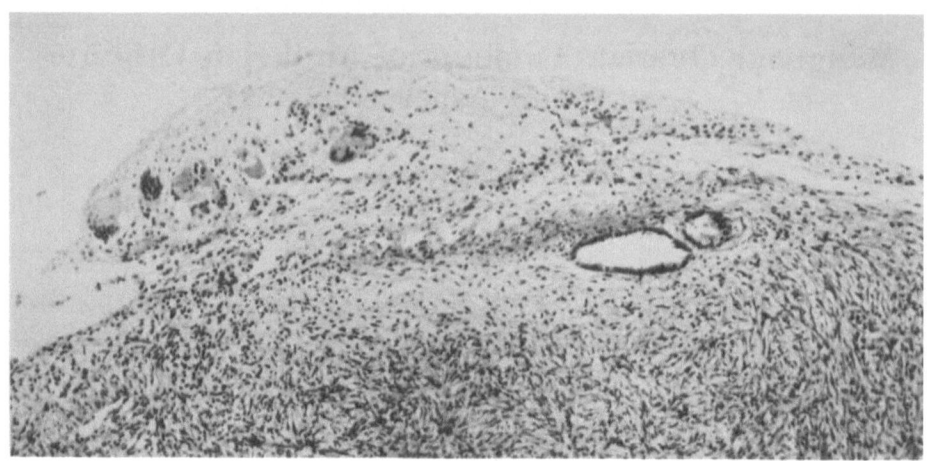

Fig. 1. Microcysts derived from the superficial ovarian epithelium, with serous and mucinous cells. The granulomatous reaction is incidental. HE

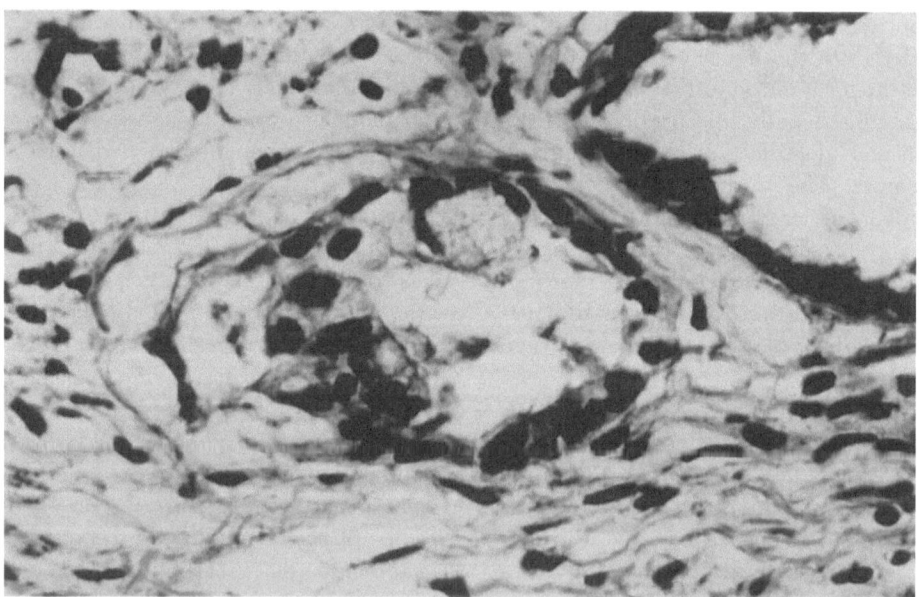

Fig. 2. Detailed aspect of the same preparation showing the serous and mucinous cells. HE

through the haematogenic route or, as advocated by Gricouroff (1939), by lymphatic embolism.

The third large group of Müllerian tumours is made up of mucinous tumours, which would embody the endocervical aspect of the potentiality of the paramesonephric ducts. The histologic

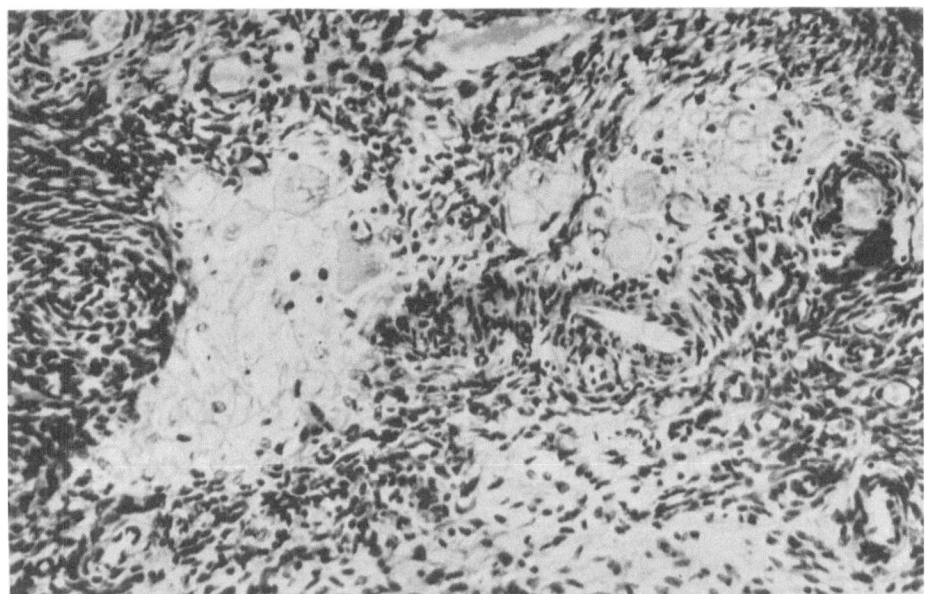

Fig. 3. Pseudo-decidual reaction of the subjacent ovarian stromal cells. HE

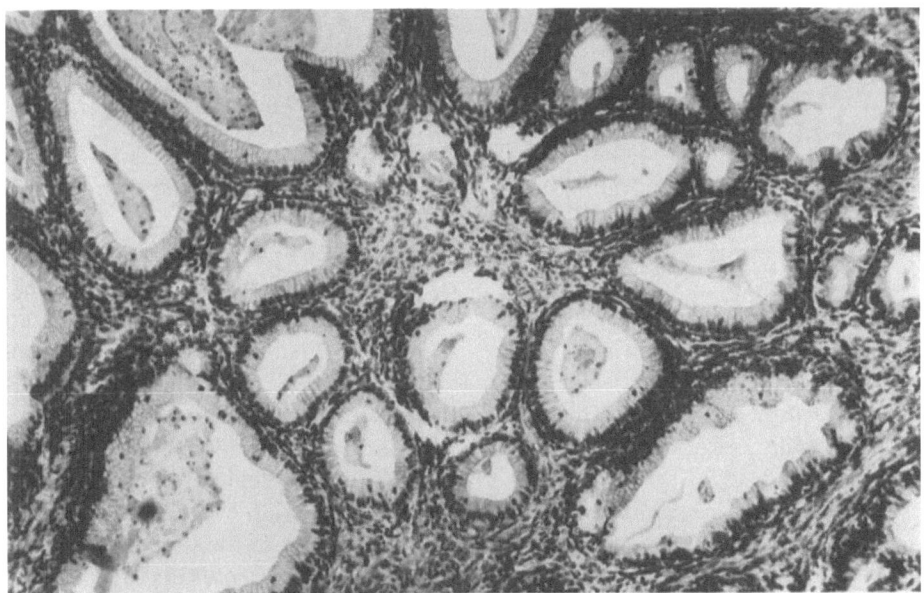

Fig. 4. Proliferating mucinous cystadenoma, possibly malignant. HE

resemblance to the endocervical epithelium is, at times, only apparent and therefore does not mean a morphological and histogenetic identity (Fig. 4).

When the argentaffin reaction is employed, some of the mucinous ovarian tumours disclose the presence of cells that spontaneously reduce the argentic salts and which are not to be found in the endocervical epithelium (Fig. 5).

Therefore, this method affords the distinction of two heterogenetic types of mucinous tumours of the ovary: one of Müllerian origin, presenting no argentaffin cells, and another including this sort of cells and consequently of different origin — the unilateral evolution of a teratoma, particularly of the intestinal

Classification

We shall review briefly some of the classifications so far presented for the Müllerian tumours of the ovary.

The first author who attempted to bring this group into a system was SCHILLER (1940). In his classification, he placed the tubal, endometrial and endo-

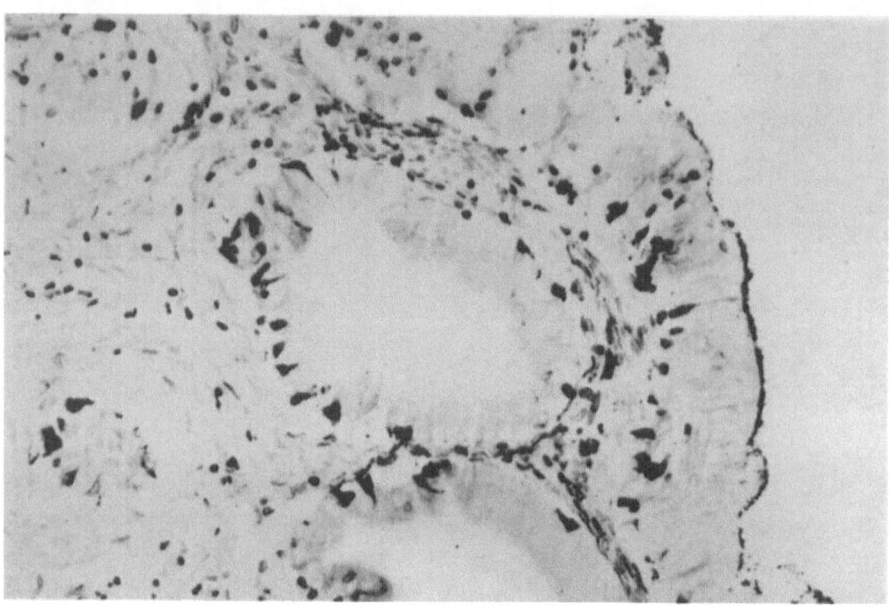

Fig. 5. Proliferating mucinous cystadenoma, possibly malignant, with argentaffin cells. Masson method. Same case of Fig. 4

type, towards the digestive epithelium. Thence it follows that a thorough study of such tumours has to be undertaken, aiming at their classification in different categories according to their microscopic structure and origin. This same view is upheld by SCHILLER (1940) in his widely-known study.

The finding of transitional forms between the serous and the mucinous types in the same tumour is not rare in histopathology. This point has considerable practical importance in the establishment of the concept under discussion. These transitional forms are recognized by GLAZUNOV (1961), who classifies them as *Dimorphus serous-pseudomucinous tumours*.

cervical types under the designations of cilioepithelial blastoma, endometrioma and mucoepithelial blastoma respectively, accepting as their original source the abnormal, Müllerian differentiation of the superficial epithelium of the ovary.

BASSIS (1960), basing himself on the theory of morphological recapitulation by the ovarian tumours of the different phases of development of the urogenital ridge, has classified the tumours that try to reproduce the structures of the Müllerian ducts. He considered first the non-neoplastic alterations such as the deciduosis, which the author names as pseudodeciduosis, the germinal inclusion cysts, the endometriosis and the Walthard cell rests. Among the neoplasms, the author listed the *adenofibroma*, which would be formed by proliferation of the cortical stroma associated to the inclusion cysts of the superficial epithelium; the *serous cystadenoma* and *carcinoma* for tubal differentiation, and the *mucinous cystadenoma* and *carcinoma* for cervical differentiation. The Brenner tumour, the adenoacanthoma and the so-called Müllerianosis complete this group. This last lesion is considered a papillary proliferation, histologically benign, diffuse, and involving superficially the uterine ligaments and internal genitalia.

HERTIG and GORE (1961) identify the following types as being of Müllerian origin:

a) Serous cystadenoma and cystadeno-carcinoma;

b) Mucinous cystadenoma and cyst-adenocarcinoma;

c) Endometrial cystoma, benign and malignant;

d) Cystadenofibroma, benign and malignant.

STERNBERG (1963) has proposed the following classification for the neoplasms arising from celomic epithelium:

A. Serous cystadenoma and malignant counterparts;

B. Mucinous cystadenoma and malignant counterparts;

C. Variants of (A) and (B). Adeno-fibroma, cystadenofibroma, surface papilloma, etc.

D. Endometrial carcinoma and adeno-acanthoma of the ovary;

E. Mixed Müllerian malignancy of the ovary;

F. Common carcinomas, many probably derived from cystomas but not histogenetically classified.

Due to its simplicity, this last classification is highly recommended.

GRAY (1963), who has analysed the problem of *Müllerian tumours*, favors the possible teratomatous origin for the mucinous ovarian tumours.

Material and Methods

In the survey of the material available up to 1963, we collected 200 cases of ovarian tumours, largely from a special hospital for neoplastic diseases, the Instituto Central A. C. Camargo, of the Associação Paulista de Combate ao Cancer.

The relatively small number of cases is easily explained for this is still a young institution, which has now reached its first decade of existence. Approximately 130 primary tumours were reviewed in the Department of Pathological Anatomy, which has a total of 45,000 specimens. The remaining cases were supplied by the Departments of Pathology of two obstetric-gynecology services, namely, the Casa Maternal, of the Legião Brasileira de Assistência, and the Associação Maternidade de São Paulo.

We studied this material by reviewing the original preparations and some pieces kept for observation, making, whenever possible and necessary, new histological sections.

Routine histological methods were employed.

We tried to study the argentaffin reaction in the mucinous tumours by Masson's method, both in slides or in blocks. Our efforts led to negative results, in spite of the excellent preparations obtained in the control material (human appendix). When the same process was applied to fresh material, recently preserved, numerous argentaffin cells were evident in 2 cases of mucinous cystadenomas, one of which presented even carcinomatous areas.

Results and Discussion

In Table I the data concerning tumours of Müllerian origin found in our survey are summarized: the type of neoplasms related to the number of cases; the age limits observed; race; unilaterality or bilaterality of the tumour, and some gross characteristics of the tumours.

GATO, 1962); in our survey, 69 per cent of the cases were in this group. GRAY (1963) estimated that approximately 81.7 per cent of the tumours in his series had their origin in Müllerian oriented epithelium; the same author observed a large number of benign and malignant lesions of the genital tract associated with such tumours, which suggests a

Table I. *Clinical-pathological data. 103 ovarian tumours of Mullerian origin*

		No. of cases	Age range Years	Race W. N. Y. ?	Side Rt. Lf. B. ?	Size range Cms.
A.	Serous cystadenoma	18	15—67	12 2 1 3	— — — —	5—25 × 12 × 9
	Proliferating serous cystadenoma	2	35—40	2 — — —	— — — —	15—22
	Serous cystadenoca	41	20—72	38 2 1 —	11 14 8 8	—
B.	Mucinous cystadenoma	16	19—63	11 4 — 2	6 8 1 1	7—38 × 30 × 18
	Proliferating mucinous cystadenoma	3	32—38	2 — — 1	1 — — 2	20—25
	Mucinous cystadenoca	5	26—61	3 1 — 1	1 1 3 —	8—22 × 17 × 10
C.	Mucinous adenofibroma	5	42—53	4 — — 1	2 2 — 1	0,6—9
	Serous adenofibroma	1	65	1 — — —	— 1 — —	17 × 13 × 18
D.	Endometrioid carcinoma	2	36—40	1 1 — —	1 1 — —	10
E.	Indifferentiated carcinoma	10	35—67	5 3 — 2	2 2 4 2	8—14 × 12 × 6

Hospital Central A. C. Camargo, A.P.C.C., São Paulo, Brasil; Casa Maternal, Legião Brasileira de Assistência; Associação Maternidade de São Paulo.

In the presentation of the common epithelial tumours, we have followed the nomenclature proposed in 1961 by the Cancer Committee of the International Federation of Gynecology and Obstetrics (HERTIG and GORE, 1966), with slight modifications.

A. Malignant Serous and Mucinous Tumours. The tumours that portray Müllerian features constitute, for many different reasons — for their frequency, in particular — the most important group of ovarian neoplasms. Tumours of the serous and mucinous types amount to 83 per cent of the malignant tumours of the ovary (ACKERMANN and DEL RE-

common stimulus proceeding from the Müllerian organs.

We used the designations *serous* or *mucinous* according to the epithelial secretory activity; quite often some areas showed a transition of epithelium, but one form always predominated. We prefer, like other authors, the designation *mucinous* because the secretion really seems to be mucin, although with some alterations.

The microscopic examination of a number of areas of this kind of tumor has demonstrated the natural existence of morphological variations; in many cases the precise determination of their benign or malignant character is quite difficult. The problem was partially by-passed by the establishment of a border-line group containing the potentially malignant neoplasms, although the cri-teria for the morphological evaluation of such cases are not uniform among the different authors (TAYLOR, 1929; KOTTMEIER, 1952; JAVERT and RASCOE, 1954; PUROLA. 1963).

The importance of an accurate histo-logic interpretation in relation to the clinical prognosis was emphasized by the studies of MUNNELL *et al.* (1957) who, reviewing several statistics on the sub-ject, disclosed a wide variation from 6,6 to 65.4 per cent.

The efforts made towards the classi-fication of these borderline tumours under a separate heading are based on the clinical behaviour of some and on the difficulty of correct evaluation of the morphological alterations responsible for this behaviour.

The criterion that takes into con-sideration the stromal invasion is sub-ject to criticism, since the evaluation of this phenomenon is not easy in the papillary tumours.

The alterations due to hyperchro-masia in the serous cystadenoma were explained by BARZILLAI (1949) as physio-logical. The anisonucleosis and the nu-clear polymorphism, as well as the nu-cleoplasmic relationship, are held as highly important by JAVERT and RASCOE (1953). The frequency of mitosis affords data which are also of relative value in the appreciation of malignancy for, as is evi-dent in the experience of WOODRUFF and NOVAK (1954), it is at times very high in benign tumours.

Based on the works of TAYLOR, PUROLA (1963) lists 5 histological grades in the ovarian serous papillary tumours:

Grade I: Benign papillary cystade-noma, inactive type;

Grade II: Benign papillary cystade-noma, hyperplastic type, with no nuclear changes;

Grade III: Borderline tumours — doubt arises regarding its benignity;

Grade IV: Well differentiated cyst-adenocarcinoma;

Grade V: Anaplastic, poorly differ-entiated cystadenocarcinoma.

PUROLA (1963) did not find any deaths due to carcinoma in patients ex-hibiting the histologically benign type, groups I and II, and the borderline type, group III, during the five-year period. In group IV, of well-differentiated carci-noma, the author attained a 5-year cure rate of 55 per cent, while in the ana-plastic group, only 15 per cent of the subjects survived that period.

However, 5 deaths due to carcinoma were registered in the borderline group after the 5-year period, i.e. from the sixth to the ninth year. After the 10-year period, no deaths from carcinoma oc-curred.

In our material we have observed a correlation between the clinical course and histologically demonstrated cancer, with two exceptions. In two cases of serous cystadenoma, the patients suf-fered a peritoneal dissemination of the process 5 and 6 years after the initial diagnosis. A histopathological re-examination of the original material sup-ported the classification of both cases within the borderline group.

Besides the cystadenocarcinomas, we observed a total of 10 cases of the inde-terminate type, so-called because they did not present any characteristics typical enough to classify them. They are con-sidered here to stress the diagnostic dif-ficulties caused by the anaplasia of some and the non-existence of a distinctive structure in others. Strictly speaking, these instances should not have been in-cluded in the present paper, since they do not show characteristics supporting Müllerian origin.

In spite of all the exhaustive and thorough work of many researchers who have devoted themselves to the elucidation of the subject, a clear appreciation of the criteria of histologic malignancy, which would explain the clinical course shown by some borderline tumours of the ovary, has not so far been established. Their classification thus depends on personal and subjective interpretations.

In the mucinous tumours, we were able to demonstrate argentaffin cells only in recently preserved material. The best preparations resulted when ammoniacal silver nitrate was employed with the block method. Reduction occurred spontaneously.

Some difference of opinions exist in regard to these cells: MASSON (1963) considers that the argentaffin cells do not reduce the silver salts spontaneously. He called the cells which do this "*cellules argento-reductrices*", the diversity being due to the different physiological condition of cells of a same nature.

LILLIE and GLENNER (1960) use the following definitions: "The term argentaffin ... designates reactions and reactive substances in which silver salts are reduced by the tissue component to the black ... without the action of any "developer" or reducing reagent ... The term "argyrophil" is used to designate those reactions and reactive substances in which a reducing agent is applied after the silver bath ..."

Such cells, argentaffins or argirophilics, present in some mucinous ovarian tumours, constitute support for the endodermal theory on the origin of these neoformations where they occur in variable numbers amongst other endodermal cells (MICHALANY, 1948).

The established existence in these tumours of enzymes physiologically produced by the large intestine, added to the demonstration of the identity between the pseudomucin and the mucin, are further elements which support this interpretation.

As variants of the sero-mucinous tumours, we must consider the mucinous fibroadenoma (Brenner tumour) and the serous fibroadenoma, or combination of both. Nevertheless, malignant forms of these tumours are very rarely found. HERTIG (1961) reported a very interesting case of bilateral ovarian cystadenofibroma, with papillary serous cystadenocarcinoma areas of low-grade malignancy.

One of our cases presented very interesting aspects. The tumour contained cystic and solid areas; the cysts were coated by serous epithelium, separated by a thick stroma with hyalinized areas. We could eventually find papillary projections with a connective center, surrounded by a single stratum of serous cells. In that tumour there were still glandular areas and stroma, with endometrial appearence and some with atypical character, as we can see in Figs. 6, 7, 8 and 9, all from the same case. This instance exemplifies once more the interrelationship between histological components reflecting the same Müllerian origin.

B. Mixed Müllerian Tumours of the Ovary. According to STERNBERG (1963), this is one of the rarest ovarian tumours, being considered as of celomatic origin and undergoing differentiation as a mixture of malignant Müllerian tissues.

We do not have personal experience with this sort of tumours arising in the ovary, but they are probably similar to those of the uterus.

Summary

The concept of "Müllerian tumours" is based on acceptance of the potentiality of the superficial ovarian epithelium and the subjacent stroma, to reproduce the morpho-functional aspects of the tubal, endometrial and endocervical types of Müllerian epithelium.

Some specimens of the mucinous tumours afford recognition of at least two distinct origins: the Müllerian and the endodermal. The endodermal source

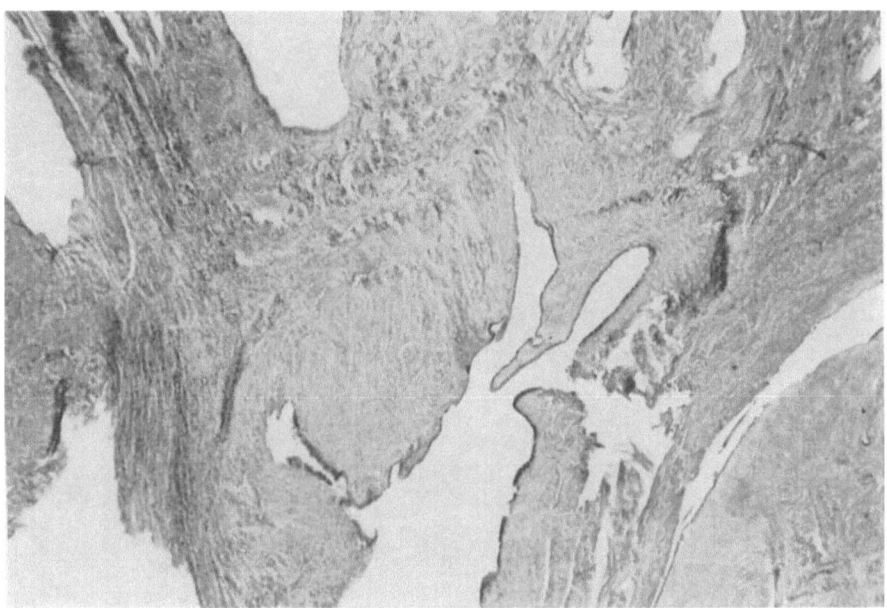

Fig. 6. Serous fibroadenoma. HE

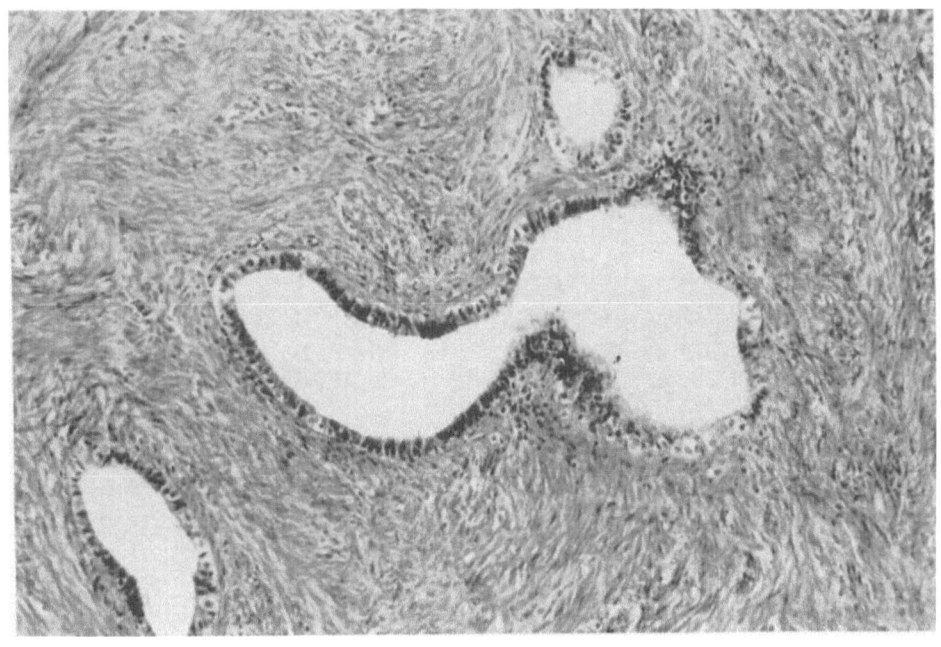

Fig. 7. Serous fibroadenoma. HE

of some mucinous tumours is substantiated by the presence of argentaffin cells, goblet cells and Paneth cells, as well as by the presence of enzymes identical to those yielded by the large intestine. These digestive enzymes are also to be found in serous cysts, but in much lower amounts (TACHIBANA cited by

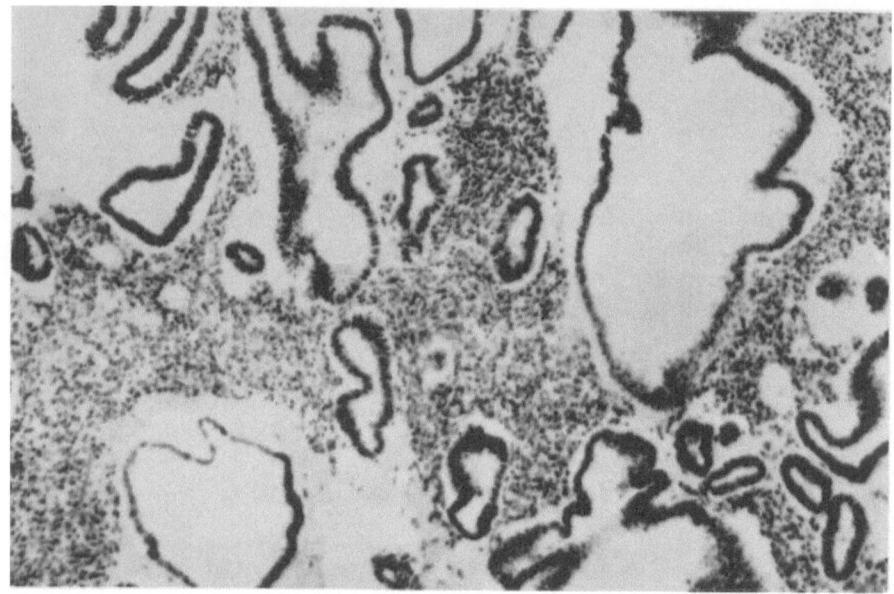

Fig. 8. Glandular structures and stroma showing endometrial appearence. HE

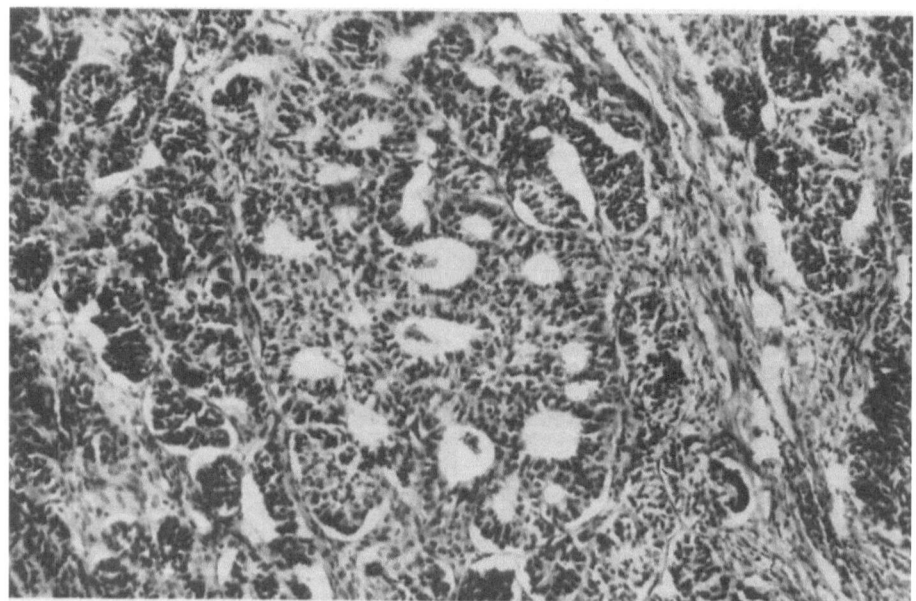

Fig. 9. Endometrioid glandular structures of low grade malignancy. The Figs. 6, 7, 8 and 9 are from the same case

MASSON, 1963). Therefore we cannot accept a single origin of the mucinous ovarian tumours, and the existence of primary ovarian enteroid tumours (MASSON, 1963) cannot be denied. This fact explains that the differential diagnosis from metastatic gastrointestinal tumours is difficult or impossible in some cases, when based only in morphological studies.

The histogenesis of some tumours which do not show in their structure morphological elements of the normal ovary is explained by the concept already described.

In this presentation only some aspects of Müllerian tumours of the ovary are discussed.

Discussion

SCULLY commented that he believed the mesonephroma, the so-called clear cell carcinoma of the ovary, was probably of Müllerian origin. He also said that he thought that this tumour might be related to endometriosis [SCULLY, R.R., RICHARDSON, G.S., and BARLOW, J.F., The development of malignancy in endometriosis. *Clin. Obstet. Gynec.* **9**, 384—411 (1966)] and showed slides which illustrated his points

(Figs. 10, 11, 12, 13). His reasons for this belief were: (1) an unusually high incidence of endometriosis is found in patients with these tumours; in the 17 cases seen in his own institution in a 15-year period, the incidence was 50 per cent (9 of 17 cases), although the incidence of endometriosis in ovarian cancer in general is only eight per cent; (2) in two specimens in his series, transitions between the clear cell or hobnail cell

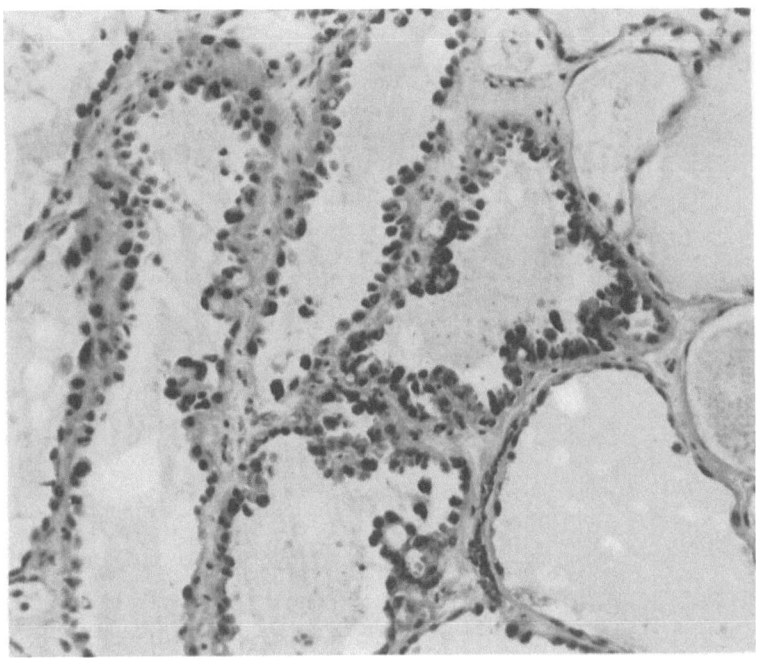

Fig. 10. Tubules lined by hobnail-shaped neoplastic cells

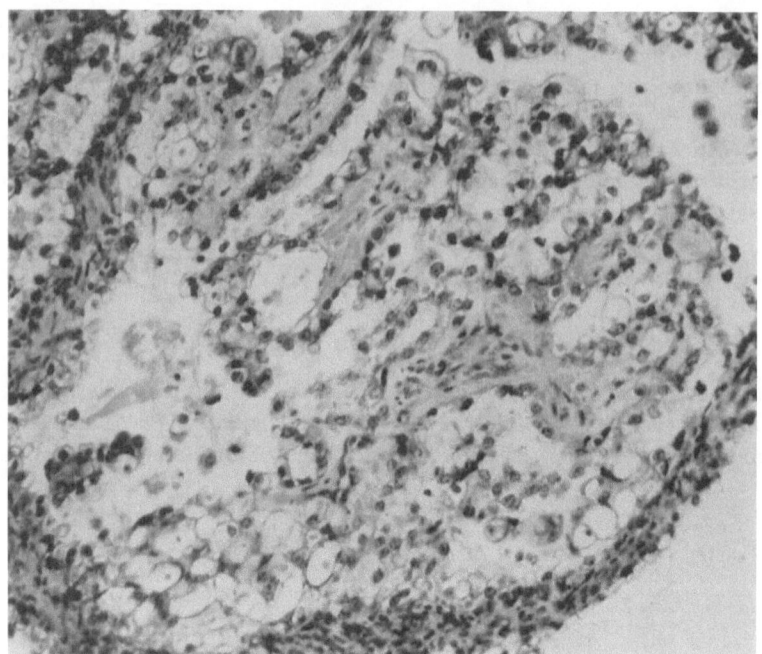

Fig. 11. Vacuolated tumour cells lining spaces

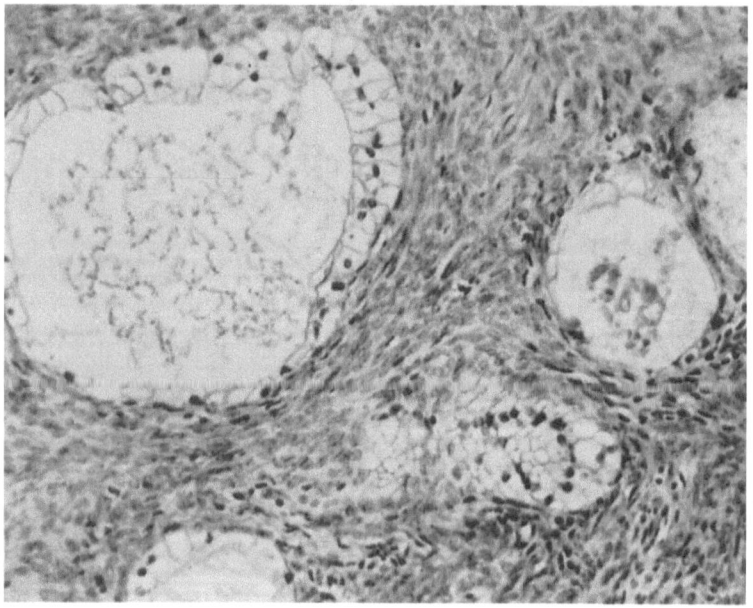

Fig. 12. Small cysts lined by clear cells and separated by stroma resembling ovarian stroma

pattern and adenoacanthoma were observed; (3) in 4 specimens, the tumour arose in an endometrial cyst; and (4) on many occasions he had observed this tumour arising in the endometrium and not involving the myometrium. He did not deny, he said, that these tumours could be differentiating in a mesonephric direction but did not believe that the majority actually arose from a meso-

tionship to endometriosis because the malignant tumours of the endometrium are hormone responsive to some extent and possibly the tumours of the clear

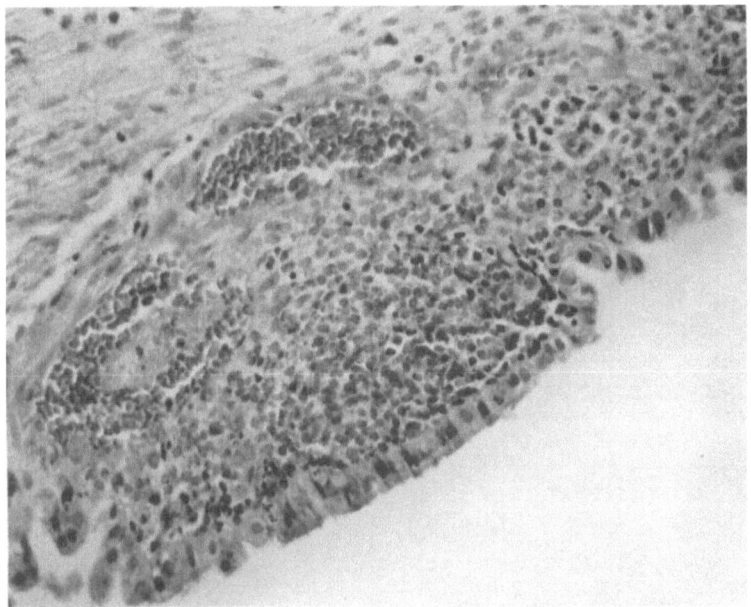

Fig. 13. Endometrial lining of large cyst from which tumour illustrated in Figs. 10 to 12 arose

nephric rest. It was important, he said, to identify tumours as having a rela-

cell type might also prove to be responsive.

References

ACKERMAN, L. V., and DEL REGATO jr., Cancer, p. 925. St. Louis: C. V. Mosby Co. 1962.

BARZILAI, G., Atlas of ovarian tumors. New York: Grune & Stratton 1949.

BASSIS, M. L., An embryologically derived classification of ovarian tumours. J. Amer. med. Ass. 174, 1316—1319 (1960).

GLAZUNOV, M. F., Ovarian tumours. Morphology, histogenesis and problems of pathogenesis, second ed. Leningrad 1961.

GRAY, L. A., Histogenesis of ovarian carcinoma. In: Progress in gynecology, vol. IV, p. 465—491. New York and London: Grune & Stratton 1963.

GRICOUROFF, G., Sur la pathologénie de l'endométriose. Ann. Anat. path. et Anat. normale med.-chir. 16, 751—760 (1939).

HERTIG, A. T., and GORE, H., Tumors of the female sex organs, sect. IX, fasc. 33, part 3. Armed Forces Institute of Pathology, Washington, U.S.A. 1961.

HERTIG, A. T., and GORE, H., In: ANDERSON's Pathology, p. 1178. St. Louis: C. V. Mosby Co. 1966.

JAVERT, C. T., and RASCOE, R. R., Serous cystadenocarcinoma of the ovary. A review of 127 cases. Surg. Clin. N. Amer. 33, 1—28 (1953).

KOTTMEIER, H. L., The classification and treatment of ovarian tumors. Acta obstet. gynec. scand. 31, 313—363 (1952).

LILLIE, R. D., and GLENNER, G. G., Histochemical reactions in carcinoid tumors of the human gastrointestinal tract. Amer. J. Path. 36, 623—651 (1960).

MASSON, P., Tumeurs humaines, deuxieme éd., p. 532. Paris: Librarie Maloine S.A. 1956.

MICHALANY, J., Sur les variations numériques des cellules argentaffines dans les kystes pseudo-mucineux de l'ovaire. Rev. biol. Canad. 7, 608—621 (1948).

MUNNELL, E. W., JACOB, H. W., and TAYLOR jr., H. C., Treatment and prognosis in cancer of the ovary, with review of new series of 143 cases treated in years 1944—1951. *Amer. J. Obstet. Gynec.* **74**, 1187—1200 (1957).

PUROLA, E., Serous papillary ovarian tumours. *Acta obstet. gynec. scand.* **42**, Suppl. 3 (1963).

SCHILLER, W., Concepts of a new classification of ovarian tumors. *Surg. Gynec. Obstet.* **70**, 773 (1940).

STERNBERG, W., Non-functionating ovarian neoplasms (GRADY, H. G., and D. E. SMITH, eds.). In: *The ovary*, p. 210. Baltimore: Williams & Wilkins Co. 1963.

TACHIBANA: Cited by MASSON, p. 714.

TAYLOR jr., H. C., Malignant and semimalignant tumors of the ovary. *Surg. Gynec. Obstet.* **48**, 204 (1929).

— LONG, M. E., and MONTGOMERY, F., Problems of cellular and tissue differentiation in papillary adenocarcinoma of the ovary. *Amer. J. Obstet. Gynec.* **70**, 753—765 (1955).

WOODRUFF, J. D., and NOVAK, E. R., Papillary serous tumors of the ovary. *Amer. J. Obstet. Gynec.* **67**, 112 (1954).

Endometrioid Tumours of the Ovary

G. GRICOUROFF

Head of the Pathological Department, Fondation Curie, Paris, France

Introduction

The substance of my presentation can be contained in two sentences:

I. The ovary can be the site of primary tumours with the histologic pattern of all the varieties of tumours found in endometrium of the uterine corpus.

II. The frequency of endometriosis in the ovary makes it reasonable to suppose that these primary ovarian endometrioid tumours originate in reality in an endometriotic lesion.

The cancer of the body of the uterus is a well-known neoplasm and the condition of endometriosis is today a familiar one. But there is much divergence in interpretation concerning the endometriotic nature of certain ovarian lesions, divergencies which at times spring from the very definition given to endometriosis and from the diversity of theories presented for explaining its histogenesis. Therefore, a definition of endometriosis in general and some observations are indicated concerning the histogenesis of this disease which has so large a place in female pathology.

Definition. Endometriosis is a displacement of the uterine body endometrium (Fig. 1). Endometriosis is *internal* when it is situated within the uterus itself but outside the corporeal mucosa, i.e. in the myometrium or beneath the peritoneum. It is *external* when it is situated outside the uterus, for example in the ovary. The majority of the endometriotic lesions are localized along the entire length of the genital tract; their frequency diminishes exponentially the further one gets from the genital tract. The pelvic-abdominal peritoneum, bladder, rectum, intestine and iliac lymph nodes are often involved; more rarely, the umbilicus and the inguinal region are affected. Far-removed sites (such as the upper or lower extremities, or the lungs) have only rarely been encountered. Lastly, endometriosis can occur in abdominal or pelvic scars, which may be of surgical origin (laparotomy, episiotomy) or accidental (perineal rent), often on a scar of long-standing, and even after an operation not involving the uterus (e.g. appendicectomy performed in childhood, treatment for hernia, etc.). The sites of endometriosis are often multiple in the same patient, but the size of the lesions varies considerably, ranging from a microscopic vesicle (Fig. 2) to voluminous masses, solid or cystic, and adhering to or infiltrating neighboring organs. Clinically, depending on the importance and site of the lesions, endometriosis can be totally asymptomatic or, contrariwise, accompanied by extremely painful periodic symptomatology.

Microscopic Characteristics. In typical cases, the histologic picture of endometriosis is one of a normal or hyperplastic uterine mucosa, with tubular glands or microcysts surrounded by endometrial stroma. The epithelial cells

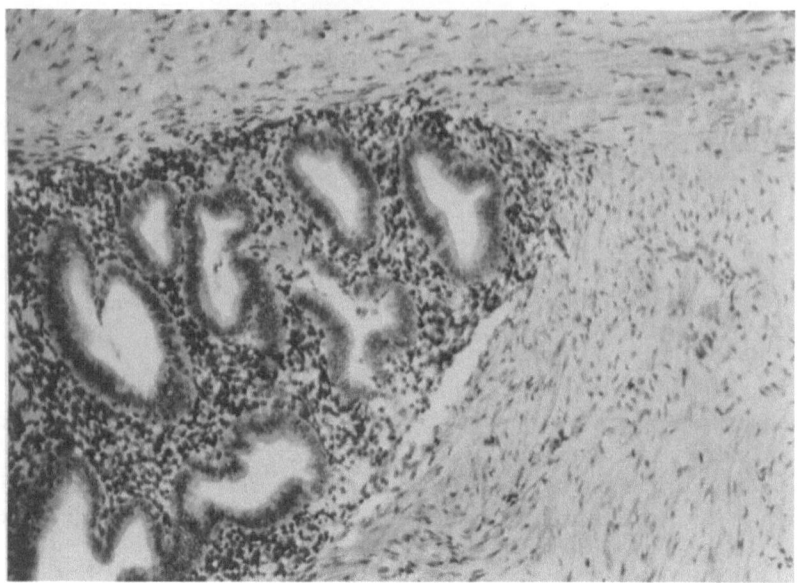

Fig. 1. Endometriosis occuring in a laparotomy scar ten years after an appendectomy. Columnar
cell glands surrounded by endometrial stroma

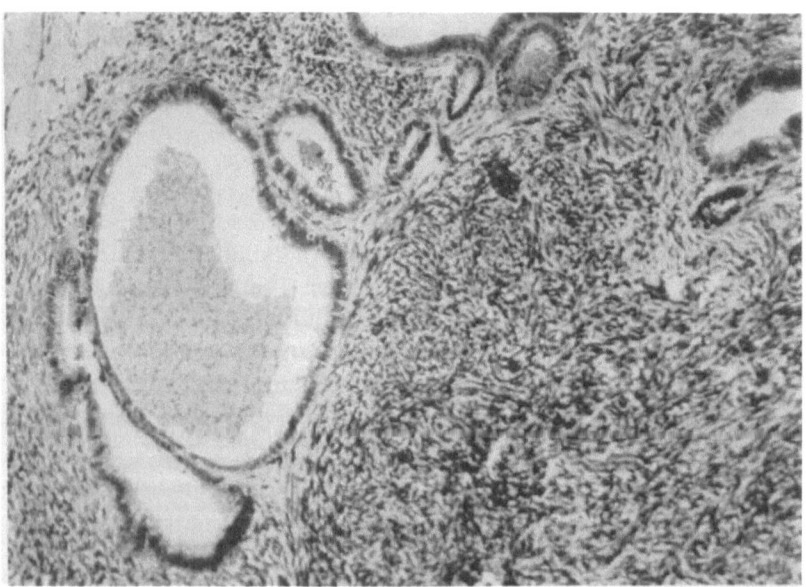

Fig. 2. Endometrial epithelial microcysts (so-called "germinal inclusion cysts") in the depth of the
ovarian cortex

are columnar and are often ciliated. The contents of the glands and cystic cavities are serous or sero-mucous. When endometriosis is situated in an organ where smooth muscle normally exists it is known as adenomyosis (as for example in the corporeal myometrium or intestine) (Fig. 3).

Usually, endometriosis shows the same cyclic changes as are seen in the uterus and the stroma undergoes decidual transformation in the course of gestation. It is thus not simply a question of morphologic appearances, but is really a heterotopic functional endometrium which reacts physiologically to hormonal incitations. The well-known

(Fig. 5), beneath the peritoneum, or in a node. It is only by virtue of the decidual transformation of pregnancy that it is possible to identify them.

Histogenesis. The histogenesis of endometriosis is still a subject of controversy. This problem must be considered as a whole since the ovary, because of its complex embryology and histology, is

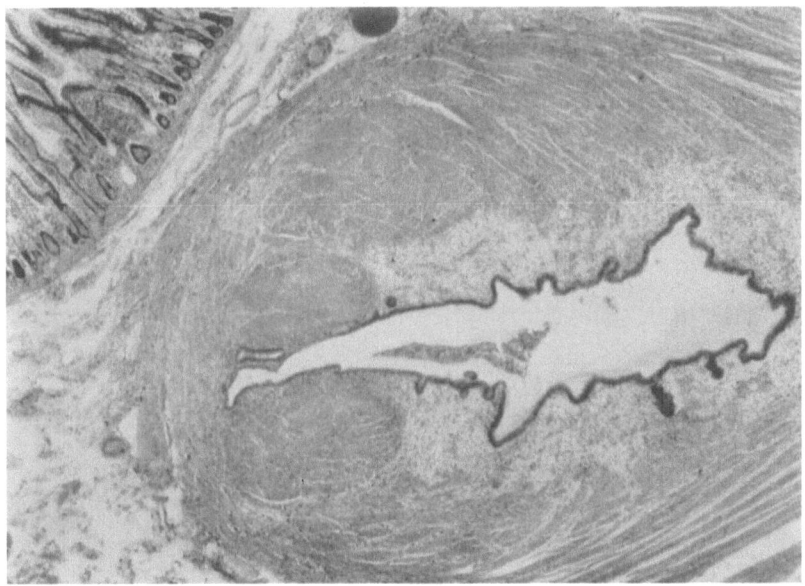

Fig. 3. "Miniature uterus" in the intestinal wall (adenomyosis). The intestinal mucosa is visible

picture of "chocolate" ovarian cysts arises from the menstrual hemorrhagic breakdown of the hypertrophied stroma.

Endometriosis does not always have this classic, complete structure. It can be purely epithelial with ciliated cell cysts, often microscopic, present in the myometrium, ovary, or lymph nodes (Fig. 4).

Lastly, endometriosis can be purely stromal, the epithelial component being absent. This stromatosis (Fig. 6) is generally situated in the myometrium. Besides it is not exceptional, during a laparotomy in a pregnant woman, to come across nests of endometrial stroma in the ovary

not a satisfactory material for investigation. Furthermore, there is no agreement as to the endometriotic nature of various lesions found in the ovary.

The histogenetic theories fall into two categories:

1. The Metaplastic Theories, according to which the origin of endometriosis is *local:* it is the outcome of a transformation of the tissues already present;

2. The Migratory Theories, which hold the origin of endometriosis to be *uterine,* the consequence of an endometrial displacement starting from the uterus itself.

The metaplastic category comprises the embryonic rests theories (Wolffian,

Müllerian) which are of purely historic interest, and above all the *celomic theory*, tive peritoneum, and the uterus, and tubes are formed from this duct. The

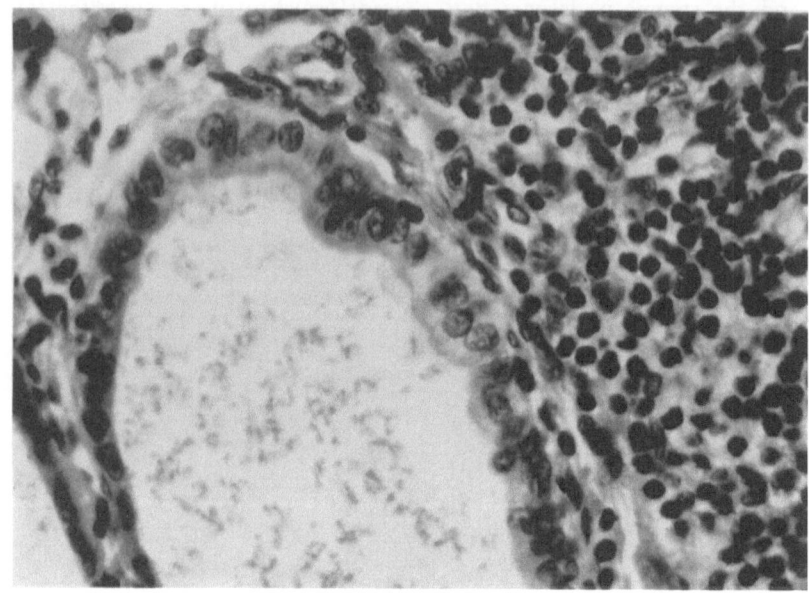

Fig. 4. Endometrial ciliated microcyst in a pelvic lymph node

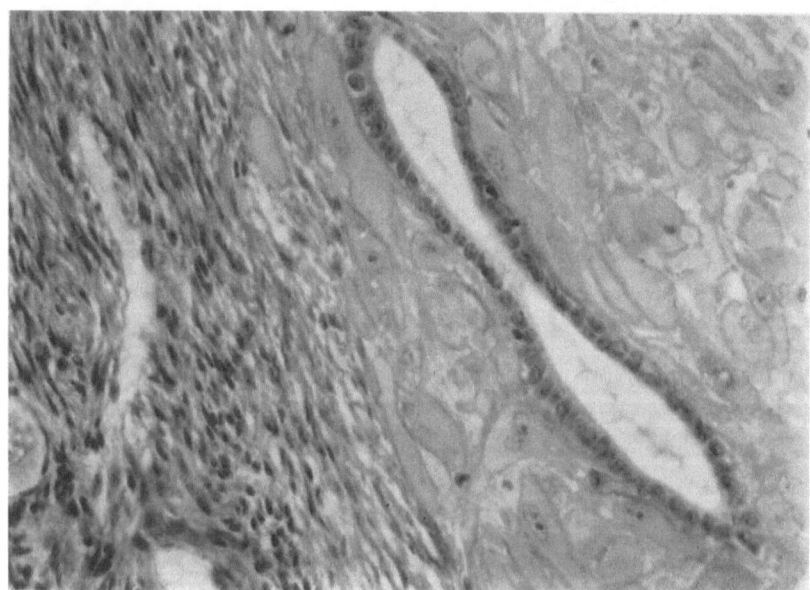

Fig. 5. Gravidic stromal reaction in an ovarian endometriosis. (A primordial follicle is visible on the edge of the photomicrograph)

based on embryonal tissue memory; as you know the Müllerian duct is the result of an invagination of the primi- peritoneal epithelium remains capable of transforming itself into an endometrium and this possibility exists in every case where the celomic epithelium or its vestiges are present, i.e. at any point over the surface of the pelvic peritoneum, the umbilicus, a hernial sac, etc. We shall be dealing further with this theory [which, since the days of IWANOFF (1898) has always had supporters of note such as HERTIG and GORE (1961)], when we come to consider the ovary.

particles fix themselves on the ovary or peritoneum. This explanation has met with considerable acceptance. But although experimentally it is possible to implant the normal endometrium, there is no clear proof that the desquamated and necrotic endometrium, carried along by the regurgitated menstrual blood, is able to implant itself and to proliferate.

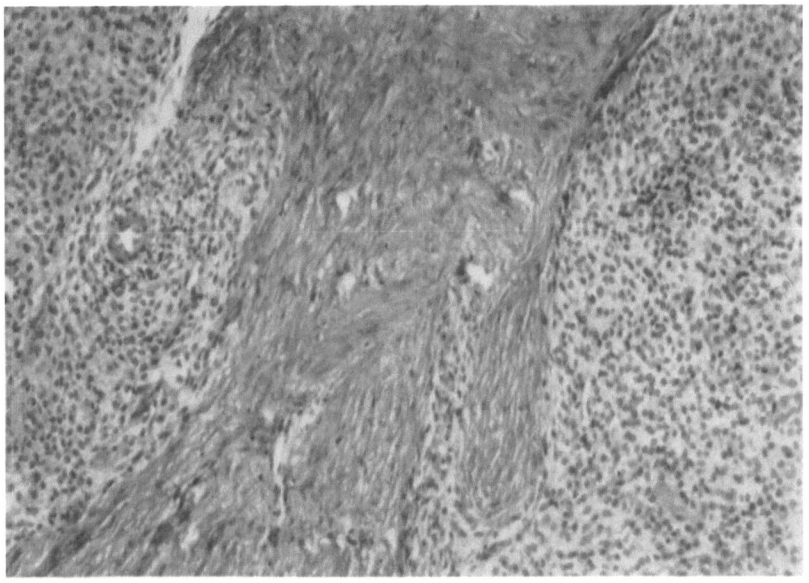

Fig. 6. Stromal endometriosis of the uterus (endolymphatic stromatosis). See Fig. 9 for its vascular propagation

The basis of the migratory theories is that the ectopic endometrium originates in the uterus itself. In this group are found:

1. The theory of interstitial progression (CULLEN, 1896) which can only account for internal endometriosis and endometriosis of the bladder or rectum;

2. SAMPSON's theory (1921) of *transtubal regurgitation* and of implantation;

3. HALBAN's theory (1925) of *migration by the lymphatic system*.

The highly original idea of SAMPSON is that retrograde tubal menstruation conveys particles of the endometrium into the peritoneal cavity and that these

The hypothesis of an implantation would not, in any case, explain the extraperitoneal cases of endometriosis.

The theory of metastasis by the lymphatic route was postulated by HALBAN in 1925. In face of the complexity and insufficiencies of all the theories hitherto put forward, he proposed a fresh one, "very simple" and "providing the clue to all the enigmas". In the course of the cyclic proliferation of the endometrium, or in the hyperplasia that is so frequent, endometrial particles could penetrate into the uterine lymphatics and be carried to just below the peritoneum, and from there outside the

uterus. The presence of characteristic inclusions in the pelvic nodes constitutes
for HALBAN a well-founded proof for
his theory of "*hysteroadenosis metastatica*",
valid for all endometriotic localizations.

It should be said here that even
before HALBAN, SAMPSON himself had
seen a particle of endometrium migrating in a vessel, but to him this patho-

in the vessels (Fig. 7, Fig. 8); I, too,
saw pelvic nodes containing benign
ciliated vesicles (Fig. 4). I have convinced only very few people. Nevertheless, the idea persisted and 12 years
later, JAVERT (1949) quite independently
proposed again the lymphatic-vascular
theory, which he combined surprisingly
with that of tubal regurgitation!

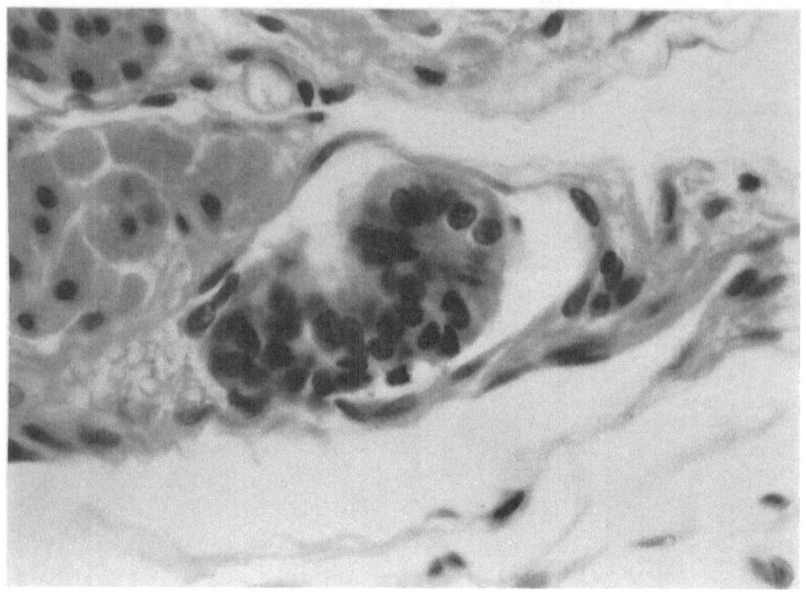

Fig. 7. Epithelial endometrial particle migrating in a capillary of the myometrium

genic mechanism was but accessory,
valid in a few cases only, whereas the
implantation in the ovary or peritoneum
of fragments conveyed by the menstrual
tubal regurgitation was for SAMPSON the
quasi-exclusive processus. HALBAN's theory of lymphatic metastasis for endometriosis in general met with little acceptance; the consensus was that only
cancer could invade the lymphatic system and give rise to metastases.

Thirty years ago, when I began to
investigate this most fascinating problem, HALBAN's hypothesis had fallen
almost completely into oblivion. I, too,
observed some particles of endometrium

Ovarian Endometriosis. In the ovary,
endometriosis occurs frequently but is
often microscopic and "silent", which
makes any statistical appraisal out of the
question. It consists principally of cystic
formations situated in the cortex or
deep down close to the hilus. The size
of these formations can vary considerably, ranging from a microscopic vesicle
to a voluminous "chocolate" cyst of
about 10-cm diameter. The epithelial
wall of the cyst is often surrounded by
an endometrial stroma of greater or lesser abundance. When the two components, ciliated epithelium and stroma,
are present, the endometrial nature is

obvious. But when the very same ciliated cysts are devoid of stroma, most authors do not consider them as endometriosis, but as "inclusion cysts" resulting from invaginations of the surface epithelium. And yet they are identical to the purely epithelial endometriosis which can be seen in the myometrium, the broad ligament, or the nodes.

depends on the surrounding stroma. According to the protagonists of celomic metaplasia (WELLER, 1935), nests of endometrial stroma exist under the peritoneum (with a regional distribution comparable to that of endometriosis!). If by chance the surface invagination occurs in the neighborhood of an islet of endometrial stroma, the "inclusion

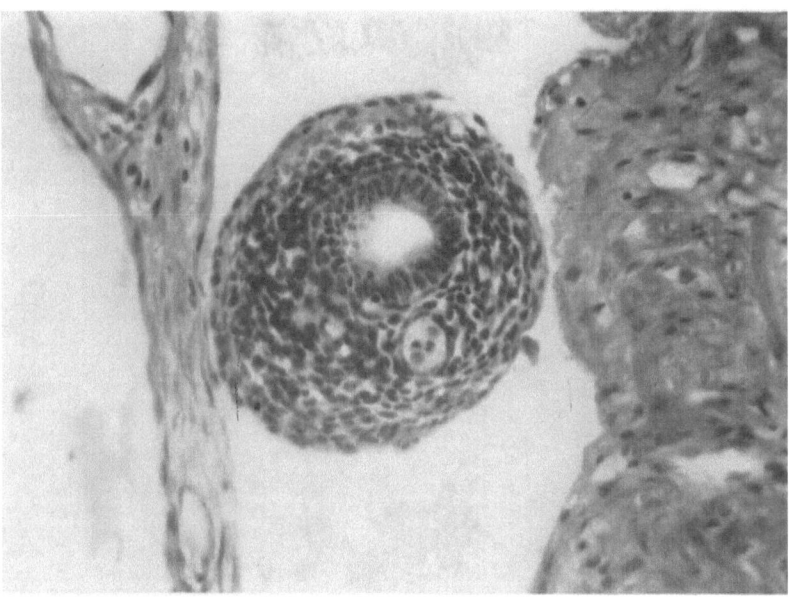

Fig. 8. Endometrial particle (gland and stroma) migrating in a subperitoneal uterine lymphatic

·In this connection it is interesting to see just what acrobatics must be performed if one adopts the celomic theory! In the adult ovary, the surface epithelium is flat and identical to the peritoneal endothelium; but it must have retained a "Müllerian potential" and a tissular memory enabling it, by means of metaplasia, to become lengthy and columnar once more, like the germinative epithelium of the young ovary, and even ciliated like that of the endometrium. After forming invaginations and inclusion cysts, the surface epithelium remains columnar or becomes flat as it was formerly. The fate of the small cyst

cyst" becomes en endometrial cyst. Otherwise, it remains a "germinal inclusion cyst".

In my opinion, all these small ciliated cysts, with or without stroma, are endometriotic lesions (Fig. 2). They do not originate in the germinative epithelium. The infoldings and invaginations of the surface of the ovary most certainly do exist, but are present mainly in elderly women after the menopause, as opposed to endometriosis which appears earlier, while the ovary is still functional.

When some parts of the covering of the ovary are cylindrical and ciliated, this could be caused by the opening of an endometrial cyst at the surface and consequent epithelial stretching.

As to the nests of endometrial stroma, it is somewhat arbitrary to declare that they pre-exist everywhere below the peritoneum. They are islets of stromal endometriosis whose origin needs an explanation, as does that of the epithelium (Fig. 9).

characteristics, since endometriosis is indeed a metastasis of the uterine mucosa itself.

2. It is applicable to all the varieties of endometriosis — epithelium and stroma, epithelium alone, or stroma alone (Fig. 9), depending on the elements which have penetrated into the lymphatics and survived the journey.

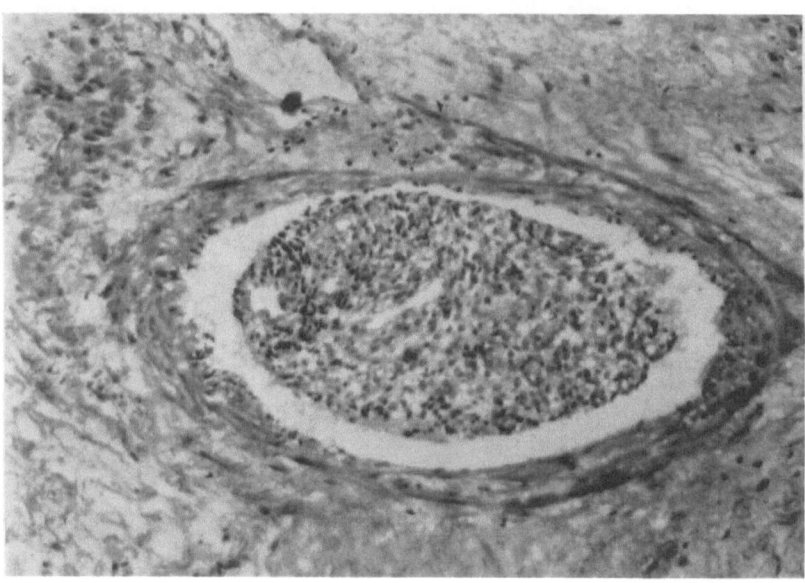

Fig. 9. Stromal endometrial particle migrating in a vessel (endolymphatic stromatosis). See Fig. 6

All in all, the celomic metaplasia theory does not seem to fit in with ovarian endometriosis; likewise for the various other sites, it is at once over-simplified and over-complex. I feel uneasy at having to invoke the Müllerian potential of a hernial sac or the endometrial memory of the umbilicus! As for SAMPSON's theories of regurgitation and implantation, their mechanism is really most unlikely and fails, furthermore, to account for extraperitoneal endometriosis.

Advantages of HALBAN's *Theory*

1. More than any other theory, HALBAN's accounts for the histophysiologic

3. It accounts for internal and external endometriosis, depending on whether the migratory particles are arrested in the myometrium or underneath the peritoneum, or whether they leave the uterus and attach themselves elsewhere, in the ovary for instance.

4. The areas where endometriosis most frequently develops are either very close to the uterus (Douglas' cul-de-sac) or else closely connected to it by lymphatics (e.g. the ovaries). When the site of endometriosis is remote from the uterus, the areas involved are always fairly accessible by the lymphatics through the internetwork anastomosis;

such is the case with certain unusual but characteristic localizations as, for instance, the inguinal region, or the umbilicus.

5. Endometriosis is most often of a regional nature and far-removed sites are rare, for the migrating endometrial particles can only survive if their passage through the lymphatics is not too prolonged.

6. Only the very tiny fragments of endometrium which permeate the lymphatics can travel far. Their migration can continue right along the finest of the networks, provided they are not held back by some natural or artificial interruption (plexus, node, operation-scar). This explains why the endometrial infiltration can at times extend to just below the mucosa (vagina, rectum, or bladder) or to underneath the skin (umbilicus). But it is above all at the level of the peritoneum that the lymphatics are superficial and lie directly under the peritoneal epithelium. In point of fact, the ectopic endometrium is situated *below* the peritoneal or ovarian epithelium. The epithelium may become pushed up, but originally it is intact. If it splits, this occurs because of the stretching and perforation of the endometrial cyst. At this point the endometriotic ciliated epithelium can spread to the surface of the ovary or peritoneum.

The occurrence of endometriotic lesions in laparotomy or episiotomy scars can be explained by the interruption of the lymphatic vessels because of the surgical incision. The hypothesis of an accidental implant of a strip of endometrium in the course of the operation has yet to be proved and is moreover valueless in the case of operations outside the genitalia (e.g. appendectomy). The umbilicus is also a scar (ligature of the cord at birth). Perineal endometriosis, which is rare, is always consecutive to a tear.

We see, therefore, that the hypothesis of a metastatic origin by the lymphatic route would explain all the known facts, even with regard to certain frequently observed peculiarities.

Arguments of Fact. What are the facts that sustain this hypothesis? Firstly, there is the presence of endometrial inclusions in the lymph nodes of the pelvis. Often they are ciliated vesicles devoid of stroma and situated in the capsule of the node, in the peripheral sinus, or in the cortex. Stroma is, at times, present in addition; at other times there is only stroma, and no epithelium. As a rule, the lesions are microscopic and discovered only by chance.

Secondly, and even more decisive, is the observation of particles of endometrium in the lymph or blood capillaries of the uterus (SAMPSON, HENRY, GRICOUROFF [Fig. 7, Fig. 8, Fig. 9], etc.). It is possible that the migration could also occur along the bloodstream, which would explain some exceptional, far-removed sites (lungs, extremities), but it is unlikely that many cells could survive the torrents of circulating blood.

Objections. The objections raised to HALBAN's theory are not of any great consequence. They are as follows: 1) As the inclusions in the lymph nodes are often devoid of stroma, this cannot be endometriosis. 2) Ovarian or peritoneal endometriotic lesions are most common at the surface and not deep inside the tissues. 3) There is at times a mixture of ciliated formations, with or without stroma, formations of the peritoneal type and a continuity between the various structures, etc.

Actually, the prejudice against the lymphatic-metastatic hypothesis is mainly doctrinal. The notions of metastasis and cancer are so bound together in our minds that it is difficult to accept the idea of a normal tissue invading the nodes and producing metastases. However, the presence of endometrial particles in the capillaries of the uterus and of inclusions in the nodes, compels us to re-examine these notions in an impartial manner. We should remember that each month, in 5 or 6 days, the thickness of the uterine mucosa in-

eral ectopic sites of the very same histophysiologically highly specific tissue, invoke regurgitation-implantation for a "chocolate" cyst, celomic metaplasia for a sub-peritoneal lesion of the tube, lymphatic metastasis for a microcyst in a node and surgical grafting for endometriosis in an appendectomy scar?

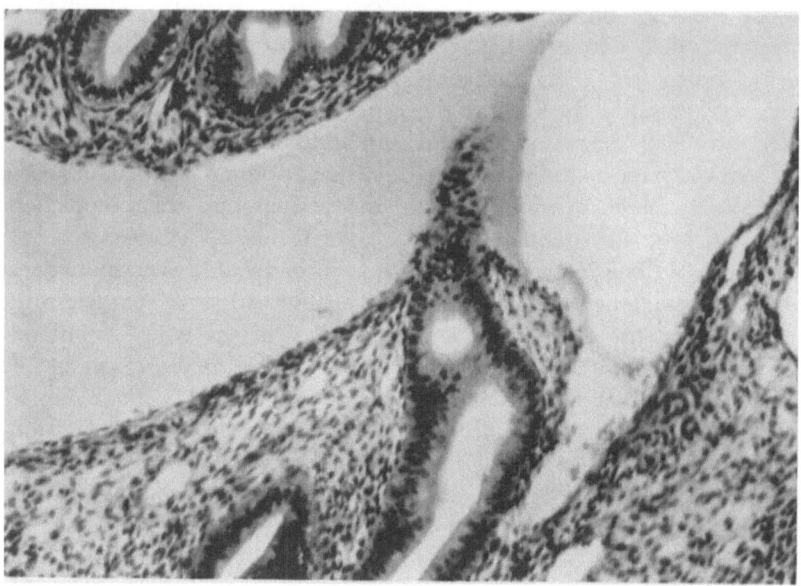

Fig. 10. Endometrial gland protruding towards a thin-walled dilated lymphatic in the uterine mucosa

creases five-fold. The screw-shaped glands lengthen considerably in a stroma, whose thin-walled lymphatic and blood capillaries are numerous and dilated (Fig. 10). The presence of intra vascular particles of endometrium is thus in no way paradoxical (Fig. 7, Fig. 8, Fig. 9)

Conclusions on Histogenesis. Many authors consider none of the theories proposed to be universal and that, depending on the site of endometriosis, one must choose the theory of histogenesis which seems best suited for the given case. But it is well known that endometriotic lesions are often multiple. Must we, therefore, when dealing with one and the same patient who has sev-

One cannot but deplore such a reasoning. It seems really necessary to adopt a single theory valid for every site. It goes without saying that the only acceptable one in my opinion is that of the lymphatic dissemination.

Endometrioid Tumours of the Ovary

It is reasonable to consider the point of departure of these tumours as being an ovarian endometriotic lesion. In many instances, the spreading of the tumour has caused the endometriotic tissue to disappear, in which case the origin is hypothetical, although probable. SAMPSON (1925), CORNER *et al.* (1950), etc., however, published a few cases in which, according to them, the origin was clearly demonstrated.

In 1961, the delegates to a Conference held at the Radiumhemmet in Stockholm, which I had the honor to attend, endeavoured to give a precise definition of endometrioid tumours of the ovary and to draw a distinction between them and serous and mucous cystomas and the neoplasms which derive from such cystomas.

Benign Endometrioid Tumours. Difficulties arose when attempts were made to define benign endometrioid tumours, because of the uncertainty or disagreement as regards the definition of endometriosis itself: benign tumour? hyperplasia? ectopic normal tissue? As a result, the place where this definition should have been inserted was left blank! But is this point of dogma really important? Nature has little regard for man's urge to categorize, erect barriers, classify ... Endometriosis exists, and we must accept it with all its pecularities. A cancer can as well develop from an ectopic normal tissue as from a heterotopic hyperplasia or from a benign tumour.

We can, then, suggest grouping under the heading of "benign" all the lesions of endometriosis in the widest sense:

1. Lesions of complete endometriosis comprising glands and stroma, and especially "chocolate" cysts.

2. Purely epithelial lesions. These are the small ciliated cysts termed germinal "inclusion cysts".

3. Purely stromal lesions.

Possibly Malignant Endometrioid Tumours

1. Papillary cystadenomas, whose glands, cystic cavities and vegetations are lined with columnar cells, which may be stratified in 2 or 3 layers, and cellular abnormalities which may be present to a greater or lesser degree. An important fact is that similar lesions in the peritoneum or in the second ovary have been observed in the course of surgical intervention. Some workers consider them to be superficial "deposits" (Sampson-type implants); for others, they are authentic metastases via the lymphatic route, which would fit in better with the rather elective spread toward the second ovary and at times deep within the hilus.

2. Fibroadenomatous solid tumours with columnar epithelium and with commonplace connective stroma. Some parts are cystic with papillary vegetations. Their appearance is reminiscent of suspect uterine tumours, often referred to as malignant adenomas.

3. Adenoacanthomas which are distinct from the preceding tumours for the presence of islets of squamous cells. They are identical to uterine adenoacanthomas.

4. If we are to remain loyal to our broad definition of endometriosis, mention must be made here of the mesenchymatous productions which are identical to stromatosis or endolymphatic stromal myosis of the uterus. No epithelial glands are present. Ovarian stromatosis is rare.

Malignant Endometroid Tumours

1. All the varieties of carcinoma of the body of the uterus, with all the grades of malignancy, can have their primary site in the ovary (Fig. 11). They are mainly adenocarcinomas, often papillary and at times cystic. The outer surface can be smooth, or covered with vegetations. The tumoural cells are columnar or cubic; all the types (ciliated, clear, muciparous) can be encountered in these tumours and often coexist in the same cancer. It must be mentioned that as with uterine adenocarcinomas, the columnar cells are not always ciliated and there is

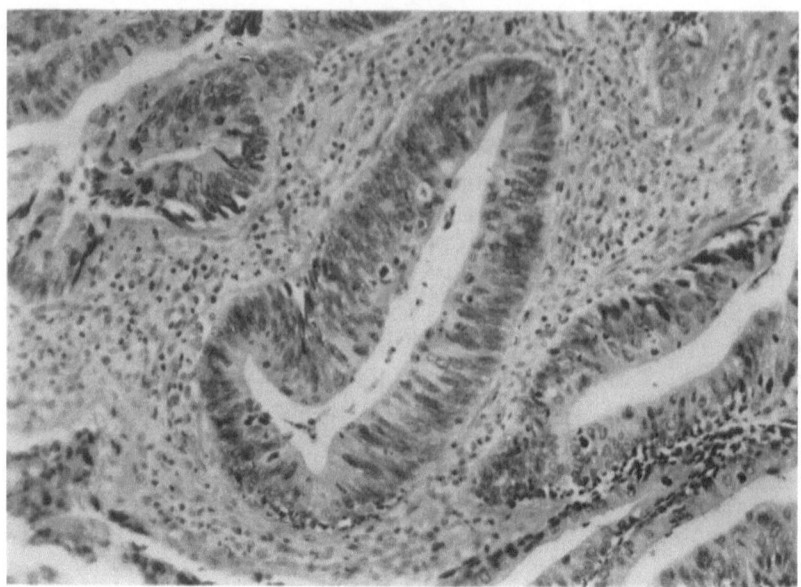

Fig. 11. Endometrioid columnar cell adenocarcinoma

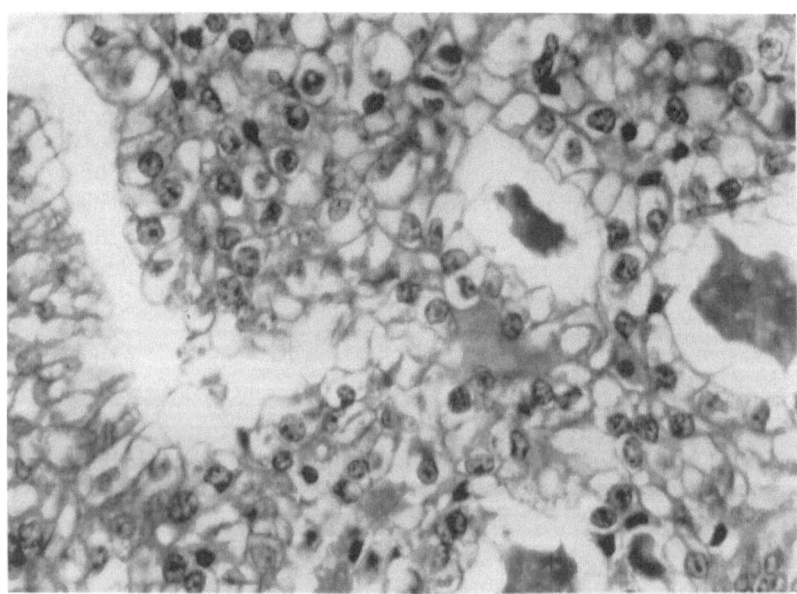

Fig. 12. Clear cell endometrioid adenocarcinoma

no endometrial stroma. Thus it is no longer possible to separate the "germinal" carcinomas from endometrioid cancers. Probably many serous, seromucous and even purely mucous (clear cell) adenocarcinomas should come under the heading of endometrioid cancers (Fig. 12), as the same types exist in cancers of the uterine body.

Not infrequent are adenoacanthotic carcinomas, with numerous squamous-cell islets mingled with the cylindric proliferation. At the extreme limit are found some purely epidermoid epitheliomas.

Certain carcinomas are formed of clear cells, with stratification giving a hypernephroid aspect. Others are highly polymorphic with pseudosarcomatous diffused zones.

2. Epithelial-mesenchymatous primary tumours (carcinosarcomas, malignant mesodermal mixed tumours) exist in the ovary as in the uterus. Their origin in an endometriosis can be accepted.

3. Lastly, primary pure sarcomas can arise from the stroma of an endometriosis.

Criteria for the Endometriotic Origin of Primary Endometrioid Adenocarcinomas of the Ovary

Obviously, it is logical to consider endometrioid cancers of the ovary as emanating from an endometriosis. But let us see to what extent this origin has been demonstrated and how far the criteria set up by SAMPSON (1925) and by CORNER et al. (1950), and others, are valid. According to SAMPSON, three conditions need to be fulfilled:

"1) the actual demonstration of both cancer and benign endometrial tissue in the same ovary; 2) the cancer and benign endometrial tissue must bear the same histologic relation to each other that cancer of the body of the uterus bears to the non-malignant portion of the endometrium; 3) it must be shown that the cancer arose in this tissue and that it has not invaded it from some other source." And CORNER et al. said that a "gradual transition from benign to malignant epithelium" can be seen in the slides.

Unfortunately, these criteria have no value at all. The images of uninterrupted continuity of connection between the normal tissue and the cancer show the invasion, the replacement of the former by the latter, but show no transition, no gradual cancerization of the normal tissue. In a cancer, there is not a permanent repeated malignant contamination of the normal cells, but proliferation starting from the first cell to be cancerized. Even in the smallest tumours, this first cell has long since disappeared and been replaced by generations of malignant daughter and granddaughter cells. In a slide, the point of contact represents the point of encounter between the cancer and the normal tissue, *not* the point of departure of the cancerization. The picture would be the same were it a case of a metastasis coming, for example, from the uterus. It is also a pity that with CORNER et al., their female patient had precisely an adenocarcinoma in the uterus too.

From all that is said above, it is logical to conclude that a very great number of benign, "borderline", or malignant tumours originate in an endometriosis and that, contrary to what is generally accepted, the malignant transformation of an endometriosis is not exceptional. Are we, then, to consider endometriosis as a pre-cancerous state? A lesion is precancerous if the chances of its transformation into cancer are great. But very discreet ovarian endometriotic lesions are present in the majority of menstruating women, whereas ovarian cancers are rare. Endometriosis is no more precancerous than is the normal or hyperplastic uterine endometrium.

Metastases from Endometrioid Adenocarcinomas

The co-existence of an ovarian cancer and a uterine cancer is not exceptional. It is always difficult to know which of the two organs was the primary site of the cancer, although it is usually the uterus because of the greater frequency of uterine cancer. But the propagation of an ovarian cancer to the uterus, by the lymphatic route, is not rare, the metastasis being sub-serous, myometrial or endometrial. The endometrial seat of the metastasis can have the aspect of a superficial deposit, which would naturally make one think of a Sampson-type direct implantation, across the tube. But the presence of neoplastic particles in the lymphatics is a cardinal point in favor of the vascular route.

The second ovary is involved in over 50% of cases. Here, too, the explanation is to be sought in a transit from one ovary to the other through the lymphatics rather than an independent bilaterality or a direct implantation. For, even when the second ovary appears to be intact, microscopic examination will often reveal the presence of cancerous cells in the lymphatics of the hilus.

The peritoneum is very often the seat of secondary localizations, even when the external surface of the ovarian tumour is smooth and there is no rupture of the capsule. The secondary peritoneal nodules are themselves in the first instance sub-serous, so it can be held that here, too, the extension has taken place by transit of the cancerous cells by the lymphatic route. Later on, vegetations may appear at the surface of the peritoneum and cancerous cells may be found in the ascites.

The nodes are invaded in a large proportion of advanced cases: iliac nodes, are the first affected; later more remote ones are invaded. And lastly, visceral metastases, which at times occur very late.

Prognosis

What, from our knowledge of endometrioid tumours of the ovary, can we say concerning the prognosis for this disease? All grades of malignancy can,

of course, exist as with uterine cancers. But it does seem as if the clinical evolution can at times produce some pleasant surprises. During laparotomy, one sometimes discovers a papillary cystadenocarcinoma of one ovary, with peritoneal metastases, which means the operation has to be incomplete. Yet patients of this type have been seen several years later and found to be in good condition. Such instances were reported long ago, and by several authors. KISTNER and HERTIG (1952) have reminded us that the prognosis seems good for adenoacanthocarcinomas originating in an ovarian endometriosis.

Among the endometrioid epitheliomas of the ovary, a certain number of tumours of low-grade malignancy (especially adenocarcinomas with no cellular abnormalities, poorly mitotic cystopapillary carcinomas, adenoacanthocarcinomas with abundant fibrous stroma) could be almost as benign as endometriosis, even when metastatic foci have been observed and when there is ascites.

Summary

Theories of the histogenesis of endometriosis are reviewed:

Primary ovarian tumours of endometrial type are numerous and it is logical to agree with Sampson's idea that they arise in an ovarian endometriosis. But the criteria for the endometriotic origin are valueless.

All grades of malignancy may exist, as they do in the adenocarcinomas of the uterine endometrium. But patients may survive years in spite of metastatic secondary growths in the peritoneum or in the opposite ovary.

Résumé

De nombreuses tumeurs primitives de l'ovaire sont histologiquement semblables aux tumeurs de l'endomètre du corps de l'utérus. Il est logique d'admettre avec SAMPSON que ces tumeurs endométrioïdes prennent naissance dans une lésion d'endométriose ovarienne. Cependant les critères proposés comme preuve de cette origine sont sans valeur.

Tous les degrés de malignité peuvent s'observer dans les adénocarcinomes endométrioïdes de l'ovaire, mais de très longues survies ont été constatées, même dans des cas où il y avait des métastases péritonéales ou dans l'autre ovaire.

L'exposé commence par une revue critique des théories histogénétiques de l'endométriose.

Discussion

TEILUM briefly reviewed the history of the term "endometrioid" from the time it was originally used in 1925. In the 1940's a few such cases were described. In 1952, KOTTMEIER reported that such tumours were more common than was usually recognized. DOCKERTY, in 1954, remarked on the histological resemblance to endometrial cancer; THOMPSON, in 1957, listed 30 cases and added 70 of his own from the Ovarian Tumour Registry file; SANTESSON, in 1961, at a conference in Stockholm, presented a study showing the frequency of the histological types in 616 primary ovarian tumours examined at the Radiumhemmet. The papillary cystadenocarcinomas constituted the largest group of tumours (39 per cent); second in frequency were the tumours with the appearance of endometrial carcinoma (24 per cent), and the third largest group was composed of the adenocarcinomas. This was the first study to indicate the relatively high incidence of primary endometrial-like lesions among the ovarian neoplasms and provided a basis for the proposals by the conference that these tumours be classified as a separate entity.

He did not agree, TEILUM said, with the theory presented by GRICOUROFF, that lymphatic spread is the sole explanation for all cases of endometriosis, because he had observed many times direct differentiation from the surface epithelium of the ovary. Stromatosis may be different, because the malignant side of stromal endometriosis behaves more like sarcoma. Under such circumstances, the spread by the lymphatic vessels and the blood stream may be of more importance. As to the so-called inclusion cyst on the surface of the ovary, he believed that the direct transition from the surface epithelium to these inclusions had been well demonstrated and, therefore, they could not be the result of lymphatic spread.

TEILUM also questioned the bases for suggesting a relationship between endometrioid tumours and tumours of the mesonephric group, since what are generally called mesonephric tumours are not usually mesonephric rest tumours. Therefore, to consider these tumours as having any special relationship to endometrioid tumours is not justified and he warned against extending the term "endometrioid" in this respect. The prognosis for the so-called clear cell tumours is much better — about 50 per cent survival in cases without spread outside the ovary and nearly 100 per cent death where there is extension outside the ovary. Therefore, the tendency to include all of these cases with the endometrioid tumour may affect the statistics. He also disagreed with the inclusion of mesoderm and mixed tumour in this group, although both the mesoderm and the mixed tumour may sometimes originate in the endometrium. Another point in differential diagnosis is that if the carcinomatous component is dominant in a carcinoma-sarcoma, the tumour may resemble endometrial carcinoma, but these tumours should be considered separately.

LUISI concurred that some cases of endometriosis can be explained by the mechanism which GRICOUROFF described but others cannot. In the case of laparotomy scars, for example, the transplantation is clearly established. In addition, the frequency of deciduosis in ovarian tumours is difficult to explain by the "embolization" of endometrial portions. He also said that in his material he had three representative cases of uterine stromatosis which were difficult to consider as sarcomatous. In one specimen, he could demonstrate the presence of glandular parts with no malignant features. In his opinion, he said, the theory of embolization explains only some cases of endometriosis; in other instances, another explanation is necessary.

SCULLY added that, in his opinion, there was occasionally a true benign neoplasm of an endometrioid type in the ovary, because he had seen adenofibromas in which the epithelium was of endometrial, rather than the serous or mucinous type. He agreed that the term "endometrioid carcinoma" should be restricted to those ovarian tumours that simulate the classic adenocarcinoma or adenoacanthoma of the uterus. He thought there was a distinction between endometrioid tumours and tumours of the ovary that may be derived from endometriosis. He agreed with GRICOUROFF that other types of malignant tumour in the ovary could be shown to originate in endometriosis, but to include these tumours in the category of endometrioid carcinoma would create a heterogeneous group, which would pose a problem in analysis.

KOTTMEIER described experimental studies done some years ago in Sweden. Endometrium was taken from pregnant rabbits and a small block applied in the muscle. After three or four weeks, changes typical of endometriosis were observed in this area. More recently, a number of therapeutic abortions have been performed in that country. The method used is to incise the fornix, dissect the bladder from the anterior wall of the cervix and remove the fetus through an incision in the cervix. A recent investigation of over 3,000 abortions showed that endometriosis occurred in the bladder and the scar for 19 per cent of these patients.

References

CORNER jr., G. W., HU, C. Y., and HERTIG, A. T., Ovarian carcinoma arising in endometriosis. *Amer. J. Obstet. Gynec.* **59**, 760—774 (1950).

CULLEN, T. S., Adenomyoma uteri diffusum benignum. *Johns Hopk. Hosp. Rep.* **6**, 133—142 (1896).

GRICOUROFF, G., Envahissement des ganglions pelviens dans le cancer du col de l'utérus et endométriose ganglionnaire. *Bull. Ass. franç. Cancer* **25**, 759—778 (1936).

— L'endométriose. Signes cliniques et théories pathogéniques. *Paris méd.* **103**, 249—262 (1937).

— Sur la pathogénie de l'endométriose. *Ann. Anat. path. et Anat. normale méd.-chir.* **16**, 751—760 (1939).

HALBAN, J., Hysteroadenosis metastatica. *Arch. Gynäk.* **124**, 457—482 (1925).

HENRY, J. S., An endometrial growth in the right labium majus. *Surg. Gynec. Obstet.* **44**, 637—647 (1927).

HERTIG, A. T., and GORE, H., Atlas of tumor pathology. *Tumors of the ovary and fallopian tube*, vol. 11, fasc. 33, part 3. Washington: A.F.I.P. 1961.

IWANOFF, N. S., Drüsiges cystenhaltiges Uterus fibromyom kompliziert durch Sarkom und Carzinom (adenofibromyoma cysticum sarcomatodes carcinomatosum). *Mschr. Geburtsh. Gynäk.* **7**, 295—300 (1898).

JAVERT, C. T., Pathogenesis of endometriosis based on endometrial homeoplasia, direct extension, exfoliation and implantation, lymphatic and hematogenous metastasis. *Cancer (Philad.)* **2**, 399—410 (1949).

— Observation on the pathology and spread of endometriosis based on the theory of benign metastasis. *Amer. J. Obstet. Gynec.* **62**, 477—487 (1951).

KISTNER, R. W., and HERTIG, A. T., Primary adenoacanthoma of the ovary. *Cancer (Philad.)* **5**, 1134—1145 (1952).

SAMPSON, J. A., Perforating hemorrhagic (chocolate) cysts of the ovary, their importance and especially their relation to pelvic adenomas of the endometrial type. *Arch. Surg.* **3**, 245—323 (1921).

— Endometrial carcinoma of ovary. *Arch. Surg.* **10**, 1—72 (1925).

WELLER, C. V., The ectopic decidual reaction and its significance in endometriosis. *Amer. J. Path.* **11**, 287—290 (1935).

Sex Cord-Mesenchyme Tumours

Pathologic Classification and its Relation to Prognosis and Treatment

Robert E. Scully, M. D.

Pathologist, Massachusetts General Hospital
Associate Clinical Professor of Pathology, Harvard Medical School
Boston, Mass., U.S.A.

Introduction

The category "sex cord-mesenchyme tumours" includes all neoplasms composed of cells that are ultimately derived from the sex cords or the mesenchyme of the embryonic gonad (Morris and Scully, 1958). These tumours may contain granulosa cells, stromal-theca cells, Sertoli cells, Leydig cells or the precursors of these elements, alone or in any combination. The term "mesenchymoma" has also been applied to this group of neoplasms (Malkasian *et al.*, 1965), but it has a less acceptable embryologic basis because there is disagreement as to whether the sex cords and their derivatives, the granulosa and Sertoli cells, develop from the mesenchyme or from the "germinal" epithelium. The designation "specialized gonadal stromal tumours" was proposed for neoplasms of the testis that contain combinations of the various cell types mentioned above (Mostofi *et al.*, 1959), and this term was subsequently adopted for the analogous ovarian tumours (Hertig and Gore, 1961; Novak and Long, 1965), but it has the same theoretical disadvantage as "mesenchymoma". The ideal name awaits a concensus among embryologists on the origins of the gonadal cell types but, whatever

term is used, authorities generally agree that the tumours in question fall into four broad categories.

1. Tumours of female cell types — granulosa cells (granulosa cell tumours), ovarian stromal and theca cells (fibroma-thecoma group of tumours) and luteinized forms of these cells (luteomas), alone or in combination (granulosa-theca cell tumours).

2. Tumours of male cell types — Sertoli cells (testicular tubular adenomas; Sertoli cell tumours) and Leydig cells (Leydig cell tumours; hilus cell tumours) alone or in combination (Sertoli-Leydig cell tumours; arrhenoblastomas; androblastomas).

3. Tumours composed of mixtures of female and male cell types (gynandroblastomas).

4. Tumours composed of cells too poorly differentiated to be identified as male or female or having morphologic features common to both.

It must be emphasized that morphology with all its limitations must remain the basis of the present-day classification of sex cord-mesenchyme tumours. Despite the great advances that have been made in steroid biochemistry, very little is known about the specific functions of the various cellular constituents of the gonads and in most cases the resemblance of the neoplastic cells to their normal counterparts is sufficiently close to warrant a specific morphologic diagnosis.

Tumours of Female Cell Types

If one excludes granulosa cell tumours, whose origin from the ovarian

inized cells (large polyhedral or rounded cells with abundant vacuolated or eosinophilic cytoplasm and round nuclei containing single prominent nucleoli) (partly luteinized fibroma, partly luteinized thecoma), the stromal luteoma (completely luteinized fibroma, completely luteinized thecoma) and the preg-

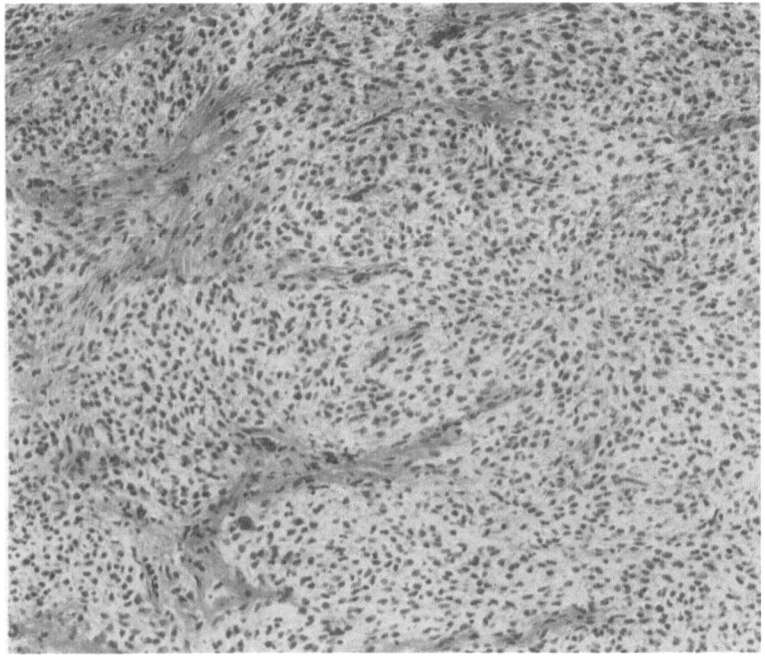

Fig. 1. Thecoma. The tumour cells have oval nuclei and abundant pale cytoplasm. Fibrous trabeculae traverse the tumour. From MORRIS, J. McL., and SCULLY, R. E., *Endocrine pathology of the ovary.* St. Louis: C. V. Mosby Co. 1958

mesenchyme has not been established with certainty, the latter can be viewed as giving rise to five types of neoplasm. The most common is the fibroma in which the neoplastic cells are collagen-producing spindle cells that may contain lipid in their cytoplasm; much less frequent is the thecoma in which many of the tumour cells are rounded and have abundant vacuolated cytoplasm laden with lipid (Fig. 1). Rarer forms of female mesenchymal tumours are the fibroma that is sprinkled with clusters of lute-

nancy luteoma. Within this category of tumours there exists no sharp morphologic distinction between the fibroma and the thecoma, and we agree with BURSLEM, *et al.* (1954) that both types of neoplasm are most satisfactorily grouped together within a fibroma-thecoma category. When the neoplasm contains little or no lipid, a diagnosis of fibroma can generally be made with confidence; when abundant fat is present in swollen vacuolated cells, the tumour is most often estrogenic and merits the designation the coma. However, when one is evaluating the transitional tumours that contain only moderate amounts of lipid, biochemical or clinicopathologic evidence of estrogen production is required before making a diagnosis of thecoma. The fibroma with clusters of luteinized cells can be identified readily, but in rare instances careful

Leydig cell tumour only by its location in the cortex or the medulla instead of the hilus of the ovary and by the absenec of crystalloids of Reinke in the cytoplasm of its constituent cells (Scully, 1964). Probably some and possibly most lipoid cell tumours of the ovary are stromal luteomas whose large size has

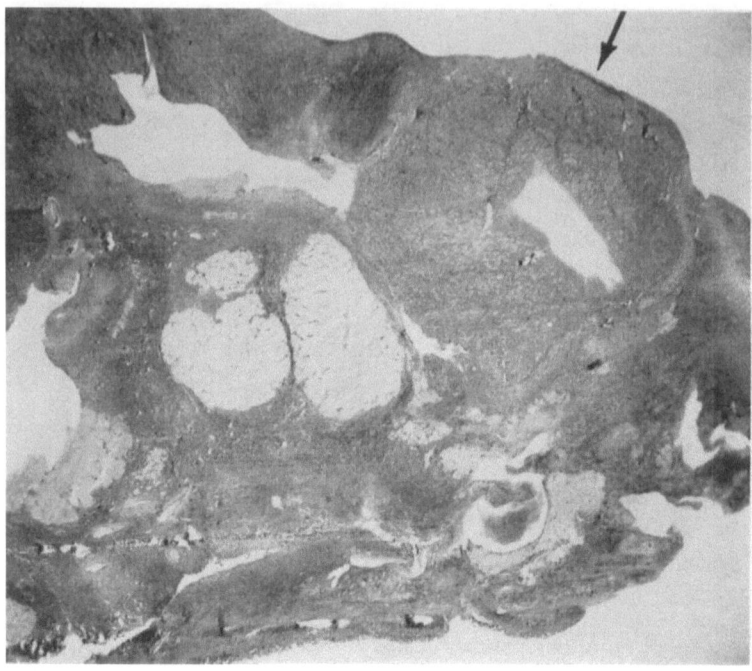

Fig. 2. Stromal luteoma. The small tumour is situated in the cortex (Arrow). From Scully, R. E., Stromal Luteoma of the Ovary. *Cancer (Philad.)* **17**, 769—778 (1964)

fied readily, but in rare instances careful study of such a tumour discloses the presence of crystalloids of Reinke in the cytoplasm of the cells that appeared on initial examination to be luteinized cells (Scully, 1953). Such a finding indicates that the cells in question are true Leydig cells and the fibromatous component is in all probability of male or hilar stromal rather than ovarian stromal origin. The stromal luteoma (Figs. 2 and 3), a tumour composed exclusively of luteinized ovarian mesenchymal cells, can be differentiated from the hilus or

erased topographical evidence of their origin within the ovarian parenchyma (Scully, 1964; Hughesdon, 1966). The pregnancy luteoma, which occurs as single or multiple tumour-like nodules composed of luteinized cells and arises in the last trimester of pregnancy, appears to be chorionic gonadotropin-dependent and not an autonomous neoplasm. It bears some resemblance to the stromal luteoma of the non-pregnant woman and may be derived from either the theca lutein or stromal lutein cell, both of which are derivatives of the ovarian mesenchyme (STERNBERG and BARCLAY, 1966).

Rare malignant tumours that resemble benign neoplasms of the fibroma-thecoma group have been reported as fibrosarcomas or malignant thecomas (FLICK and BANFIELD, 1956; FODA et al., 1961); the illustrations suggest that some

component of cells of mesenchymal origin. Just as it can difficult to distinguish a fibroma from a thecoma, so it may be impossible to decide in some cases whether the mesenchymal element of a granulosa cell tumour is a truly neoplastic fibromatous or thecomatous component or merely an ovarian stromal

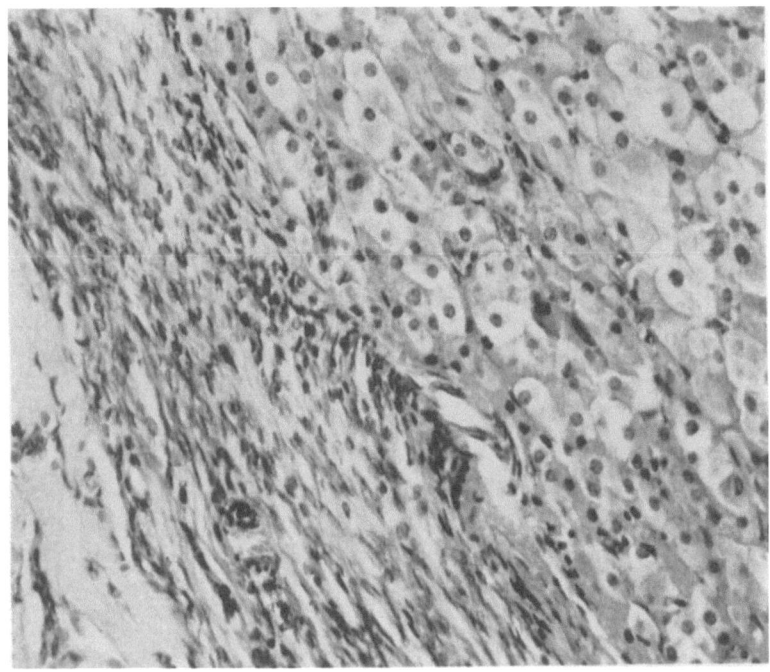

Fig. 3. Stromal luteoma and adjacent ovarian stroma. The neoplastic cells are large and rounded with central nuclei. From SCULLY, R. E., Stromal luteoma of the ovary. Cancer (Philad.) 17, 769—778 (1964)

of these neoplasms are sarcomatoid granulosa cell tumours, while others may be banal fibrosarcomas not proven to have originated from the ovarian mesenchyme; we are not aware of any such tumours that have been associated with conclusive evidence of estrogen production and deserve the diagnosis of malignant thecoma.

The terms "granulosa cell tumour" and "granulosa-theca cell tumour" have been used interchangeably for neoplasms that contain more than a rare nest of granulosa cells and a variable

reaction of the type elicited by other ovarian epithelial tumours, benign and malignant, primary or metastatic (MORRIS and SCULLY, 1958).

The granulosa cell tumour has been subdivided according to its manner of growth into several types: macrofollicular, microfollicular, insular, trabecular, cylindromatous, tubular, moiré-silk, and diffuse or sarcomatoid; these patterns are commonly mixed in the same neoplasm. The follicular form is the best differentiated. The macrofollicular pattern is characterized by the presence of large follicles resembling Graafian follicles, and rare examples of neoplastic cysts lined by granulosa and theca cells can be differentiated from physiologic follicular cysts only by their enormous size (SHER and MARSH, 1963; PALLADINO, *et al.*, 1965; TAYLOR, 1966). The hallmark of the microfollicular pattern is the Call-Exner

clinical malignancy. The insular, trabecular and cylindromatous patterns are characterized by sharply demarcated groups of well-differentiated granulosa cells that are not forming follicles. The so-called tubular form can be subdivided into two categories: the true tubular and the pseudotubular. Neoplasms contain-

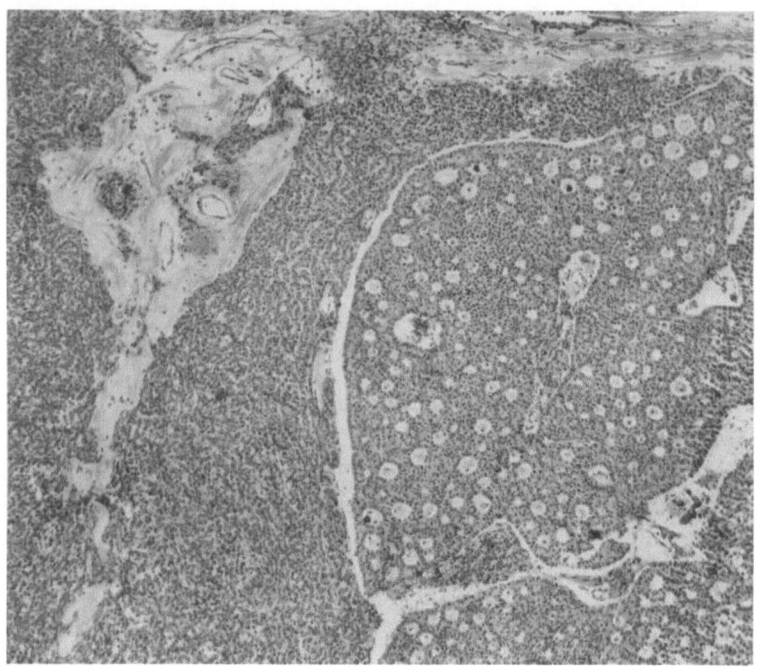

Fig. 4. Granulosa cell tumour. A microfollicular pattern is seen at the right; a moiré-silk pattern, at the left. From MORRIS, J. McL., and SCULLY, R. E., *Endocrine pathology of the ovary*. St. Louis: C. V. Mosby Co. 1958

body, a small round cavity filled with eosinophilic material and often one or two shrunken nuclei, and surrounded by well-differentiated granulosa cells whose irregular nuclei have a haphazard orientation (Fig. 4). The misinterpretation of carcinomatous glands lined by anaplastic cells vaguely resembling granulosa cells and of the acini encountered in carcinoids as Call-Exner bodies has often led to an erroneous diagnosis of granulosa cell tumour and a higher than deserved reputation of the latter for

ing true tubules with lumens were originally considered to be tubular granulosa cell tumors when they were associated with estrogenic manifestations, but are now more generally regarded as estrogenic Sertoli cell tumours or Sertoli-Leydig cell tumours (androblastoma tubulare lipoides) (TEILUM, 1958). The pseudotubular pattern is one in which the architecture is similar to that seen in the true tubular form, but the centers of the tubules, rather than being empty, are filled with the pale cytoplasm of the

Sertoli cells, which may be laden with lipid. Pseudotubular areas are common in otherwise typical granulosa cell tumours, but when they form the predominant element of the neoplasm, a diagnosis of Sertoli cell tumour or Sertoli-Leydig cell tumour is generally made since the pseudotubular pattern is more culum is present among granulosa cells, but an abundant network invests theca cells individually. When the granulosa cells acquire abundant cytoplasm and resemble granulosa lutein cells, the term "luteinized granulosa cell tumour" is often used, but the presence of "luteinization" cannot be correlated with evi-

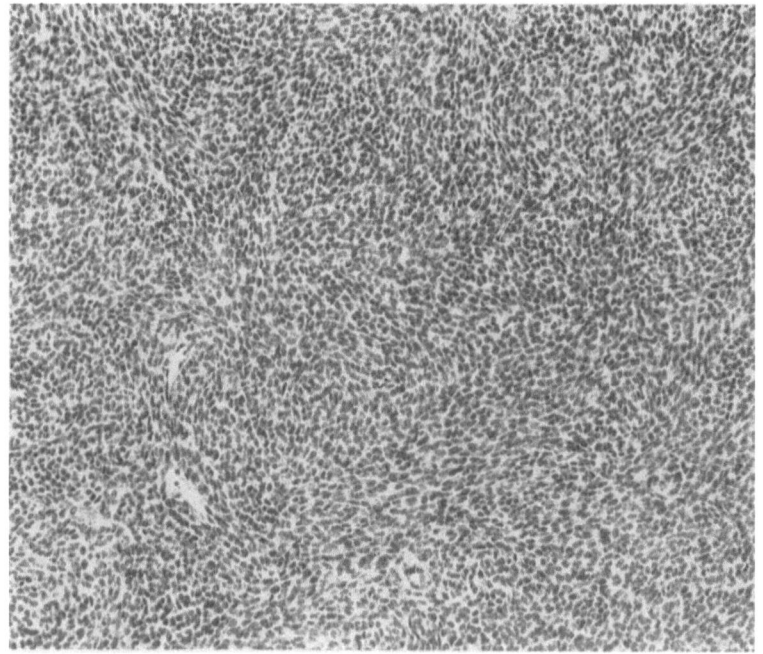

Fig. 5. Granulosa cell tumour, sarcomatoid pattern. From MORRIS, J. McL., and SCULLY, R. E., *Endocrine pathology of the ovary*. St. Louis: C. V. Mosby Co. 1958

characteristic of male than female sex cord derivatives. The moiré-silk pattern, in which the granulosa cells are arranged in slender zigzag columns (Fig. 4), often merges with the sarcomatoid pattern in which the tumour cells are growing diffusely and the nuclei are generally round and closely packed (Fig. 5). The sarcomatoid form of granulosa cell tumour is sometimes confused with the thecoma, and in making the distinction the reticulum stain is most helpful — typically little or no reti-

dence of progesterone secretion by the tumour.

There is a difference of opinion in regard to the correlation of the microscopic appearance of granulosa cell tumours with their prognosis. BUSBY and ANDERSON (1954) found grading useful, reporting a 10 per cent five-year mortality in patients with Grade 1 and Grade 2 tumours, but a 63 per cent mortality when the neoplasm was Grade 3 or Grade 4. Similarly, KOTTMEIER (1953) recorded a 13 per cent rate of

clinical malignancy in five years among
the patients with follicular or cylindromatous forms of granulosa cell tumour,
as opposed to a 36 per cent rate among
those with the sarcomatoid type. In
opposition to these views, BURSLEM and
his associates (1954), who reported a
28 per cent incidence of clinical malignancy, TAYLOR (1966), who stated that
less than 5 per cent of granulosa cell
tumours are malignant and SJÖSTEDT
and WAHLEN (1961), who recorded a
five-year cure rate of 84 per cent, were
unable to distinguish the benign and the
malignant cases by microscopic examination. These differences of opinion may
reflect in part variations in the interpretation of poorly differentiated carcinomas that bear an incomplete resemblance
to typical granulosa cell tumours. We
believe that whether or not one considers such tumours to be of granulosa
cell origin they should be placed in a
separate category because of their obviously high degree of malignancy. Although microscopic evaluation of prognosis may have statistical validity in
large series of cases, it probably is of
limited help in individual patients, except
perhaps when one is dealing with tumours at either extreme of differentiation. The gross extent of the tumour at
the time of operation appears to be the
best guide to prognosis and treatment.
BUSBY and ANDERSON (1954) reported
that only 3 per cent of the patients in
whom the tumour was confined to one
ovary died of spread of the tumour
within 5 years, whereas over half of
those with extension beyond the ovary
at the time of operation died of metastatic tumour. Similarly, SJÖSTEDT and
WAHLEN (1961) recorded an 88 per cent
five-year survival if no metastases were
found at operation in contrast to a 43
per cent survival in women with metastatic spread. Fixation of the tumour,
per se, was not a highly significant prognostic factor, since the patients with
adherent tumours had a 75 per cent survival; also, those whose tumours had
ruptured (20 per cent of the total number) had an 80 per cent five-year survival.

There are several facts regarding the
spread and biological behavior of granulosa cell tumours that are of importance
in determining the choice of therapy:
1. Less than 5 per cent of the neoplasms
are bilateral (but before a decision is
made to conserve the ovary opposite
the tumour in a young woman, that
ovary should be bisected and, if feasible,
biopsied to exclude involvement). The
results achieved with unilateral operation are not significantly worse than
those obtained by bilateral oophorectomy followed by radiation therapy in
young women according to SJÖSTEDT
and WAHLEN (1961). 2. The tumour
tends to spread locally and distant metastases are rare. 3. Recurrences, which
frequently appear more than 5 years
after the initial operation, can often be
successfully treated by a second operation or radiation (KOTTMEIER, 1953;
SJÖSTEDT and WAHLEN, 1961); (MALKA-
SIAN, et al., 1965).

Tumours of Male Cell Types

These neoplasms are composed of
Sertoli cells, Leydig cells or the precursors of either, alone or in any combination. The mixed forms were chris-
tened "arrhenoblastomas" or "androblastomas" by MEYER, but MORRIS and
SCULLY (1958) preferred the designation
"Sertoli-Leydig cell tumours", which
is in agreement with the terminology
that is used for the tumours of female
cell types and avoids the connotation
of masculinization, which may be absent
in patients with these tumours.

The most mature form of Sertoli-
Leydig cell tumour is the tubular ade-

noma of PICK, composed of hollow tubules lined by well differentiated Sertoli cells and separated by typical Leydig cells, which occasionally contain crystalloids of REINKE in their cytoplasm. At the opposite extreme of differentiation is the sarcomatoid tumour (Fig. 6), which resembles a banal sarcoma, but cytoplasm or as indifferent-appearing spindle cells. Perplexing heterologous elements are present in a minority of these tumours. Exceptionally one encounters smooth muscle, skeletal muscle, fat, cartilage or bone (HUGHESDON, 1953); more often, glands lined by mucus-secreting cells (Fig. 7) and occa-

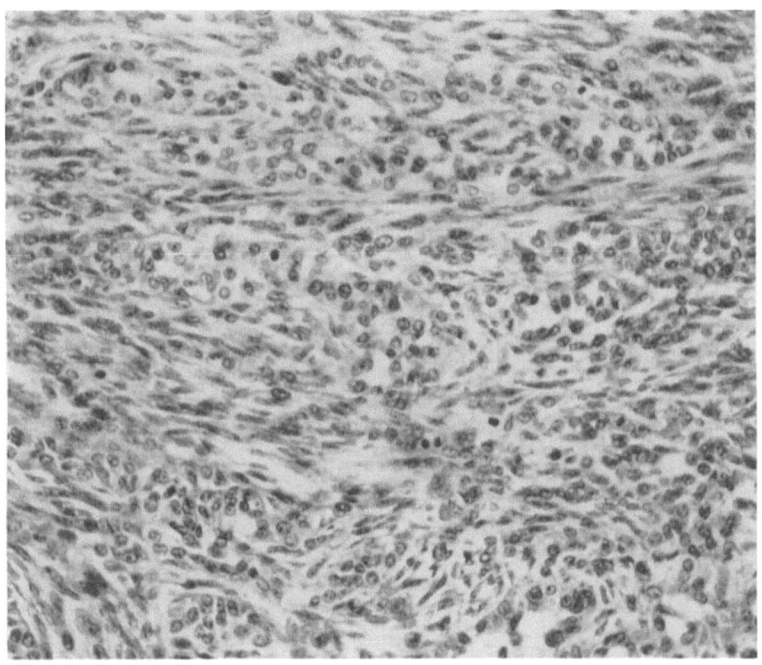

Fig. 6. Sertoli-Leydig cell tumour, sarcomatoid pattern. Many mitoses are visible

contains cords of Sertoli cells, aggregates of Leydig cells or other elements, the presence of which betrays the nature of the tumour. Between the tubular and the sarcomatoid varieties is the intermediate form of Sertoli-Leydig cell tumour (Fig. 7), which exhibits a wide range of microscopic patterns. The Sertoli cells may line true tubules, retiform channels or cysts or may form solid tubules, trabeculae, islands, or slender columns resembling sex cords. The Leydig element may appear as mature cells with rare crystalloids of REINKE, as large rounded cells with spongy lipid-laden sional argentaffin cells are seen (HARTZ, 1945; SCULLY, 1966). We have encountered one case in which a small tumour of the intermediate variety lay adjacent to a rhabdomyosarcoma; metastases were composed of neuroblastomatous elements and embryonal cartilage.

A small number of Sertoli-Leydig cell tumours are comprised entirely or almost entirely of Sertoli cells. The best differentiated form of Sertoli cell tumour is the tubular adenoma in which the tubules have lumens and intertubular Leydig cells are scant or absent. When this type of tumour is accompanied by estrogenic manifestations it has been traditionally interpreted as a tubular granulosa cell tumour but, with the more recent evidence that Sertoli cells may be capable of estrogen production and the realization that true tubule formation is not an architectural feature of granulosa cell proliferation, it has appeared more

have a pseudotubular architecture and a cellular composition that justifies placing them in the Sertoli cell category.

Pure or almost pure Leydig cell tumours fall into two categories — the hilus (hilar Leydig) cell tumour and a spindle cell tumour presumably arising from the male, or hilar, stroma and dif-

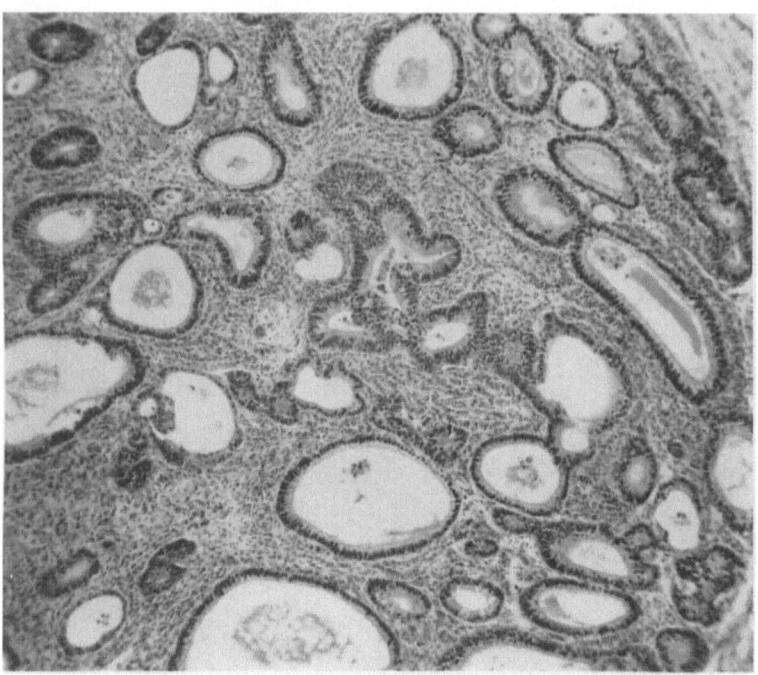

Fig. 7. Sertoli-Leydig cell tumour. Mucus-secreting tubular structures are separated by a sarcomatoid proliferation. From Case Records of The Massachusetts General Hospital, Case 8—1965. *New Engl. J. Med.* **272**, 365—371 (1965)

logical to make the diagnosis of an estrogenic Sertoli cell tumour (androblastoma tubulare lipoides) (TEILUM, 1958). Another well differentiated sex cord neoplasm that has been recently reclassified in the Sertoli cell group (TEILUM, 1958) is the estrogenic "folliculome lipidique" of Lecene, a tumour composed of winding solid tubules containing cells rich in lipid; this neoplasm resembles, to some extent, the estrogenic Sertoli cell tumour of the canine testis. Finally, occasional ovarian carcinomas

ferentiating focally into Leydig cells (SCULLY, 1953). Since hilus cells cannot be differentiated from luteinized stromal cells, theca lutein cells or the cells of adrenal cortical rests, except by the occasional presence of crystalloids of REINKE in their cytoplasm, hilus cell tumours that do not contain these inclusions cannot be diagnosed specifically, but only suspected with varying degrees of confidence. Such tumours of inconclusive nature have to be placed in the general category of lipoid cell tumours, which also includes neoplasms that may arise from the cells of adrenal cortical rests or lutein cells. If one requires the presence of crystalloids for a positive diagnosis there have been less than 20 acceptable cases of hilus cell tumour reported to date. The rare spindle cell tumour with focal differentiation into Leydig cells likewise cannot be distinguished from the fibroma with clusters of lutein cells unless crystalloids of REINKE are identified.

The incidence of clinical malignancy of Sertoli-Leydig cell tumours is unknown because their rarity has prevented the acquisition of a significantly large series of unselected cases. The literature contains figures ranging from under 5 to over 30 per cent of the cases (MATHET, 1956; O'HERN and NEUBECKER, 1962; TAYLOR, 1966). NOVAK and LONG (1965), who reported a 34 per cent death rate in patients who were followed for at least 5 years, were unable to correlate the degree of differentiation of the tumour with the prognosis in a series of 111 cases from the Ovarian Tumour Registry. Important facts to bear in mind in the treatment of Sertoli-Leydig cell tumours are that less than 5 per cent are bilateral (NOVAK and LONG, 1965) and their spread is mainly intraabdominal with distant metastases uncommon. Unlike the granulosa cell tumour, the Sertoli-Leydig cell tumour rarely recurs after 5 years (NOVAK and LONG, 1965). No convincing case of clinically malignant hilus cell tumour has been reported although it is conceivable that some of the malignant lipoid cell tumours that have been described are of hilus cell origin.

Sex Cord-Mesenchyme Tumours of Indeterminate and Mixed Cell Types

The patterns of growth and the types of cells that are encountered in about 10 per cent of sex cord-mesenchyme tumours are compatible with neoplasia of either female or male cell types; in such cases, examination of the tumour by various experts generally results in widely varying opinions. Our approach to these tumours is as follows: when a nondiagnostic growth pattern is seen in a part of the tumour, and a much more characteristic pattern elsewhere, the diagnosis is based on the latter; when the entire neoplasm is non-specific morphologically, a diagnosis of "sex cord-mesenchyme tumour of indeterminate cell types" is made.

Many otherwise typical Sertoli-Leydig cell tumours contain small areas that, considered alone, would undoubtedly evoke a diagnosis of granulosa cell tumour; similarly, the typical granulosa cell tumour may have pseudotubular formations that are, by themselves, more characteristic of the Sertoli cell tumour. While an argument might be advanced for regarding such neoplasms as mixed tumours, or gynandroblastomas, the transitional morphological zone between granulosa cell tumours and Sertoli cell tumours is so vaguely delimited that we prefer to restrict the diagnosis of gynandroblastoma to cases where mature granulosa cells with typical Call-Exner bodies coexist with typical hollow tubules or with Leydig cells containing crystalloids of REINKE (Figs. 8 and 9). Unless one requires the presence of these highly specific features, diagnostic chaos results in this area and the designation "gynandroblastoma" becomes meaningless. Since female cells are capable of androgen production and male cells can secrete estrogens, the hormonal manifestations of these tumours are not reliable criteria for identifying the neoplastic cell types and consequently are of no value in making a diagnosis of gynandroblastoma. There are only rare

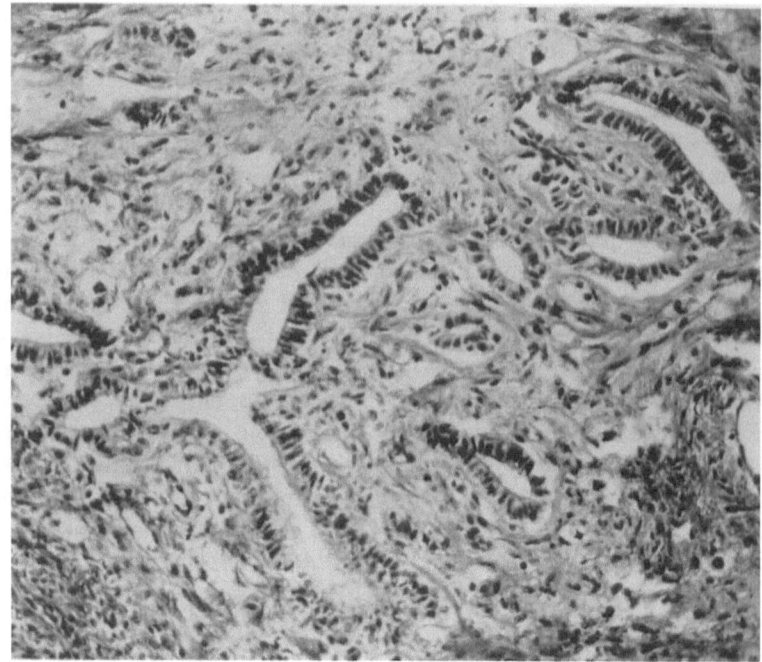

Fig. 8. Mixed sex cord-mesenchyme tumour (gynandroblastoma) showing tubule formation. Published with the permission of ROBERT L. BERGGREN, M.D.

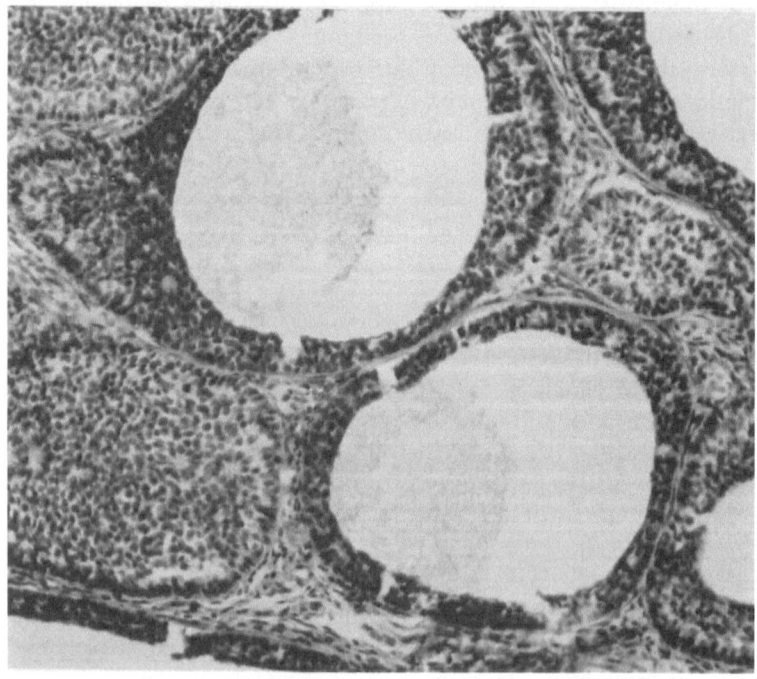

Fig. 9. Granulosa cell portion of gynandroblastoma illustrated in Fig. 8

cases in the literature that fulfill the rigid criteria for gynandroblastoma given above (MORRIS and SCULLY, 1958).

Since no large series of cases of either mixed or indeterminate sex cord-mesenchyme tumours has been reported, little can be said about their prognosis and

are generally present in the form of nests or solid tubules, in which cells with small oval or round nuclei (Sertoli or granulosa cells) are disposed peripherally in single file, in coronal fashion about the germ cells or around eosinophilic deposits that resemble Call-Exner

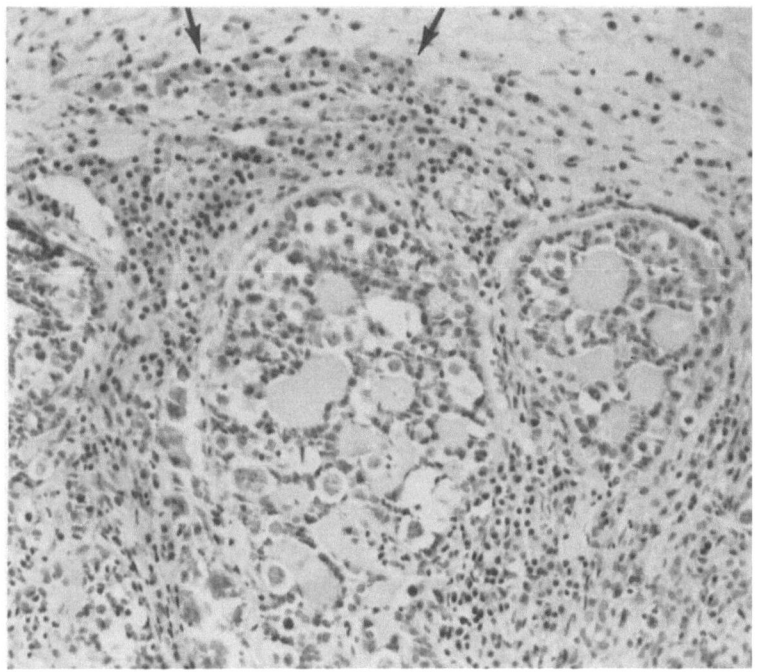

Fig. 10. Gonadoblastoma. Solid nests composed of large germ cells and smaller epithelial cells are separated by elements resembling both Leydig and theca cells (Arrows). Numerous hyaline bodies resembling Call-Exner bodies are present within the solid nests. From SCULLY, R. E., Androgenic lesions of the ovary, chapter 9 in: GRADY, H. G., and SMITH, D. E. (eds.), *The ovary*. Baltimore: Williams & Wilkins Co. 1963

treatment, but there is no reason to believe that they differ from those of tumours of pure male or female cell types.

Gonadoblastomas

Gonadoblastomas are sex cord-mesenchyme tumours of indeterminate cell types that also contain germ cells (SCULLY, 1953). We are aware of over 60 cases (SCULLY, 1966), about a third of them unreported. The sex cord and germ cell components of the tumour

bodies (Fig. 10). Laminated calcific concretions are commonly encountered within the nests and often fuse to form irregular confluent masses (Fig. 11), which may be so large and extensive that the calcification is detectable on an x-ray film of the pelvis (MELICOW and USON, 1959; TETER, 1960). Mesenchymal elements may or may not be present; when they are, they resemble both lutein cells and Leydig cells (Fig. 10); they may contain lipochrome granules, but crystalloids of REINKE have not been identified in them. The germinal element is composed of cells that resemble those of the germinoma (dysgerminoma; seminoma); even in neoplasms of microscopic size they commonly exhibit mitotic activity; often they overgrow the other components of the tumor to form typical germinomas; indeed, a rare nest of sex cord elements and germ cells or a small focus of calcification may be the only clue that a large germinoma arose as a one-sided germ cell overgrowth of a gonadoblastoma. Occasionally, a gonadoblastoma may be mixed with other forms of germ cell neoplasia such as endodermal sinus tumour, choriocarcinoma or solid teratoma (SANTESSON and MARRUBINI, 1957; FRASIER et al., 1964). The gonadoblastoma is found most often in intersexual individuals who are chromatin-negative phenotypic females with primary amenorrhea; more often than not they are virilized to varying degrees. In the few patients from whom they have been obtained, karyotypes have generally shown a 46 XY pattern or XO-XY mosaicism (SIEBENMANN, 1961; FRASIER et al., 1964; ROBINSON et al., 1964; TETER et al., Acta Endocrinol., 1964; TETER et al., Am. J. Obst. & Gynec. 1964; MILLER, 1964; COHEN and SHAW, 1965; STRUMPF, 1965). Often the tumour has replaced the involved gonad so that its nature cannot be determined, but in those cases in which a gonadal remnant has been identified it has proved to be a streak gonad composed of ovarian-type stroma (Fig. 12) or a testis, which is usually abdominal, but occasionally inguinal. In over one-third of the cases bilateral involvement has been demonstrated. The gonad opposite the neoplasm has usually proved to be a streak or

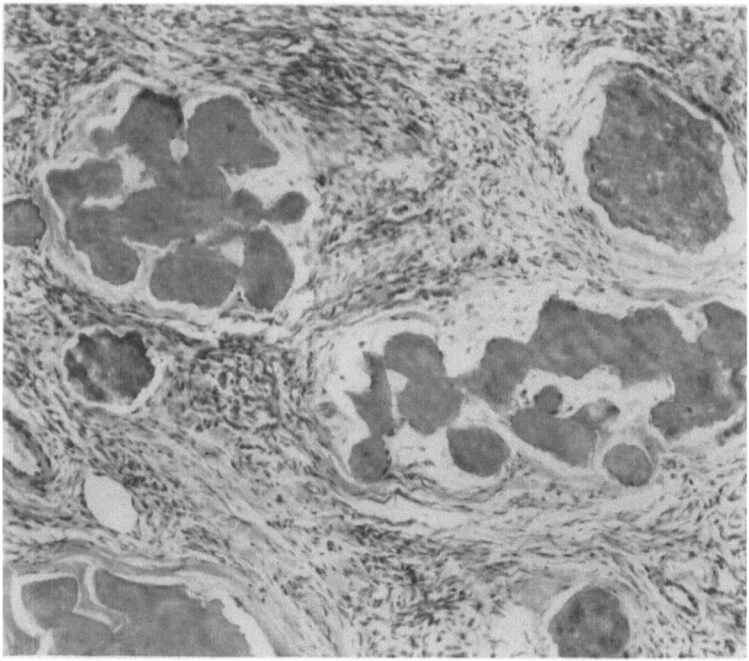

Fig. 11. Gonadoblastoma. Irregular calcified masses are separated by stroma resembling ovarian stroma

rudiment, but often a testis. Although often the exact nature of the patient's intersexual state was in doubt because the tumour had entirely replaced one gonad, many patients apparently had pure gonadal dysgenesis or mixed gonadal dysgenesis (asymmetrical gonadal differentiation). One patient had gonadoblastoma has produced androgens, because virilizing manifestations have improved after the removal of the tumour (SCULLY, 1953; USIZIMA, 1956; GIUSTI et al., 1962; SCULLY, 1966).

No case of gonadoblastoma has as yet been reported to metastasize, but many have been discovered incidentally

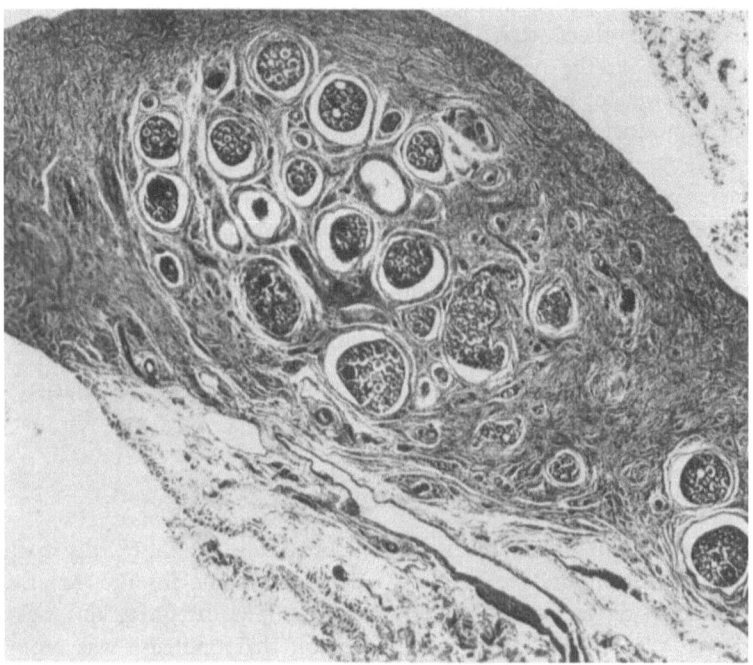

Fig. 12. Gonadoblastoma arising in a gonadal streak

atypical testicular feminization (FLOR et al., 1962) and another, classical Turner's syndrome (DOMINGUEZ and GREENBLATT, 1962). Even though most patients with gonadoblastomas have been clearly intersexual on the basis of the findings on physical examination or operation, a few, who did not have karyotypes, appeared to be relatively normal females with periods of amenorrhea alternating with apparently normal cycles; one patient had two pregnancies (SCULLY, 1966). In occasional women there has been strong evidence that the during the surgical investigation of intersexual patients and have been small and often microscopic in size; few have had a long-term follow-up. Since the germ cell element commonly overgrows to form a germinoma, the gonadoblastoma is a potentially dangerous neoplasm, and its identification in a biopsy specimen of a gonad justifies its removal. When germinomatous overgrowth is present the patient should be treated as though she had an uncomplicated dysgerminoma; because the opposite gonad is almost always abnormal and commonly contains a microscopic, if not a gross neoplasm, the question of its conservation rarely arises.

Summary

Sex cord-mesenchyme tumours are neoplasms composed of cells that are ultimately derived from the sex cords or the mesenchyme of the embryonic gonad. These tumours may contain granulosa cells, stromal-theca cells, Sertoli cells, Leydig cells or the precursors of these elements, alone or in any combination. Of the tumours of female cell types, the thecoma is rarely, if ever, malignant, but neoplasms containing granulosa cells with or without theca cells may exhibit a low grade of malignancy. There is disagreement as to whether the microscopic pattern of such tumours bears any relationship to their prognosis. Among the tumours of male cell types, no convincing case of malignant hilus cell tumour has been reported. The Sertoli-Leydig cell tumours (arrhenoblastomas) may show a form of malignancy similar to that of the granulosa-theca cell tumours. There does not appear to be any relationship between the microscopic appearance of these neoplasms and their clinical course. Little is known of the prognosis of the sex cord-mesenchyme tumours of indeterminate or mixed cell types, but it is probably similar to that of the pure female or male tumours.

The gonadoblastoma is a tumour composed of germ cells as well as sex cord and mesenchyme elements. It is encountered chiefly in intersexual patients, who are usually phenotypic females; although it has not been reported to metastasize as such, it often gives rise to a germinoma, which is a malignant tumour capable of metastasis.

Discussion

GRICOUROFF commented that some of the lipoidic cell tumours were closely related to tumours of the ovarian mesenchyme and to the so-called pregnancy luteomas. He did not know, he said, whether the pregnancy luteomas were true neoplasms or reactive proliferations, but he favored the latter. Metastases from granulosa cell tumours are rare early in the course of this disease, but late metastases are fairly frequent. He inquired as to the malignant potential of the polycystic folliculomas, which he believes are benign tumours, or "granulosa cell adenomas".

LUISI agreed with SCULLY that the hilus cell tumours can be diagnosed only by the demonstration of Reinke's crystalloids, which are the only structures permitting differentiation from luteinized stromal cells, theca lutein cells, and adrenal rest cells. This difficulty in distinction is the rationale for the generic lipoidic cell tumour category, and was also the reason that one case was reported as a malignant hilar cell tumour, a diagnosis with which he did not agree.

Misinterpretation of granulosa cell tumours is common. There are some highly malignant forms, LUISI said; he himself had one in which the diagnosis was made only because of the observation of a little focus of follicular differentiation but it was questionable whether some of the so-called malignant granulosa cell tumours in the literature really belonged in this category. He added that he had seen two specimens in which an ovarian lymphoma was confused with a granulosa cell tumour because of the presence of small rounded cavities surrounded by homogeneous cellular proliferation. He demonstrated the presence of reticular cells in these supposedly empty rounded spaces in new sections of the tumours.

Opinions differ, he said, as to whether there really exists a mixed granulosa theca cell tumour, or if the fibrothecomatous component is merely an ovarian stromal reaction. Resolution of this point would help in the interpretation of some controversial points about the embryology of the gonads. Possibly, the intimate relationship between granulosa and theca cells favors the theory of a common mesenchymal genesis.

The designation of Sertoli-Leydig cell tumours avoids the implication of masculinization. In his four cases, he could not demonstrate the presence of Reinke's crystalloids in the interstitial eosinophilic lipid-containing cells. This group included one patient with progressive masculinization of four years' duration. At operation, the surgeon removed a voluminous ovarian tumour with an adenocarcinomatous structure, which he believed, justified the diagnosis of a Sertoli cell tumour with marked cellular anaplasia. In 50 blocks he could not demonstrate Leydig cells or a stromal reaction that could explain the masculinization, although it had partially regressed after removal of the tumour.

KOTTMEIER emphasized that it was misleading to designate granulosa cell tumours as granulosa cell carcinomas and to include patients with these tumours in statistics on therapeutic results in ovarian carcinoma. He agreed that the five-year cure rate does not give much information about granulosa cell tumours. If patients are followed for 15 or 20 years, however, more recurrences will be noted. At the Radiumhemmet, of 165 cases observed for 14 or more years, about 70 per cent of the sarcomatoid granulosa cell tumours recurred;

but there were recurrences of the other types in only 14 per cent.

As for therapy, at the Radiumhemmet, patients under 45 years of age with granulosa cell tumours are treated only by unilateral oophorectomy and irradiation is not given. If the patient is postmenopausal, however, radiation is given in addition to surgery, for sarcomatoid tumours, since they are probably more radiosensitive than the other types.

KOTTMEIER then inquired as to the frequency of endometrial carcinoma in association with granulosa and theca cell tumours.

TEILUM said that no objection could be made to the common heading of "Sex Cord-Mesenchyme Tumours" but this was not a distinctive term for a specific tumour type. He did not consider it practical to call the tumour formerly known as "arrhenoblastoma" a "Sertoli-Leydig cell tumour" since such a tumour does not always contain identifiable Sertoli or Leydig cells. MEYER used the term "arrhenoblastoma" originally to indicate mainly the virilizing effect. Since, in his own earlier studies, he found tumours with the morphology of the arrhenoblastoma associated with feminization, both in the male and the female, he suggested the term "androblastoma", a morphological definition that is more comprehensive and does not apply only to virilizing tumours. In his own classification, androblastoma includes both the virilizing arrhenoblastomas and the feminizing tumours. As to GRICOUROFF's question about the so-called polycystic folliculoma, he agreed that this type was benign and thought there was no doubt that it was a well-differentiated granulosa cell tumour.

SCULLY agreed with GRICOUROFF that cystic well-differentiated granulosa cell tumours are almost always benign, but there are rare exceptions to this statement. In regard to the reported malignant hilar cell tumour, he personally had examined the slides and was not convinced that it was indeed a hilar cell tumour. As to KOTTMEIER's remark about the incidence of carcinoma of the endometrium with granulosa cell tumours, SCULLY did not have a large enough series to be statistically significant. The problem revolves around the ability of the pathologist to distinguish severe atypical hyperplasia from Grade 1 adenocarcinoma of the endometrium and the points of distinction are fuzzy and controversial.

As to the frequency of arrhenoblastomas, he commented that, at one time, the diagnosis was made in many cases on the basis of clinical history alone. It was believed, he said, that a virilizing tumour had to be either an arrhenoblastoma or a lipoid cell tumour. Today, it is known that there are tumours in which the neoplastic cells are not in themselves functioning, but they may stimulate the stroma of the ovary, which produces the tumour stroma, to secrete steroid hormones, including androgens. Carcinomas of the ovary, both primary and metastatic, can be virilizing on occasion. Such tumours were probably diagnosed at one time as arrhenoblastomas. As to TEILUM's argument in favor of the term "androblastoma" to include the whole range of tumours of the male type, SCULLY still preferred the term "Sertoli-Leydig cell tumour". He has named the tumours according to the directions in which he believes they are differentiating, while TEILUM has done so on the basis of the blastema from which they are arising. Both terms had already been discussed in a World Health Organization meeting and, in the final classification, both were used.

References

BURSLEM, R. W., LANGLEY, F. A., and WOODCOCK, A. S., A clinicopathological study of oestrogenic ovarian tumours. *Cancer (Philad.)* 7, 522—538 (1954).

BUSBY, T., and ANDERSON, G. W., Feminizing mesenchymomas of the ovary. *Amer. J. Obstet. Gynec.* 68, 1391—1420 (1954).

COHEN, M., and SHAW, M. W., Two XY siblings with gonadal dysgenesis and a female phenotype. *New Engl. J. Med.* 272, 1083—1088 (1965).

DOMINGUEZ, C. J., and GREENBLATT, R. B., Dysgerminoma of the ovary in a patient with Turner's syndrome. *Amer. J. Obstet. Gynec.* 83, 674—677 (1962).

FLICK, F. H., and BANFIELD jr., R. S., Malignant theca-cell tumors. Two new case reports and review of the eight published cases. *Cancer (Philad.)* 9, 731—735 (1956).

FLOR, F. S., SCHADT, D. C., and BENZ, E. S., Gonadal dysgenesis with male chromatin pattern: testicular feminization syndrome. Clinical and pathological findings in two cases in siblings. *J. Amer. med. Ass.* 181, 375—379 (1962).

FODA, M. S., YOUSSEF, A. J., and SHAFEEK, M. A., Malignant theca cell tumour of the ovary. *J. Obstet. Gynaec. Brit. Emp.* 68, 982—985 (1961).

FRASIER, S. D., BASHORE, R. A., and MOSIER, H. D., Gonadoblastoma associated with pure gonadal dysgenesis in monozygous twins. *J. Pediat.* 64, 740—745 (1964).

GIUSTI, G., BORGHI, A., BIGOZZI, U., NEGRI, L., and TOCCAFONDI, R., Ovarian dysgerminoma with precocious isosexual puberty followed by virilization. *Obstet. and Gynec.* 20, 755—760 (1962).

HARTZ, P. H., Giant cystic arrhenoblastoma of ovary containing entodermal epithelium and carcinoid. *Amer. J. Path.* 21, 1167—1191 (1945).

HERTIG, A. T., and GORE, H., *Tumors of the ovary and Fallopian tube*, p. 9—176. Armed Forces Instiute of Pathology, Washington 1961.

HUGHESDON, P. E., Ovarian lipoid and theca cell tumors; their origins and interrelations. *Obstet. and Gynec.* 21, 245—288 (1966).

—, and FRASER, I. T., Arrhenoblastoma of ovary. Case report and histological review. *Acta obstet. gynec. scand.* (Suppl. 4) 32, 1—78 (1953).

KOTTMEIER, H. L., *Carcinoma of the female genitalia*, p. 174—192. Baltimore: Williams & Wilkins Co. 1953.

MALKASIAN, G. D., DOCKERTY, M. B., WILSON, R. B., and FABER, J. E., Functioning tumors of the ovary in women under 40. *Obstet. and Gynec.* 26, 669—675 (1965).

MATHET, P., *Les tumeurs masculinisantes de l'ovaire.* Paris These 114 p. Paris: Libraire Arnette 1956.

MELICOW, M. M., and USON, A. C., Dysgenetic gonadomas and other gonadal neoplasms in intersexes. Report of 5 cases and review of the literature. *Cancer (Philad.)* 12, 552—572 (1959).

MILLER, O. J., The sex chromosome anomalies. *Amer. J. Obstet. Gynec.* 90, 1078—1138 (1964).

MORRIS, J. McL., and SCULLY, R. E., *Endocrine pathology of the ovary*, p. 15—138. St. Louis: C. V. Mosby Co. 1958.

MOSTOFI, F. K., THEISS, E. A., and ASHLEY, D. J. B, Tumors of specialized gonadal stroma in human male patients. Androblastoma, Sertoli cell tumor, granulosa-theca cell tumor of the testis, and gonadal stromal tumor. *Cancer (Philad.)* 12, 944—957 (1959).

NOVAK, E. R., and LONG, J. H., Arrhenoblastoma of the ovary. *Amer. J. Obstet. Gynec.* 92, 1082—1093 (1965).

O'HERN, T. M., and NEUBECKER, R. D., Arrhenoblastoma. *Obstet. and Gynec.* 19, 758-770 (1962).

PALLADINO, V. S., DUFFY, S. L., and BURES, G. S., Probable true cystic granulosa cell tumor. Report of a case. *Obstet and Gynec.* 25, 729—733 (1965).

ROBINSON, A., PRIEST, R. E., and BIGLER, P. C., Male pseudohermaphrodite with XY/XO mosaicism and bilateral gonadoblastomas. Letter to the editor. *Lancet* 1964 I, 111—112.

SANTESSON, L., and MARRUBINI, G., Clinical and pathological survey of ovarian embryonal carcinomas, including so-called "mesonephromas" (SCHILLER), or "mesoblastomas" (TEILUM), treated at the Radiumhemmet. *Acta obstet. gynec. scand.* 36, 399—419 (1957).

SCULLY, R. E., Gonadoblastoma. A gonadal tumor related to the dysgerminoma (seminoma) and capable of sex-hormone production. *Cancer (Philad.)* 6, 455—463 (1953).

SCULLY, R. E., An unusual ovarian tumor containing Leydig cells, but associated with endometrial hyperplasia, in a postmenopausal woman. *J. clin. Endocr.* 13, 1254—1263 (1953).

— Stromal luteoma of the ovary. A distinctive type of lipoidcell tumor. *Cancer (Philad.)* 17, 769—778 (1964).

— Unpublished observations 1966.

SIEBENMANN, R. B., Pseudohermaphroditismus masculinus mit Gonadoblastom-line besondere Intersexform. *Path. et Microbiol. (Basel)* 24, 233—238 (1961).

SHER, J., and MARSH, M., Multilocular cystic granulosa cell tumor. Report of a case. *Amer. J. clin. Path.* 40, 72—77 (1963).

SJÖSTEDT, S., and WAHLEN, T., Prognosis of granulosa cell tumours. *Acta obstet. gynec. scand.* 40, 1—26 (Suppl. 6) (1961).

STERNBERG, W. H., and BARCLAY, D. L., Luteoma of pregnancy. *Amer. J. Obstet. Gynec.* 95, 165—184 (1966).

STRUMPF, I. J., Gonadoblastoma in a patient with gonadal dysgenesis. *Amer. J. Obstet. Gynec.* 92, 992—995 (1965).

TAYLOR, H. B., In: *Pathology annual*, vol. 1, ed. by S. C. SOMMERS, p. 127—147. New York: Appleton-Century-Crofts 1966.

TEILUM, G., Classification of testicular and ovarian androblastoma and Sertoli cell tumors. A survey of comparative studies with consideration of histogenesis, endocrinology, and embryological theories. *Cancer (Philad.)* 11, 769—782 (1958).

TETER, J., An usual gonadal tumour (gonadoblastoma) in a male pseudo-hermaphrodite with testicular dysgenesis. *J. Obstet. Gynaec. Brit. Emp.* 67, 238—242 (1960).

— PHILIP, J., WEÇEVICZ, G., and POTOCKI, J., A masculinizing mixed germ cell tumour (Gonocytoma III). *Acta endocr. (Kbh.)* 46, 1—11 (1964).

— PHILIP, J., and WEÇEVICZ, G., "Mixed" gonadal dysgenesis with gonadoblastoma in situ. *Amer. J. Obstet. Gynec.* 90, 929—935 (1964).

USIZIMA, H., Ovarian dysgerminoma associated with masculinization. Report of a case. *Cancer (Philad.)* 9, 736—739 (1956).

Tumours of Germinal Origin

GUNNAR TEILUM, M. D.

Professor i Patologisk Anatomi
Director of Universitetets patologisk-anatomiske institut, Copenhagen, Denmark

Introduction

Tumours of germ cell origin constitute more than 95 per cent of testicular tumours, but are relatively infrequent in the ovary. Although it was well known that dysgerminomas and teratomas, as well as very rare cases of teratomatous choriocarcinomas occurred in the ovary, the development of counterparts of the so-called embryonal carcinomas of the testis was less widely appreciated. Such neoplasms had not been characterized histologically and had not found an appropriate place in any previous classifications. The concept of classifying identical gonadal tumours is relatively new. About 25 years ago I initiated investigations in this field and, principally on a histogenetic basis, set up a general classification of "homologous" ovarian and testicular tumours characterized by their origin from early stages of germ cells in the gonads (TEILUM, 1946, 1950, and 1952). A specific ovarian tumour of germ cell origin showing a close histologic resemblance to certain types of testicular so-called "embryonal carcinomas" was recognized and distinguished from ovarian tumours of entirely different origin. This tumour was previously misinterpreted as "mesonephroma ovarii" (SCHILLER). At the same time it was confused with different tumour entities, such as mesonephric tumours of "hob-nail" or *"clear cell"* *type*, or was considered e.g. an "endo

thelioma of ovarian anlage" (KAZANCIGIL *et al.*, 1940), angiosarcoma, angiorecticuloma or unspecific carcinoma.

The *histogenesis and interrelationship* of the "homologous" ovarian and testicular tumours of germinal origin are shown in the Fig. 1. The dysgerminoma is a monocellular tumour type composed of cells resembling the undifferentiated germ cells in the early gonad, and it is considered to arise from primordial germ cells. In contrast to the germinomas the teratoid tumours of the gonads are derived from totipotential cells and may follow various lines of development leading to:

1. Teratomas (immature or adult somatic structures or a mixture of both).

2. Endodermal Sinus Tumour (Mesoblastoma vitellinum) (tumours showing a unilateral overgrowth of the extraembryonic mesoblast intimately associated with yolk sac endoderm).

3. Choriocarcinoma (Neoplasms showing trophoblastic differentiation).

Combinations of the characteristic patterns of two or more of these types are occasionally present.

The term "embryonal carcinoma" has been subject to criticism as it lacks clarity and leads often to confusion by its ambivalent use. "Embryonal carcinoma" in the testis has been considered as much a conceptual as a morphologic entity; this category has also included

tumours showing early differentiation toward somatic (epithelial or mesodermal)
or trophoblastic cell forms. Tumours
showing areas of glandular formations
have sometimes been designated "embryonal adenocarcinomas" without a
more specific interpretation. The term
"embryonal" would also imply somatic

sufficient basis for the histologic char-
acterization of the ovarian counterparts.
These are usually large tumours exhibiting a selective, unilateral overgrowth of
extra-embryonic primitive mesoblast connected with derivatives of yolk sac endoderm lining sinusoid spaces or veritable
endodermal vesicles or small cysts.

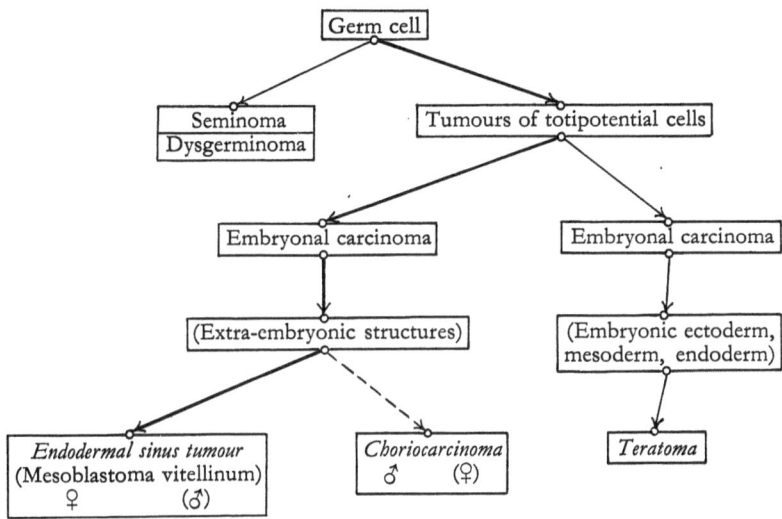

Fig. 1. Histogenesis and interrelationship of ovarian and testicular tumours of germ cell origin.
In this classification the term "embryonal carcinoma" is restricted to tumours composed of undifferentiated neoplastic embryonal cells (cf. STEVENS) representing the undifferentiated form of
extra-embryonic as well as embryonic types

origin although the majority of the neoplasms in the ovary show a selective development of *extra-embryonic* structures.
When the multiplicity of ovarian tumours, which may display great variations
in histological pattern, is considered, it is
not surprising that the nature of these
ovarian neoplasms of germinal origin remained unrecognized for a long time.
Although the designation "embryonal
carcinoma", for practical use, is applicable to these complex germ cell tumours *in the testis*, which comprise a fairly
homogeneous *clinical* group, it is not a

In the present classification the term
"embryonal carcinoma" (Fig. 1) is therefore — in agreement with STEVENS (1962)
— restricted to tumours composed of
undifferentiated neoplastic embryonal
cells.

Series of testicular germinal tumours
have been studied by various investigators (FRIEDMAN and MOORE, 1946; TEI-
LUM, 1946; DIXON and MOORE, 1952;
PEYRON, 1939; MELICOW, 1955; GAIL-
LARD, 1961). The presented concepts of
the nature and histogenesis of *ovarian*
counterparts of "embryonal" testicular

tumours are in basic agreement with later investigators. Santesson and Marrubini (1957) reported the first large series of 17 cases of the "mesoblastomas" and Cabanne (1954 and 1957), Martin *et al.* (1954), Saphir (1958), Masson (1956), Neubecker and Breen (1962), Scully (1963), and Sternberg (1963) have reported studies or observations of this type of ovarian germ cell tumours.

There are clear histological and biological differences between tumours of the dysgerminoma-seminoma types and the other units of the group of germ cell tumours. The 20 dysgerminomas of the ovary studied by Theiss *et al.* (1960) were all of female nuclear sex, while testicular seminoma, the male counterpart, is always chromatin-negative, suggesting that these tumours arise from diploid germ cells before meiosis. Nuclear sexing of teratoid tumours showed that ovarian teratoma are chromatin-positive, while the nuclei in most testicular teratomas were chromatin-negative and in half as many cases they were chromatin-positive (Theiss *et al.*, 1960). The remaining few cases showed areas both of male and female nuclear sex, suggesting a multicentric origin for some of

Table I. *Classification of ovarian tumours of germ cell origin*

1, Dysgerminoma
2. Endodermal sinus tumour (Mesoblastoma vitellinum)
3. Choriocarcinoma

4. Polyembryoma (Peyron, Simard)
5. Polyvesicular vitelline tumour (showing multiple yolk sac [endoblast] vesicles)
6. Solid teratoma (immature and adult)
7. Cystic teratoma (dermoid cyst)
8. Gonadoblastoma (dysgenetic gonadoma)

9. The term "*embryonal carcinoma*" is restricted to tumours entirely composed of undifferentiated neoplastic embryonal cells. Such areas are often combined with other forms of germ cell tumours.

these tumours. It was believed that the 2:1 proportion of chromatin-negative to chromatin-positive tumours (2XY:1XX) could be hypothetically explained by a fusion of two haploid daughter cells, a phenomenon which is known to occur in the ovary in certain types of parthenogenesis in lower animals. This presupposes that the cells of genotype YY are not viable. The problem of the genesis of teratoid tumours has not yet been solved, but preliminary studies would suggest that teratoid tumours of the testis and, by inference, also their ovarian counterparts are derived from germ cells after meiotic division.

1. Dysgerminoma

An ovarian tumour duplicating the seminoma of the testis was described by Chevassu (1906) as a special type, and later termed "disgerminoma" (R.Meyer, 1930), because the same tumour originates from the male and female gonads (dis = two). The "*dysgerminomas*", as these tumours were generally termed later, are characterized histologically by fairly uniform undifferentiated cells with large nuclei, one or two nucleoli and poorly defined cytoplasmic outlines. The stroma varies in amount and is characteristically infiltrated with lymphocytes. Focal necrosis and areas of pseudotubercle formation with foreign body giant cells are occasionally seen. Santesson (1947) reported a series of 37 cases of pure dysgerminomas radiologically treated at the Radiumhemmet, Stockholm, and reviewed the data of an additional 192 cases from the literature. In the entire series of 229 cases, the age incidence was 81 per cent under thirty and 44 per cent under twenty years of age. The neoplasm predominately affected the right ovary. The location, mentioned in 196 cases, was in 51 per cent in the right ovary and in 17 per cent bilateral. Histologic criteria related to the degree of malignancy were not found. However, a rather reliable prognostic judgement could be based on the extension of the tumour observed at operation. In 107 cases the five-year survival rate was 51.4 per cent, and for the cases at Radiumhemmet it was 66.7 per cent. Like the seminoma, the dysgerminoma is very radiosensitive. Surgery followed by radiotherapy is the treatment of choice. Only small or moderate doses and never massive doses should be administered (KOTTMEIER, 1952). The prognosis in cases with bilateral tumours is very serious. While the dysgerminoma in the majority of cases is a pure monocellular entity, combination with elements of other types of germ cell tumours is sometimes present.

In several instances dysgerminomas arise in the gonads of intersexes, and may be combined with gonadoblastoma. Some reported cases classified as dysgerminoma may possibly represent gonadoblastoma (SCULLY, 1953).

2. Endodermal Sinus Tumour (Mesoblastoma vitellinum)

Synonyms and Related Terms. Extraembryonic (endo-mesodermal) membrane tumour, yolk sac carcinoma, so-called "mesonephroma ovarii" (SCHILLER).

Definition. A highly malignant germ cell tumour showing as essential elements a selective (unilateral) overgrowth of the extra-embryonic mesoblast associated with yolk sac endoderm lining characteristic sinusoid spaces or endodermal small cystic cavities or (vitelline) vesicles.

Clinical Features. All cases of this ovarian tumour occur in young patients. In Santesson and Marrubini's series (1957) comprising 17 cases, the age range was from $2^1/_2$ to 35 years, including nine cases occurring in the second decade and four in the third. The mean

age was 17.9 years. In the series of 27 cases reported by NEUBECKER and BREEN (1962) the average age was 20.3 years: 85 per cent (23) of the patients were less than 26 years old and 56 per cent (15) were in the age group of 16 to 25 years. The tumour is not sensitive to radiation. Regardless of the treatment all cases had a malignant course. Within a period of from few months to one year, recurrence of pelvic and abdominal masses appear. The manner of propagation is different from the chiefly vascular invasion of trophoblastic tumours.

Since endodermal sinus tumours have often been misdiagnosed and, until recently, not included in even larger registry materials, the real incidence is not known. Even though it is rare, like other malignant germ cell tumours of the ovary, my own experience and additional unpublished cases seen in consultation suggest that the endodermal sinus tumour, as well as the dysgerminoma, may represent a characteristic and, by no means uncommon germinal tumour type.

Grossly the tumours may vary in size from about 15 cm up to 25 cm in diameter. In several cases the finding of a large abdominal mass has warranted the consideration of pregnancy. In most cases the tumour is firm, globular and unilateral with a smooth surface, but there may be extension of the tumour. The cut surface is soft and friable, and variable in color. It may be cystic with foci of necrosis.

The following specific *microscopic patterns* are encountered:

1. Areas of stellate mesodermal cells forming a *loose* vacuolated network with wide meshes or cystic spaces (Fig. 10), sometimes lined by flat mesothelial cells and showing foci of active hemopoiesis in the underlying capillary spaces. The meshes often contain hyaline, acidophilic and PAS-positive globules or mucoid

precipitates. The more compact areas may show star-like halos or mantles of cells surrounding the larger capillaries. The characteristic loose pattern resembling the "magma reticulare" or the extra-embryonic mesoderm of the exocoelom (cf. Figs. 8 and 9) led first to the recognition of the *mesoblastic* nature of the tumour, i.e. "mesoblastoma extraembryonale" (TEILUM, 1950).

2. Endodermal Sinus Pattern. In more differentiated areas are seen groups of peculiar perivascular formations (Figs. 2 to 5) consisting of a mesodermal core with a capillary in its centre and covered with a visceral layer of cylindric cells of epithelial appearance. The surrounding capsular sinusoid space is lined by a single (parietal) layer of flat cells with prominent nuclei. The general patterns often resemble a complicated labyrinth of communicating cavities or channels with papillary processes. The perivascular sinusoid structures — regarding the general architecture, appearance in cross and longitudinal sections and the type of lining cells — were found to recapitulate the so-called endodermal sinuses (TEILUM, 1959) (Fig. 6), i.e. embryologically well-defined structures, which are prominent in the rat placenta. Obviously, in the rodent placenta as in the human tumour, these formations are diverticula of yolk sac endoderm that expand and dissect around the vessels of the extra-embryonic mesenchyme. Whereas the endodermal sinuses in the placenta have been considered as an accidental phenomenon without general significance, the mantling of vessels by yolk sac endoderm in the tumour will simply result in the formation of identical structures. This would, of course, not imply a specific capacity of the tumour to reproduce stages in the embryological development of the extra-embryonic membranes in the rodent.

3. Compact aggregates of small *undifferentiated neoplastic embryonal cells*, which are considered analogous to the masses of undifferentiated cells visible during the early stage of development of the embryo. Certain sections of the tumour show such areas merging with the reticular network of extra-embryonic mesoblast (Fig. 2) or with the endodermal sinus pattern (Fig. 3).

4. Cystic structures may form a regular arrangement of small cavities lined by a layer of flat cells with protruding nuclei continuous with the parietal lining of the endodermal sinuses; or individual cysts showing a clear, columnar, partly mucinous epithelium may occur in the loose myxoid stroma with mesoblastic mesothelial-like elements and early differentiation of yolk sac endoderm forming characteristic festoon-shaped configurations (Fig. 8). I consider these endodermal cysts (Fig. 8) equivalent to the yolk sac (endoblast) vesicle of the early embryo (Fig. 9), and this part of the tumour demonstrates clearly the intimate relationship between the extra-embryonic mesoblast and the yolk sac endoderm.

5. Occasionally the predominant part of these vitelline tumours show a myriad of yolk sac (endoblast) vesicles (Fig. 12) lined with a columnar or cuboidal epithelium showing transition to a layer of flat mesothelial-like cells. The individual cavities are varying in form and size and show invaginated processes and protrusions into the lumen. Often the distal parts of the vesicles covered with mesothelial cells are constricted off from the portion covered with partly mucinous epithelium — thus making a smaller vesicle — reflecting the embryologic conversion of the primary yolk sac into the secondary sac.

Obviously the nature of this pattern (Fig. 12) showing a myriad of yolk sac (endoblast) vesicles — different from the

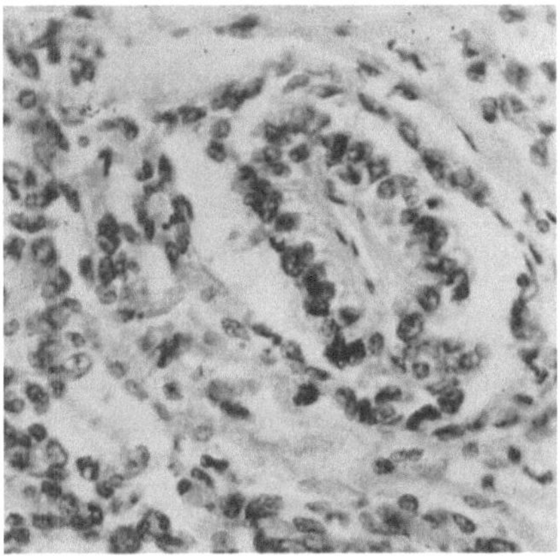

Fig. 2

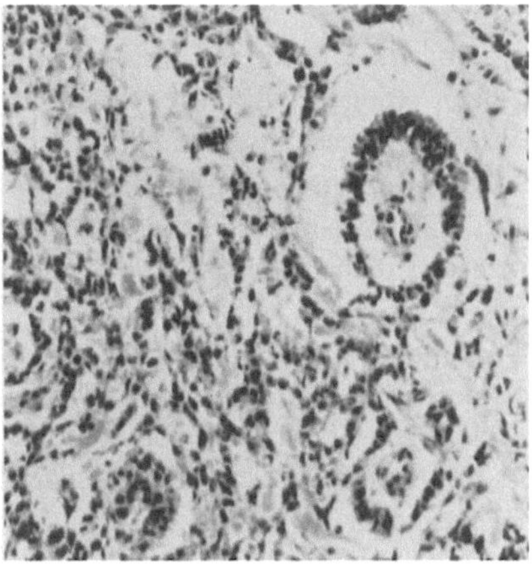

Fig. 3

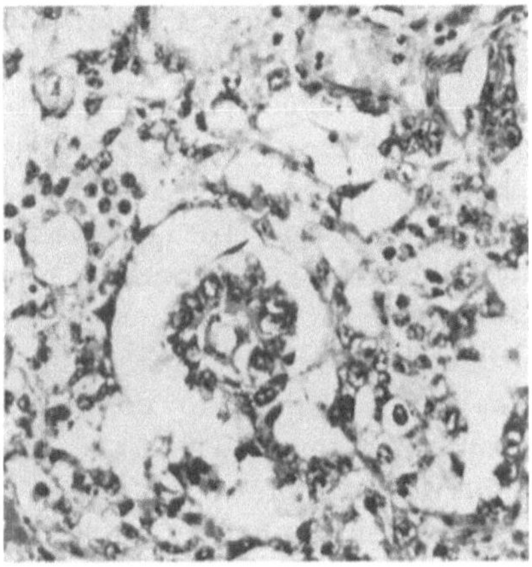

Fig. 4

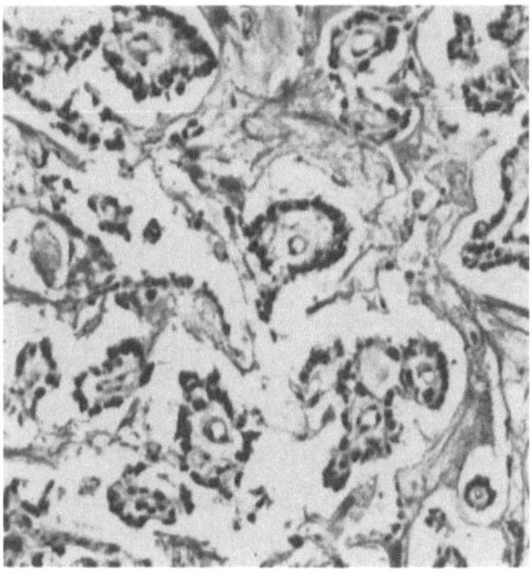

Fig. 5

Figs. 2—5. *Endodermal sinus tumour* of the ovary (Fig. 2), adult testis (Fig. 3), anterior mediastinum in 35-year old man (Fig. 4) and ovary in 3-year old girl (Fig. 5)

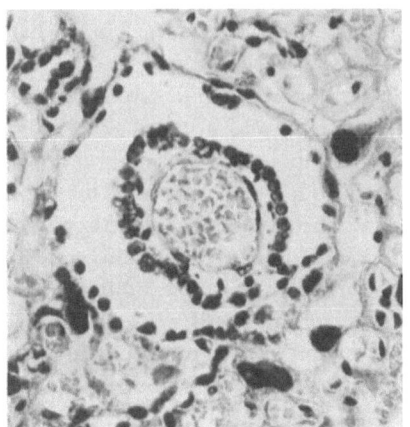

Fig. 6. Endodermal sinus of the rat placenta

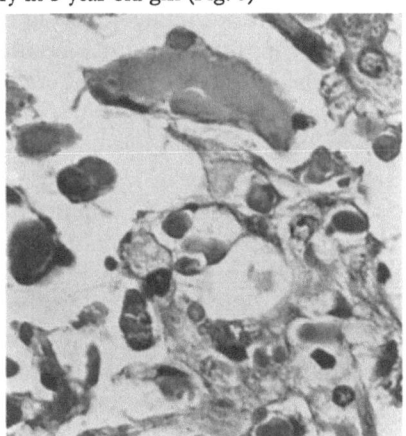

Fig. 7. Endodermal sinus tumour of the ovary showing tumour cells resting on bands of hyalin and focal accumulation of PAS-positive hyaline globules

polyembryoma described below — has not been recognized before. At any rate an identical case is depicted (1963) in Novak et al.'s paper on unclassified tumours in the Ovarian Tumour Registry, 1942—1962. The tumour was "originally believed by OTR to represent a cystic edematous ovary or old retrogressed endometriosis, although one pathologist mentioned metastatic adenocarcinoma". The 30-year-old patient died 14 months after operation.

Histogenesis

The interpretation of this type of ovarian germ cell tumour has been based on: 1. The histologic identity with certain "embryonal" tumours in the adult testis (Figs. 2—3). 2. The loose reticulated network analogous to the extra-embryonic mesoblast (Figs. 8—9). 3. The characteristic perivascular structures formed by invaginated mantled blood vessels, recapitulating the embryologically well-defined endodermal sinuses (Figs. 2 to 6). 4. A demonstrable continuity between the cells lining these structures and those covering veritable yolk sac (endoblast) vesicles. 5. The presence of intracellular PAS-positive, diastase-resistant hyaline bodies in the lining cells (Fig. 7).

Further support to the interpretation is lent by the recent experimental studies by Pierce and Dixon (1959), who during conversion of a transplantable testicular teratocarcinoma of the mouse to the ascites form found a simplification of the tumour pattern containing many elements of a yolk sac carcinoma intermingled with areas of well formed visceral yolk sac arranged in small cystic spaces and sometimes in papillary tufts.

The teratocarcinoma employed was LS 402 VI. The tumour arose spontaneously in the testis of a strain 129 mouse and was developed as a transplantable line by L. C. Stevens of the Roscoe B.

Jackson Laboratory. Also an ovarian teratocarcinoma in mice underwent ascitic conversion. Once the tumour had lost the ability to produce certain differentiated tissues as a result of the conversion, the tumour never regained the ability to produce the tissue.

Fawcett et al. showed, as a result of growing fertilized mouse ova beneath the renal capsule, the presence of cells embedded in hyalin that looked remarkably similar to those described by Pierce and Dixon, and they considered them to be parietal yolk sac in origin.

The significance of the differences in morphologic differentiation of ovarian and testicular "embryonal carcinomas" in human subjects is not clear.

It is of interest that a testicular tumour type, that has been reported in early childhood under a variety of names and histogenetic concepts, and called "distinctive adenocarcinoma of the infants testis" ascribed to nongerminal testicular parenchyma (Teoh et al., 1960), exhibits the pattern characteristic of endodermal sinus tumours in the ovary (Huntington et al., 1963).

Cases of extragonadal endodermal sinus tumour originating in the sacrococcygeal region (Rao et al., 1964) or the anterior mediastinum (Teilmann, cf. Fig. 4) have recently been observed. Friedman (1951) studied the comparative morphogenesis of extragenital and gonadal teratoid tumours, and there are several observations of the various types of germ cell tumour in the anterior mediastinum (thymic region), including germinoma, choriocarcinoma and teratoma similar to the tumours in the gonads.

In several of the reported cases the endodermal sinus tumour in the ovary was combined with a benign cystic teratoma (dermoid). More infrequently areas of dysgerminoma or choriocarcinoma have been observed. Of interest also is

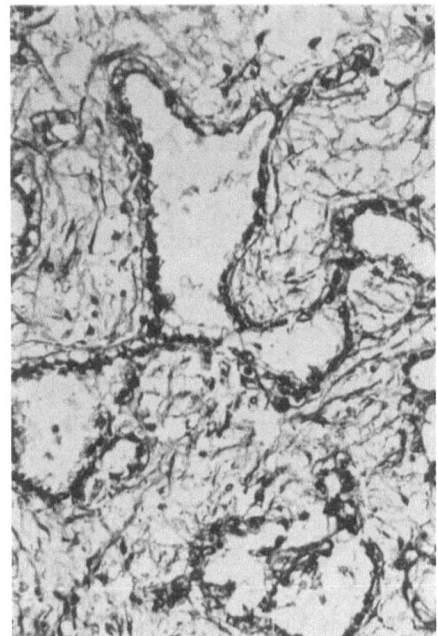

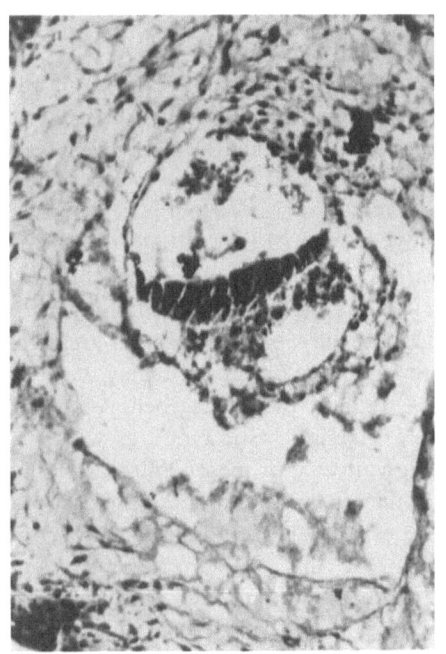

Fig. 8. Endodermal sinus tumour of the ovary. Areas showing characteristic yolk sac (endoblast) vesicles in loose reticulum resembling the "magma reticulare" or extra-embryonic mesoderm of the exocoelom (cf. Fig. 9)

Fig. 9. Human embryo in early stage. The extraembryonic mesoderm forms a loose reticulum, the magma reticulare (cf. the ovarian tumour Fig. 8)

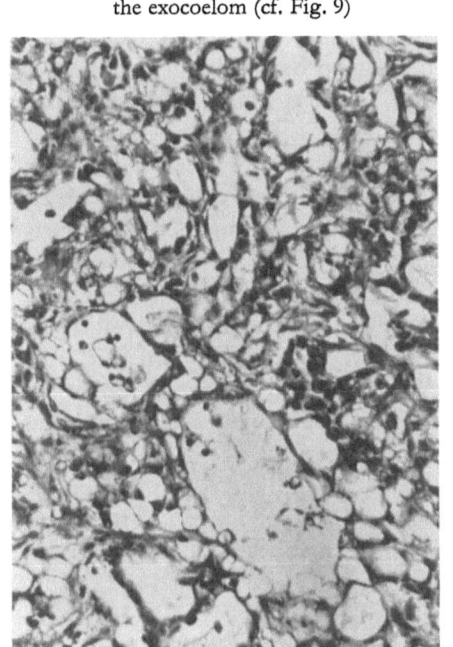

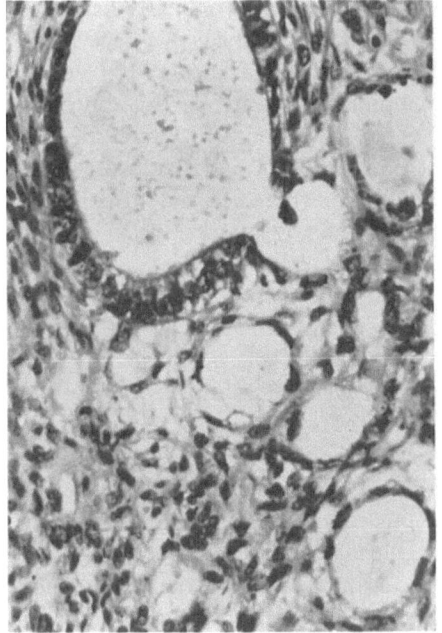

Fig. 10. Areas of endodermal sinus tumour of the ovary showing a markedly vacuolated meshwork with honeycomb appearance with developed microcysts. A similar vacuolated pattern is prominent in the analogous testicular vitelline tumour occurring in infancy

Fig. 11. Polyvesicular vitelline tumour of the ovary showing a multiplication of small vesicles from the basal vacuolated cytoplasm of the cells lining the larger vesicle (cf. Fig. 10)

the association of endodermal sinus tumour with gonadoblastoma (dysgenetic gonadoma) observed by Santesson and Marrubini, 1957.

Differential Diagnosis. It is evident that tumours referred to as "mesonephroma ovarii" (Schiller) comprise two different entities having nothing in common with regard to histogenesis, general architecture, incidence or clinical behaviour.

Originally Schiller believed there was a "benign cystic type" as well as a malignant type of mesonephroma showing the characteristic perivascular cell mantles, but later he admitted that a confusion of his "mesonephroma" and "parvilocular cystomas" has occurred. However, the first type, containing Schiller's "glomerulus-like structures", were later recognized as a highly malignant germ cell tumour (Teilum, 1946), whereas the parvilocular types, showing a more regular tubular pattern and often low epithelium of "hobnail" character (Fig. 14) was classified as a true mesonephric tumour. The so-called adenocarcinoma with clear cells (hypernephroid) of the ovary (Fig. 15), which was later described (Saphir and Lackner, 1944), represents a characteristic form of this (non-germinal) mesonephric tumour (Teilum, 1952).

Tumours of the mesonephric type occur at all ages and may be found along the line of the mesonephric duct and Gartner duct (Teilum, 1954, Novak *et al.*, 1954). The majority of the true mesonephric tumours of the ovary arise in the fifth and sixth decades. Clinically this tumour in the ovary is simular to any other malignant ovarian tumour. When apparently confined to the ovary, mortality is 50%; with spread beyond, it approaches 100% (Novak and Woodruff, 1959). However, several cases of this type have had a benign course (Teilum, 1954; Wade-Evans and Langley, 1961).

Tumours composed of clear cells are not necessarily of mesonephric origin. Certain tumour-varieties of e.g. the salivary glands [oxyphil adenoma ("oncocytoma"), carcinoma of clear cell type] may show a similar appearance.

3. Choriocarcinoma

Primary choriocarcinoma of the ovary is extremely rare, and there are only about 40 recorded cases. The tumour is usually solid and hemorrhagic with the typical histological appearance. Areas indicating teratoma or other type of germinal tumour may be present in some cases.

4. Polyembryoma

Peyron (1939) first discovered and described in detail embryoid structures, morphologically similar to early human embryos in a human testicular teratoma. These embryoid bodies, like human blastocysts, were composed of ectodermal and endodermal vesicles with mesodermal cells between them. He considered them to be homologous to normal human embryos and to be the result of parthenogenesis (polyembryonic parthenogenesis) of the germ cells. Since Peyron's original discovery many workers have observed embryoid bodies in teratomas of the human testis, whereas these are more infrequently present in ovarian teratomas. A polyembryonic embryoma of the ovary containing literally hundreds of these early embryonic formations — similar to Peyron's observation in the testicular teratoma — was first reported by Simard, 1957, and recently embryoid structures have been found in metastatic and transplantable testicular teratomas in mice (Stevens, 1958; Pierce and Dixon, 1959).

In the case observed by Simard of the ovarian tumour, except for the blastocysts, the greater part was made up of a mixture of almost all the tissues of the human body.

5. Polyvesicular Vitelline Tumour

This term refers to the characteristic histological pattern, which occasionally was found as a predominant part of vitelline tumours in the ovary (TEILUM, 1965).

The tumour contained in these areas a myriad of blastocyst-like yolk sac (endoblast) vesicles (Fig. 12) showing great variation in form, size and degree of development. Most of the vesicles are lined with a layer of flat mesothelial-like cells, which may show transition to a columnar or cuboidal epithelium. Frequently the cells showed conspicuous basal or paraluminal cytoplasmic vacuoles, and in some areas vacuolated cells and stroma were scrambled together (Fig. 11). Here clumps of markedly vacuolated cells formed delicate cobweb-like structures with developed microcysts. I find that this picture in ovarian vitelline tumours (Figs. 10 and 11) is quite analogous to the process observed by MAGNER et al. (1951 and 1956) during the development of the distinct type of testicular adenocarcinom occurring in infancy. This observations lends further support to the later recognition of the specific *vitelline* nature of this tumor type, which in other parts may show the classic and unequivocal pattern of endodermal sinus tumor (HUNTINGTON et al., 1963).

6. Solid Teratoma

Ovarian teratomas which are not dermoid cysts are solid teratomas. They are relatively more common in childhood and young adult life, with a peak incidence in the second decade. Histologically these neoplasms may be composed entirely of mature (adult) tissues or show a variable mixture of immature embryonic and mature tissues. Areas of dysgerminoma, endodermal sinus tumour, choriocarcinoma or polyembryoma may be present.

Metastases to pelvic and abdominal cavities are common.

THURLBECK and SCULLY (1960) recently reviewed the subject and stated that although commonly equated to malignant teratomas, these tumours may behave in a benign fashion. According to these authors a grading of solid teratomas has proved of definite prognostic value in their series of 9 cases.

It is generally believed that teratomas arise from germ cells. However, how the germ cell accomplishes the formation of teratomas is not clear (cf. STEVENS, 1962).

7. Cystic Teratoma (Dermoid Cyst)

About 99% of ovarian teratomas are well-differentiated benign tumours composed of mature (adult) tissues. The adult teratoma is rather common in the ovary and rare in the testis. It has been suggested that something in the environment of the female gonad predisposes germ cell neoplasms to somatic differentiation, whereas in the male undifferentiated malignant growth is more frequent (DIXON and MOORE, 1950). The pathologic features of dermoid cysts are well known. Cases showing a unilateral preponderance of thyreoid tissue are called struma ovarii. These tumours may resemble nodular goiters, and evidence of thyrotoxicosis has been present in some of these cases.

Also cases of primary carcinoid tumours (argentaffinomas) of the ovary may arise in the wall of dermoid cysts either from intestinal or from bronchial epithelium. Malignant transformation of a dermoid cyst has been found in ca. 1.8% (PETERSON, 1957; KELLEY and SCULLY, 1961).

8. Gonadoblastoma

SCULLY (1953) first described this rare tumour which is composed of a mixture of large germ cells, like those of

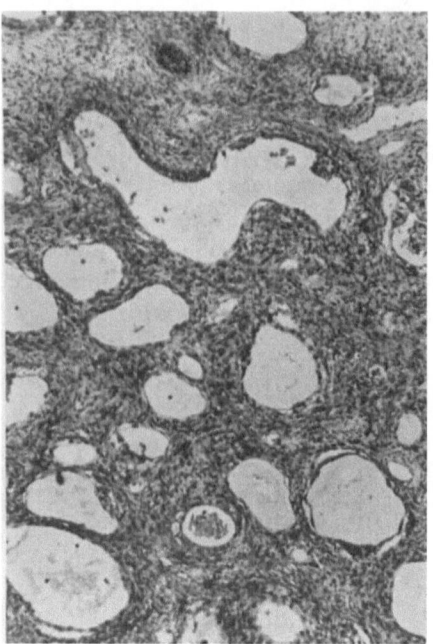

Fig. 12. Polyvesicular vitelline tumour of the ovary showing yolk sac (endoblast) vesicles lined with cells of columnar or mesothelioid type with transitions from one to another

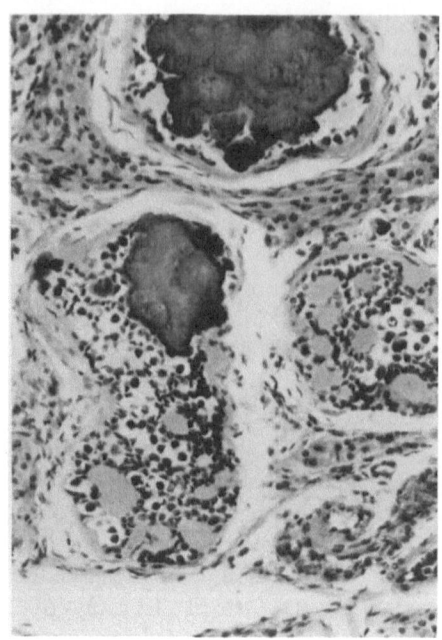

Fig. 13. Gonadoblastoma

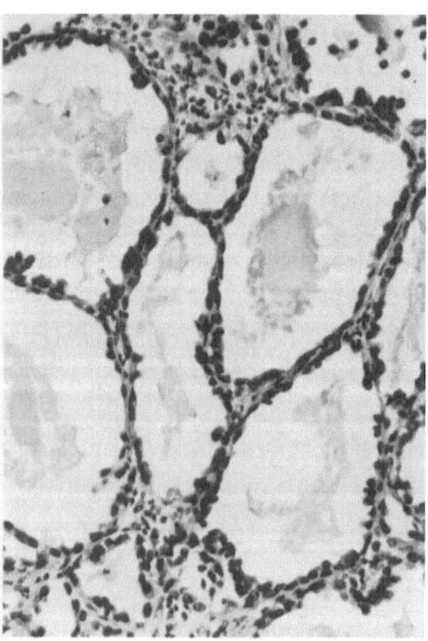

Fig. 14. Mesonephric tumour showing a regular tubular pattern and a low epithelium of "hobnail" character

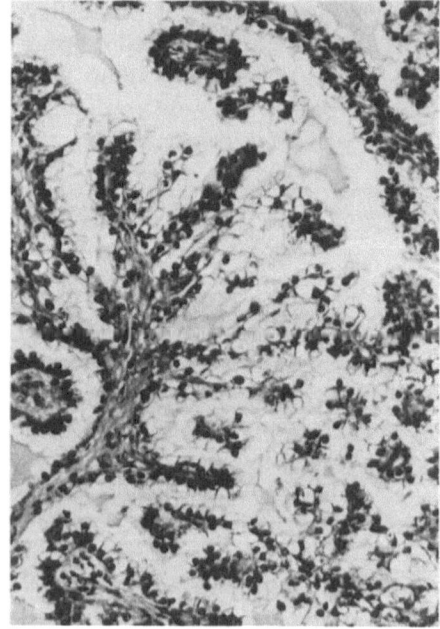

Fig. 15. Mesonephric tumour of clear cell type

the dysgerminoma and small epithelial cells of the granulosa-Sertoli cell type, that may be arranged in three types of pattern: in coronal fashion around individual germinoma cells, 2) at the periphery of nests of germ cells, or 3) about round spaces filled with eosinophilic colloid-like material, resembling a microfollicular granulosa cell tumour. In addition the stroma often contains Leydig cells as a third type. Scully drew attention to the fact that these tumours may be capable of sex-hormone production. The arrangement of the sex cord cells was found consistent with either granulosa or Sertoli cells similar to the pattern of these cells in fetal gonads of both sexes.

Grossly, the tumour may be similar to dysgerminoma or to a firm fibrous mass. A characteristic feature is the presence of disseminated or diffuse and extensive calcification, which may be visible on an x-ray film of the pelvis. The growth of the tumour usually obscures the nature of one gonad; the opposite gonad may be testicular or dysgenetic and may show microscopic gonadoblastoma that is not grossly evident. Most patients with gonadoblastoma are intersexual and phenotypically female, and complain of primary amenorrhoea. The patients have a male sex chromatine pattern, 46 (XY) or sex chromosome mosaicisme, XO/XY (TETER et al., 1964; PHILIP and TETER, 1964) and reveal eunuchoidal features or signs of Turner's syndrome. From the histologic, clinical, and endocrinologic points of view, TETER (1960) has made a distinction between this type containing Leydig cells and associated with masculinization (gonocytoma III) and a type (gonocytoma II) composed of only two types of cells (germ cells and Sertoli-granulosa cells, but not Leydig cells) and occurring in patients with normal somato-sexual development and often

precocious puberty due to the feminizing activity of the tumor. In these cases the sex chromatin pattern is in accordance with phenotype (positive in girls). TETER (1962) reported 6 cases of this type, all in girls in the age of 7—16 years.

Since the dysgenetic gonads in Turner's syndrome typically contain groups of Leydig cells (hilus cells), while no follicles or germ cells are seen in the cortex, the possibility exists that the component of Leydig cells in cases of gonadoblastoma associated with gonadal dysgenesis should be considered a manifestation of this typical finding rather than an essential cellular component of the tumour. This would explain the histological variations and their relation to the clinical characteristics.

The malignant potential of gonadoblastoma has not been established. Probably it is mainly determined by the development of a malignant germ cell tumour of other type, such as dysgerminoma or endodermal sinus tumour from the germinal component of the tumour.

Summary

The subject of ovarian tumours of germinal origin is reviewed with emphasis on a systemic classification based on histogenesis and demonstrated interrelationship existing between tumours of widely different histologic structure, but all being of germ cell origin.

Comparative studies have shown that ovarian and testicular tumours of germ cell origin are in great part homologous. However, several differences exist between the female and male tumours in reference to form of differentiation. The ovarian counterparts of testicular "embryonal carcinomas" show a more uniform histologic pattern with a unilateral development of extra-embryonic mesoblast-yolk sac structures, i.e. endodermal-sinus tumour. Such neoplasms were previously misdiagnosed under a variety of names and confused with ovarian neoplasms of different origin. Trophoblastic elements and great variations of immature embryonic tissues are far more characteristic of the male "teratoid" tumours.

The so-called "distinctive adenocarcinoma of the infant's testis", which previously had been ascribed to nongerminal testicular parenchyma, exhibits the same selective differentiation of vitelline structures characteristic for endodermal sinus tumour in the ovary, and there have been recently several observations of highly malignant extragonadal teratoid tumours originating in the anterior mediastinum or the sacro-coccygeal region showing the typical pattern of endodermal sinus tumour (or mesoblastoma vitellinum) in the ovary.

Discussion

Luisi reported that in his material he had nine specimens which were apparently the pure type of dysgerminoma with large nuclei and cytoplasmic lines, but he did not know whether there were any embryonal or extra-embryonal structures in these tumours. In addition, he had examined several specimens, sent to him by other investigators, which had the characteristics described by Teilum: (1) loose vacuolated network with the cystic spaces; (2) aggregates of undifferentiated embryonal cells; (3) characteristic perivascular formations connected with the large, vacuolated exocoelomic mesoblasts. He agreed with Teilum, he said, that the diagnosis of endodermal sinus tumours was missed in many instances, and said that he himself knew of two such tumours which were reported as mesonephroma of the ovary, which is an entirely different tumour. He described experience with one patient who had a tumour with an unusually large teratomatous component in the sacro-coccygeal region. The patient was referred to his institution because of recurrence after operation for what was diagnosed histologically as malignant teratoma. At the second operation, the histological diagnosis was teratomatous endodermal sinus tumour.

Scully discussed the gonadoblastoma, the so-called solid teratoma of the ovary, cancer arising in a dermoid cyst, and the carcinoid tumour of the ovary. A number of cases of gonadoblastomas arising in an undescended testis, usually abdominal but occasionally inguinal, have been recorded. None has been reported in a descended testicle. This type of tumour also seems to arise in the streak gonad or gonadal dysgenesis. It is often difficult, he said, to tell just what type of gonadal abnormality these patients have. The majority, however, are phenotypic females with amenorrhea and some virilism; a smaller group have amenorrhea without virilism. An even smaller group is composed of phenotypic males who have hypospadias, cryptorchidism, and usually, if the abdomen is explored, some internal female genitalia. No gonadoblastoma, to his knowledge, has been known to metastasize, but germinomas, whether dysgerminous or seminomas, frequently arise from underlying gonadoblastomas. He believed (he said) that careful study would show that a high percentage of the germinomas arising in intersexual individuals arose in gonadoblastomas.

The so-called solid teratoma of the ovary is generally predominantly solid and shows a variegated appearance on the section surface with small cysts and solid tumours of various varieties. The term "solid teratoma" is in some respects a misnomer because these tumours also may develop large cysts. Many appear highly malignant microscopically and are sometimes called malignant teratoma of the ovary. However, in perhaps one third to one half of cases, the tumour consisted of widely differentiated tissue. In his own series of nine cases, those patients with low-grade tumours usually did well; those who had tumours of a higher histological grade generally did poorly. Other investigators, he said, reported that the differentiation of the tumours is a reasonable guide to prognosis. He added that, in his opinion, since patients with the endodermal sinus tumour or the solid teratomas are usually young women or children, and the tumours are rarely bilateral, conservative treatment with simple oophorectomy is indicated, if there is no evidence of involvement of the opposite ovary. In most reported series, the treatment for most of the "cured" patients with malignant teratomas or embryonal cancers had been simple oophorectomy. He knew, (he said,) of only one five-year survivor with endodermal sinus tumour, although one patient treated at his own institution had survived for 18 months. In both instances, the treatment was simple oophorectomy.

Cancer arising in a dermoid cyst is rare since this occurs only in from one to two per cent of dermoid cysts. However, it is important that this possibility be recognized, because if the surgeon is cognizant of the fact that the tumour is malignant at the time of operation, he might be more aggressive in his attempts to remove the tumour. Cancers arising in dermoid cysts are usually squamous cell carcinomas, but an occasional sarcoma has been reported.

The carcinoid tumour has been confused with the granulosa cell tumours in some reports but is an entirely different neoplasm. The possibility of a primary carcinoid of the ovary should be considered when a patient has the carcinoid syndrome; about one third of the 30 or more cases of "*coronary*" carcinomas of the ovary reported in the literature have been associated with the carcinoid syndrome. If cardiac damage is not already present, cure can be achieved by removal of the carcinoid tumour. None of these tumours had metastasized, according to his knowledge, (Scully said.).

KOTTMEIER commented that in the Radiumhemmet series, patients with germ cell tumours have all been younger than 25 years of age. In the experience at this institution (he said), it had been impossible to determine histologically if the dysgerminoma was benign or malignant. Some patients with tumours which appeared benign histologically had had distant metastasis; some who had had cellular tumours had recovered. In most instances, the tumour involves only one ovary, usually the right. The opposite ovary is seldom affected but metastases to the retroperitoneal nodes are common. Because the tumours are radiosensitive, the preferred treatment at the Radiumhemmet is to remove the affected ovary and give x-ray treatment to the retroperitoneal nodes but not to the remaining ovary. Some of his colleagues, Professor SANTESSON for one, disagreed and thought that bilateral oophorectomy should be performed for dysgerminomas. However, said KOTTMEIER, he thought that although there was a slight risk of undetected tumour in the other ovary, the physiological value of retaining ovarian function outweighed this risk.

TEILUM commented that although the various types of germ cell tumour may be found in combination occasionally, the endodermal sinus tumour shows a more specific and uniform pattern. In various reports, this tumour has been confused with other tumours and not classified as a characteristic type of ovarian germ cell tumour. The term endodermal sinus tumour defines the characteristic structures of yolk sac endoderm mantling vessels of the extraembryonic mesoderm similar — although

accidentally — to the embryologically well-defined endodermal sinuses of the rat placenta and composed of the same extra-embryonic layers.

References

CABANNE, F., Étude d'une tumeur du ligament large chez une fillette; mésonéphrome? *Bull. Ass. franç. Cancer* **41**, 139—148 (1954).
— Les dysembryomes du testicule. *Sem. Hôp. Paris (pathologie-biologie 5)*, **33**, 517—534 (1957).
CHEVASSU, M., *Tumeurs du testicule*. Thèse de Paris 1906.
DIXON, F. J., and MORRE, R. A., *Tumors of the male sex organs; Atlas of tumor pathology*, sect. VIII, fasc. 31b and 32. Armed Forces Institute of Pathology, Washington, D. C. 1952.
EVANS, R. W., Developmental stages of embryolike bodies in teratoma testis. *J. clin. Path.* **10**, 31—39 (1957).
FAWCETT, D. W., Development of mouse ova under capsule of kidney. *Anat. Rec.* **108**, 71—91 (1950).
FRIEDMAN, N. B., The comparative morphogenesis of extragenital and gonadal teratoid tumors. *Cancer (Philad.)* **4**, 265—276 (1951).
—, and MOORE, R. A., Tumors of the testis. A report on 922 cases. *Milit. Surg.* **99**, 573—593 (1946).
GAILLARD, J.-A., La polyembryonie dans les tumeurs. Sciences et l'enseignement des sciences. *Revue franç. Sci. et Techn.* **16**, 7—16 (1961).
HUNTINGTON jr., R. W., MORGENSTERN, N. L., SARGENT, J. A., GIEM, R. N., RICHARDS, A., and HANFORD, K. C., Germinal tumors exhibiting the endodermal sinus pattern of Teilum in young children. *Cancer (Philad.)* **16**, 34—47 (1963).
KAZANCIGIL, T. R., LAQUEUR, W., and LADEWIG, P., Papillo-endothelioma ovarii; report of 3 cases and discussion of Schiller's "mesonephroma ovarii". *Amer. J. Cancer* **40**, 199—212 (1940).
KELLEY, R. R., and SCULLY, R. E., Cancer developing in dermoid cysts of the ovary. A report of 8 cases, including a carcinoid and a leiomyosarcoma. *Cancer (Philad.)* **14**, 989—1000 (1961).
KOTTMEIER, H.-L., The classification and treatment of ovarian tumours. *Acta obstet. gynec. scand.* **31**, 313—363 (1952).
MAGNER, D., CAMPBELL, J. S., and WIGLESWORTH, F. W., Testicular adenocarcinoma

with clear cells, occurring in infancy. *Cancer (Philad.)* **9**, 165—175 (1956).
MARTIN, J. F., CABANNE, F., and FEROLDI, J., Il mesoblastoma dell'ovaio (mesonefroma di Schiller); studio d'insieme con tre osservazioni personali. *Arch. De Vecchi Anat. pat.* **22**, 1—35 (1954).
MASSON, P., *Tumeurs humaines*, 2ᵉ éd. Paris: Maloine 1956.
MELICOW, M. M., Classification of tumors of testis. *J. Urol. (Baltimore)* **73**, 547—574 (1955).
MEYER, R., The pathology of some special ovarian tumors and their relation to sex characteristics. *Amer. J. Obstet. Gynec.* **22**, 697—713 (1931).
NEUBECKER, R. D., and BREEN, J. L., Embryonal carcinoma of the ovary. *Cancer (Philad.)* **15**, 546—556 (1962).
NOVAK, E., WOODRUFF, J. D., and NOVAK, E.R., Probable mesonephric origin of certain female genital tumors. *Amer. J. Obstet. Gynec.* **68**, 1222—1242 (1954).
NOVAK, E. R., and WOODRUFF, J. D., Mesonephroma of the ovary, thirty-five cases from the ovarian tumor registry of the American Gynecological Society. *Amer. J. Obstet. Gynec.* **77**, 632—644 (1959).
— —, and LINTHICUM, J. M., Evaluation of the unclassified tumors of the ovarian tumor registry 1942—1962. *Amer. J. Obstet. Gynec.* **87**, 999—1007 (1963).
PETERSON, W. F., Malignant degeneration of benign cystic teratomas of ovary; collective review of literature. *Obstet. gynec. Surv.* **12**, 793—830 (1957).
PEYRON, A., Faits nouveaux relatifs à l'origine et à l'histogénèse des embryomes. *Bull. Ass. franç. Cancer* **28**, 658—681 (1939).
— Bibliographie de ses travaux. In: R. DUFAU, *Les tumeurs du testicule et les syndromes de masculinisation (Thèse)*. Le François 1941.
PHILIP, J., and TETER, J., Significance of chromosomal investigation of somatic cells to determine the genetic origin of gonadoblastoma (Gonocytoma III). *Acta path. microbiol. scand.* **61**, 543—550 (1964).
PIERCE, G. B., and DIXON, F. J., Testicular teratomas. I. Demonstration of teratogenesis

by metamorphosis of multipotential cells. *Cancer (Philad.)* **12**, 573—583 (1959).

PIERCE, G. B., and DIXON, F. J., Testicular teratomas. II. Teratocarcinoma as ascitic tumor. *Cancer (Philad.)* **12**, 584—589 (1959).

RAO, N. R., VELIATH, G. D., and SRINIVASAN, M., An unusual case of sacrococcygeal mesonephroma (SCHILLER). *Cancer (Philad.)* **17**, 1604—1609 (1964).

SANTESSON, L., Clinical and pathological survey of ovarian tumors treated at the Radiumhemmet; dysgerminomas. *Acta radiol. (Stockh.)* **28**, 644—668 (1947).

—, and MARRUBINI, G., Clinical and pathological survey of ovarian embryonal carcinomas, including so-called "mesonephromas" (SCHILLER), or "mesoblastomas" (TEILUM), treated at Radiumhemmet. *Acta obstet. gynec. scand.* **36**, 399—419 (1957).

SAPHIR, O., A text on systemic pathology, vol. I, p. 612. New York and London: Grune & Stratton 1958.

—, and LACKNER, J. E., Adenocarcinoma with clear cells (hypernephroid) of ovary. *Surg. Gynec. Obstet.* **79**, 539—543 (1944).

SCHILLER, W., Mesonephroma ovarii. *Amer. J. Cancer* **35**, 1—21 (1939).

— Histogenesis of ovarian mesonephroma *Arch. Path.* **33**, 443—451 (1942).

SCULLY, R. E., Gonadoblastoma; gonadal tumor related to dysgerminoma (seminoma) and capable of sex-hormone production *Cancer (Philad.)* **6**, 455—463 (1953).

— Germ cell tumors of the ovary and Fallopian tube. In: J. V. MEIGS and S. H. STURGIS (eds.), *Progress in gynecology*, vol. IV, p. 335—347. New York: Grune & Stratton 1963.

SIMARD, L.-C., Polyembryonic embryoma of the ovary of parthenogenetic origin. *Cancer (Philad.)* **10**, 215—223 (1957).

STERNBERG, W. H., Nonfunctioning ovarian neoplasms. In: H. G. GRADY and D. E. SMITH, *The ovary*. Internat. Acad. Path. Monograph. Baltimore: Williams & Wilkins Co. 1963.

STEVENS, L. C., The biology of teratomas including evidence indicating their origin from primordial germ cells. *Ann. Biol.* **1**, 585—610 (1962).

TEILMANN, I., KASSIS, H., and PIETRA, G., Primary germcell tumour of the anterior mediastinum with features of endodermalsinus tumour (Mesoblastoma vitellinum). Acta path. microbiol. scand. (in press) 1967.

TEILUM, G., Gonocytoma; homologous ovarian and testicular tumors; I; with discussion of "mesonephroma ovarii" (SCHILLER: Amer. J. Cancer 1939). *Acta path. microbiol. scand.* **23**, 242—251 (1946).

— "Mesonephroma ovarii" (SCHILLER); extra-embryonic mesoblastoma of germ cell origin in ovary and testis. *Acta path. microbiol. scand.* **27**, 249—261 (1950).

— Classification of ovarian tumours. *Acta obstet. gynec. scand.* **31**, 292—312 (1952).

— Histogenesis and classification of mesonephric tumors of female and male genital system and relationship to benign so-called adenomatoid tumors (mesotheliomas); comparative histological study. *Acta path. microbiol. scand.* **34**, 431—481 (1954).

— Endodermal sinus tumors of the ovary and testis. Comparative morphogenesis of the so-called mesonephroma ovarii (SCHILLER) and extra-embryonic (yolk sac-allantoic) structures of the rat's placenta. *Cancer (Philad.)* **12**, 1092—1105 (1959).

— Classification of endodermal sinus tumour (Mesoblastoma vitellinum) and so-called "embryonal carcinoma" of the ovary. *Acta path. microbiol. scand.* **64**, 407—429 (1965).

TEOH, T. B., STEWARD, J. K., and WILLIS, R. A., The distinctive adenocarcinoma of the infants testis: an account of 15 cases. *J. Path. Bact.* **80**, 147—156 (1960).

TETER, J., A new concept of classification of gonadal tumours arising from germ cells (gonocytoma) and their histogenesis. *Gynaecologia (Basel)* **150**, 84—102 (1960).

— A mixed form of feminizing germ cell tumor (gonocytoma II). *Amer. J. Obstet. Gynec.* **84**, 722—730 (1962).

— PHILIP, J., WECEWICZ, GR., and POTOCKI, J., A masculinizing mixed germ cell tumour (gonocytoma III). *Acta endocr. (Kbh.)* **46**, 1—11 (1964)

THEISS, E. A., ASHLEY, D. J. B., and MOSTOFI, F. K., Nuclear sex of testicular tumors and some related ovarian and extragonadal neoplasms. *Cancer (Philad.)* **13**, 323—327 (1960).

THURLBECK, W. M., and SCULLY, R. E., Solid teratoma of the ovary; a clinicopathological analysis of 9 cases. *Cancer (Philad.)* **13**, 804—811 (1960).

WADE-EVANS, T., and LANGLEY, F. A., Mesonephric tumors of the female genital tract. *Cancer (Philad.)* **14**, 711—725 (1961).

I am indebted to Dr. I. TEILMANN *et al.*, Chicago, and Dr. J. TETER, Warsaw, for having contributed Figs. 4 and 13, respectively.

Figs. 1—2, 6—8, and 10—12 were previously published in the author's paper in Acta path. microbiol. scand. **64**, 407—429 (1965).

Lipoidic Cell Tumors of the Ovary

G. Gricouroff

Head of the Pathological Department, Fondation Curie, Paris, France

F. Veith

Assistant Pathologist, Pathological Department, Fondation Curie, Paris, France

Introduction

The category of lipoidic cell tumours includes rare ovarian tumours which until recently have been given a variety of names and which have in common the following histologic characteristics (Fig. 1):

1. endocrine architecture with full cords, almost joined, and well irrigated by a slender capillary-type stroma;

2. voluminous oval or polyhedral tumour cells, whose cytoplasm contains a greater or lesser quantity of lipids.

On staining with the standard stains, the lipids appear in the form of intra-cytoplasmic vacuoles, which are isolated or confluent (Fig. 2). Histochemical methods confirm their fatty nature and show that they are lipids in the liquid phase.

These lipoidic cells emanate from the hilar or cortical mesenchyme of the ovary. They have the same embryologic origin. They possess common biological and biochemical properties: under the influence of various stimuli, such as hor-

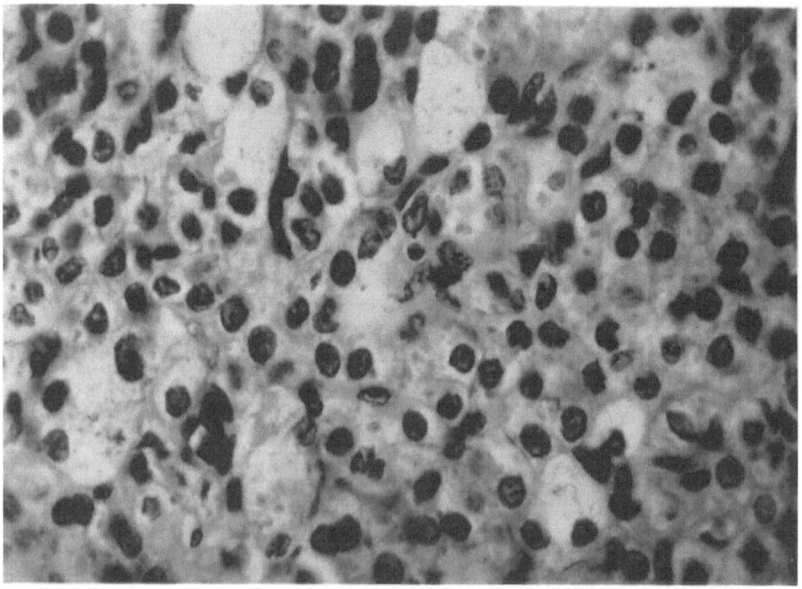

Fig. 1. Lipoidic cell tumour of the ovary. Endocrine architecture. Cells containing a greater or lesser quantity of lipids

monal incitations, which are most often of hypophyseal or placental origin, they are able to multiply and acquire an endocrine secretory function which is regulated by enzymatic mechanisms. The hormones they are thus able to produce are sex steroids. Depending on their abundance, their chemical structure and

ovarian tumour presenting these hilar cells (Fig. 3). In 1949, STERNBERG published 2 similar cases with virilism. Since then, other reports have appeared, although incomplete, of virilized or, contrariwise, hyperfeminized patients, operated upon for hilar cell tumours of this type.

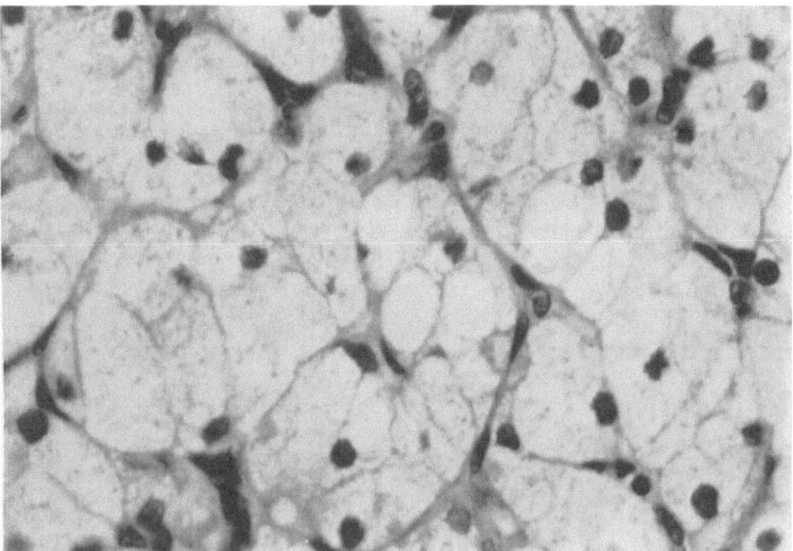

Fig. 2. Adrenocortical-like cell tumour. Spongiocyte-like cells riddled with confluent lipidic vacuoles

their hormonal "potency", these steroids will have clinical repercussions that can be masculinizing, feminizing, or inapparent.

These cells can resemble the Leydig cells present in the hilus of the normal ovary, the luteinized cells of the corpus luteum in activity, or the adreno-cortical spongiocytes.

In 1923, BERGER identified in the ovarian hilus in contact with the vessels, small clusters of cells that were identical with the testicular Leydig cells and which he termed "sympathicotropes", as he found them mostly situated in the vicinity of nerve fibers. In 1942 he described the case of a female patient suffering from masculinization, who presented an

The term "luteoma" denotes ovarian neoplasms bearing lipoidic cells which resemble the luteinized cells. STERNBERG (1963) was the first to publish a major description of "luteomas" found in the course of pregnancy ("pregnancy luteomas"). He considered these neoplasms to be a clinicopathologic entity (Fig. 4).

At present, the case reports of the more frequent type of tumours, consisting of cells resembling those of the zona glomerulosa and zona fasciculata of the adrenocortical gland (BRUKHANOV, 1899; PEHAM, 1899), are more than 70 (Figs. 1, 2) in number.

Great confusion has arisen concerning these lipoidic cell ovarian tumours, because of the various names given to them. These diverse appelations were not only often erroneous, but had the drawback of relying on a certain secretory specificity, a particular histogenesis, or an initial anatomic localization of the proliferated lipoidic cells.

Barzilai was the first in 1949 to insist on the fact that such tumours always show the same morphologic feature, i.e. their lipidic aspect. Hence she used the term "lipidic cell tumours" for these neoplasms. It would be even

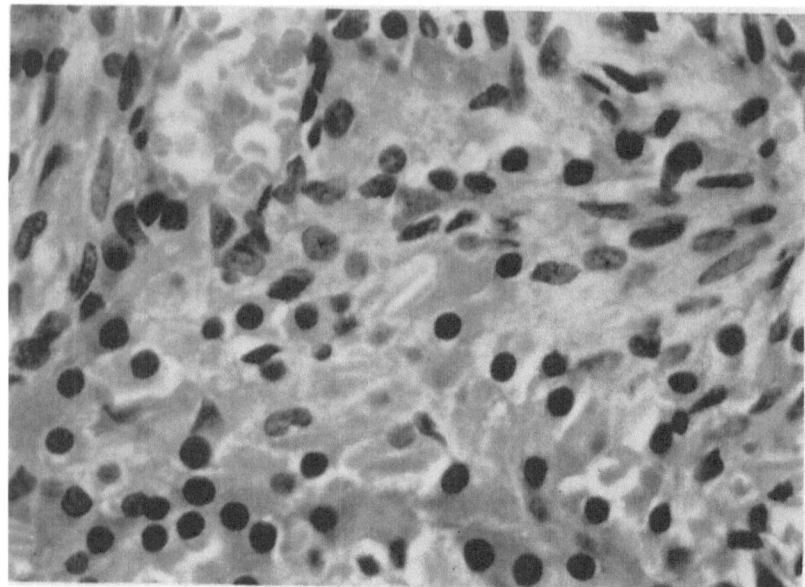

Fig. 3. Hilar cell tumour

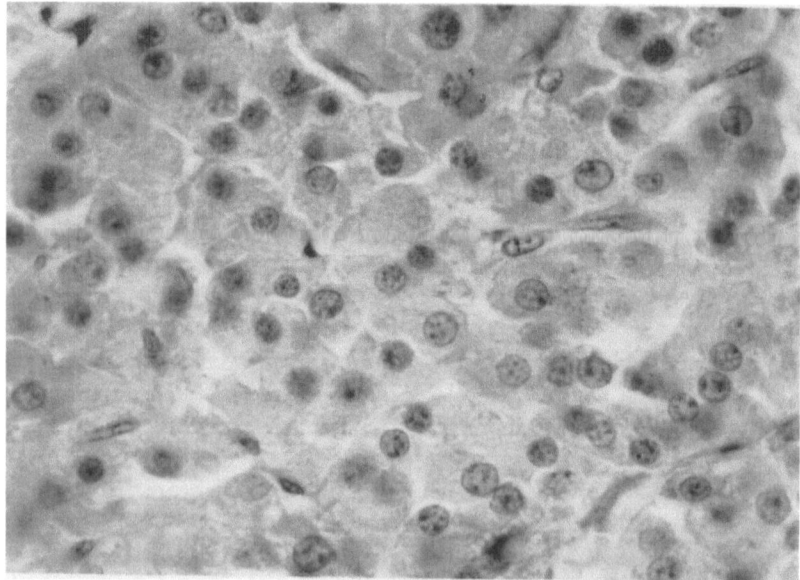

Fig. 4. Pregnancy luteoma

more prudent to use the term "lipoidic" for cells in whose cytoplasm fatty inclusions appear to be present, as we know nowadays that such cells are not always soudanophile. This is the term adopted, at least for the time being, by the W.H.O. scientific group on the histopathologic nomenclature of ovarian tumours, thereby leaving the way open for a study of these neoplasms without any preconceived ideas.

But as SCULLY (1963) pointed out recently, the term is nonetheless inadequate; it is not even strictly generic. Some tumours belonging to this group are wholly made up of non-soudanophile elements, and have a cytoplasm that is homogeneous or granular. Thecomas, however, which are classified separately in the ovarian mesenchymal tumour group of which they constitute by far the greatest subgroup, contain, when they are secretory, numerous cells packed with lipids.

Therefore, we should adopt the term "lipoidic cell tumour" only tentatively, as a temporary term to designate the sub-group of *mesenchymal endocrine tumours having no theca cell component*.

The study of these neoplasms is not an easy task.

They are relatively rare, and a review of the 106 cases published up to the present[1] time discloses the incompleteness of many observations. Hormone determinations and the histochemical detection of intracellular lipids are described only in the most recent publications.

The main difficulty is that what we are concerned with is an endocrine tumour pathology. The criteria for identifying by routine purely morphological histologic techniques are inadequate. Unfortunately, the histochemical techniques available at the present time also give disappointing results. True, they make it possible to detect endoplasmic

lipids and to discover whether the lipoidic cells are secretory. But none make it possible to decide whether the cellular lipids are corticoids or sex steroids, or to what type of sex steroid they might belong.

The method of sex steroid and corticoid determination through measurement of their excretion in urine over a 24-hour period has its value. It provides objective confirmation of the masculinization or feminization already observed clinically and a means whereby to appreciate the existence or non-existence of signs of adrenocortical hyperfunction. But nothing as yet allows us to state categorically the adrenocortical or ovarian origin of the male- or female-type sex steroids detected in the urine. As H. SERMENT and L. PIANA (1964) pointed out: "It seems as if each glandular system (capable of manufacturing sex hormones under normal physiological conditions) is unable to secrete any one steroid to the exclusion of the others. If it produces more of one, it necessarily produces a certain amount of the others. Thus it has been established (ZANDER, 1958) that DHA is not only of adrenal origin, any more than testosterone is necessarily gonadal". This is even more true in the case of a tumour secretion. Everything would be quite simple if each cellular type always produced the same hormonal substances, with female cells giving rise to feminization and male cells to masculinization. It would all be very easy if a considerable proportion of the androgens of adrenal origin were eliminated in the form of DHA and those secreted by the ovary were excreted mainly in the form of androsterone. But with the sex steroids, "we know that one and the same cell can secrete serveal

---

[1] These cases covered: "Hilar" cell tumours: 28; "Adrenocortical" cell tumours: 71; "Luteomas": 7.

hormones and that one and the same hormone can be secreted by different varieties of cells. Thus in certain cases a lipoidic cell tumour, morphologically non-thecomatous, can, clinically, produce a virilism, while another one produces hyperestrogenism"... And lastly, "the metabolic intrication of the various androgens is such that it would be illusory to take the elimination products as a basis for a qualitative hypothesis concerning their precursors. Androsterone and etiocholanolone, for instance, can arise either from DHA or from testosterone..."[1]

Fortunately, there are the adrenocortical restraining tests, by means of which injections of dexamethasone depress the level of the urinary 17-ketosteroids, where there is virilizing adrenal hyperplasia, but have no effect on them when the tumour has a Leydig-type component, these tests are of great value for diagnostic purposes. But as far as we know, only one case has been reported in the literature of a virilizing lipoidic cell ovarian tumour for which these tests were applied[2].

With these facts in mind, we might admit that the traditional anatomo-clinical method is still largely the best. Histologic examination of the ovarian tumour, a thorough clinical examination, and the various hormonal explorations practised at frequent intervals should be undertaken in a correlative manner for each case. Only by such a combination of the anatomo-clinical and histobiochemical data can we come to an understanding of these lipidic non-theca cell bearing tumours.

Materials and Method

As the materials available in our Laboratory at the Fondation Curie were insufficient for our study, Drs R. Scully, G. Teilum, L. Przybora and A. Luisi

were kind enough to provide us with the means of personally examining 26 cases of endocrine ovarian non-theca cell bearing tumours, by letting us have the microscopic preparations and corresponding clinical observations for these cases.

The material comprised:
11 lipoidic cell tumours, of which
5 were the hilar cell variety (Figs. 3, 5),
3 were the luteinic cell variety (Fig. 4), and
3 were the adrenal-like cell variety (Figs. 1, 2);
10 arrhenoblastomas;
5 diverse ovarian tumours with functioning stroma.

Our investigation of the two last categories as well as of one case of hilar cell hyperplasia revealed, in the functioning stroma of these tumours, the presence of the various types of lipid cells that were observed in the 11 purely lipoidic tumours.

After a study of the existing descriptions, we compared our observations with those recorded in the literature, particularly with those giving the *description princeps* of the three types, hilar, luteinic, and adrenal-like, which had appeared in the most recent monographs published in 1963 and 1964[3,4]. In order to understand the significance of these tumours, we undertook a further detailed review of all the recent data concerning the embryology, histology, and endocrinology of the ovary and adrenals under normal physiological condi-

---

[1] According to the following schema taken from Serment and Piana:

Testo-   ↗ Androsterone
sterone → Δ₄ androstenedione → Etiochol-
D.H.A. ↗   anolone

[2] H. Serment and L. Piana (1964).

[3] "The Ovary". International Academy of Pathology Monograph, 1933.

[4] "Tumeurs endocrines sexuelles de l'ovaire". Serment et Piana, 1964.

tions. In discovering the progress achieved in these disciplines, we were struck by the unity and the morphological resemblance of the mesenchymal cells capable of secreting the sex steroids, their great degree of plasticity, their functional omnipotence, and the close chemical kinship of the sex hormones they produce from a single starting material derived from cholesterol: progesterone.

Anatomo-Clinical Study

Our 11 cases showed the following characteristics:

Clinical

Age. Four of the five hilar cell cases had been operated upon after the menopause (at 53, 53, 61 and 69 years of age) and one case had been discovered in a young pregnant girl of 15. The three "luteomas" had been operated upon in young women aged 25, 33, and 35 years, at the end of pregnancy. The three cases of adrenal-like tumours had been operated upon in patients aged 21, 23, and 50 years.

Endocrine Syndrome. All 8 hilar and adrenal-like tumours were virilizing. There were distinct signs of masculinization (hirsutism, increase in size of clitoris, deepening voice, etc.). These signs had appeared progressively in 2 cases during the final month of pregnancy, and in 3 instances, following an initial period of defeminization. The patients were operated upon during the period of reproductive functions. In no case was a Cushing-like syndrome observed. It is interesting to note that the three pregnant women operated upon for a "luteoma" were multiparous and had shown signs of gravidic toxemia toward the end of pregnancy.

Hormone Determinations. The level of the 17-ketosteroids was measured in 5 of the 8 virilized patients. In four of them, it was high before the operation. In 2 cases, recently communicated to us by SCULLY, fractionation of the 17-ketosteroids, which had risen to 140 mg and 200 mg per 24 hours, showed high levels of androsterone and androstenedione. Unfortunately, in none of the cases were the F.S.H., L.H., and corticosteroid levels determined.

Tumour Syndrome. Nine times out of ten the small-sized tumour could not be diagnosed clinically, but was discovered in the course of an exploratory laparotomy, during a Caesarian section, or at necropsy. The two clinically-detected pelvic tumours, which were voluminous, were diagnosed in the 2 patients who had by far the highest levels of 17-ketosteroids. Ascites is not mentioned in any of the case reports.

Gross Characteristics

These tumours were solid, unilateral in 10 cases out of 11, small-sized (1 to 8 cm in diameter) 9 times out of 10, oval shaped, well limited, pushing back the intact ovarian tissue to the periphery, and with a smooth surface. On section, the cut surface was yellow or orange-yellow with only occasional cystic or hemorrhagic areas.

Histologic Characteristics

All the cases presented the same over-all endocrine architecture, with the lipoidic tumour cells grouped in cords around vascular connective axes.

1. In the cases of "*hilar cell tumours*" (Fig. 3), the cells were polyhedral, medium-sized (d = 12 to 20 microns), with hyperchromatic spherical nuclei. The cytoplasm was eosinophilic, most often finely granular, at times vacuolized and lipoidic in the largest elements. We saw only one case of crystalloids of Reinke (Fig. 5), which were intracytoplasmic,

stick-shaped, and as long as the cell. An endoplasmic brownish pigment was more frequently encountered.

2. The three cases of "*luteomas*" (Fig. 4) had the aspect described by STERNBERG, of a voluminous tumour corpus luteum, quite distinct from the true corpus luteum of pregnancy visible in the ovary at a distance from the luteinic

first, were spongiocyte-like and their cytoplasm was clear, abundant, and riddled with confluent lipidic vacuoles (Fig. 2).

An interesting fact is that none of the 11 cases we investigated was of one of the three pure cytological types, i.e. Leydig-type, luteinic, or spongiocyte-like. The hilar cell tumours seemed to

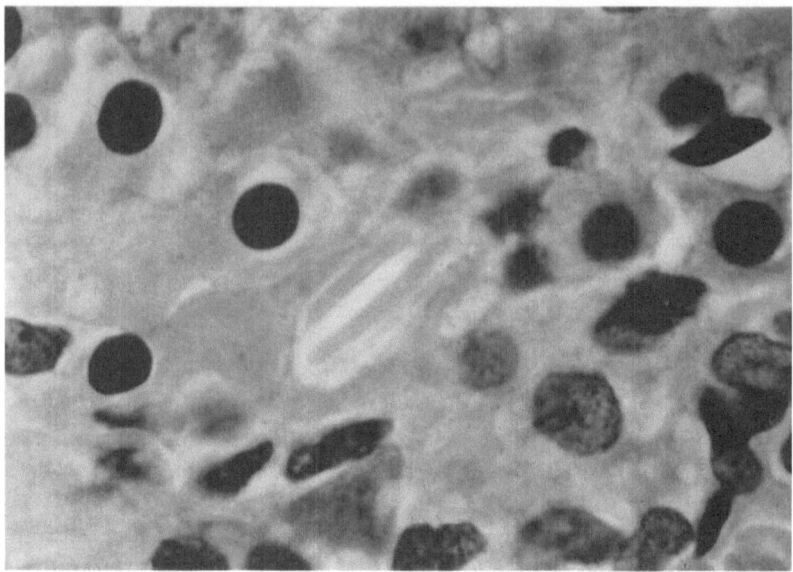

Fig. 5. Hilar cell tumour. One cell contains two stick-shaped crystalloids of REINKE

neoplasm. The large-sized cells had a finely granular cytoplasm, containing in the largest elements small lipoidic vacuoles and a vesicular central nucleus containing one or two nucleoli within a blurred chromatin.

3. The three "*adrenal-like tumours*" (Figs. 1, 2) were identical to cortical adenomas of the adrenal, with well structured cell cords consisting of elements resembling the zona glomerulosa and zona fasciculata cells of that gland. The first type, less voluminous and with an eosinophilic and granular cytoplasm (Fig. 1), looked extraordinarily like the hilar cells of the normal ovary. The second type, closely mingled with the

contain, depending on the area, medium-sized eosinophilic Leydig-like cells, looking very much like the glomerulosa cells visible in the "adrenal-like tumours", and other larger ones which, with their spumous cytoplasm, had a spongiocyte-like aspect. Some of the lipoidic cells of the "luteomas" were likewise spongiocyte-like in appearance; the others, with their granular and finely vacuolized cytoplasm, were difficult to distinguish from certain elements found in the "hilar cell tumours". Furthermore, the simultaneous presence in several tumours of two or three of the main cell varieties and their close relationship gave us the impression that all these elements belong to the same cellular family, of which they most probably represent various stages — or various modes — of secretory activity.

Lastly, the mitotic activity of the majority of these neoplasms was weak. In only one case did the normal. or atypical mitoses and the numerous cellular anomalies leave no doubt as to the malignancy which, however, was confirmed by necropsy at the end of the 14-month period which followed surgical intervention.

The postoperative course was known in only 4 cases. The one woman who had a malignant lipoidic cell tumour died with what was, clinically, generalized cancer despite intensive high-voltage radiotherapy. Another, who had a histologically benign "luteoma", died from gravidic nephropathy which was also confirmed at necropsy. There was no recurrence of the tumours of the 3 other virilized women; their level of 17-ketosteroids returned to normal but there was only incomplete regression of the signs of masculinization.

Discussion

It is pertinent to recall here the recently acquired information concerning the embryology, histology and endocrine biochemistry of the normal ovary and adrenal cortex. With this information and our study of 11 new cases, we can come to a clearer understanding of the common biology of lipoidic cell ovarian tumours than was possible only a few years ago. And indeed we wonder whether, despite the different circumstances of their development and their at times paradoxical clinical behavior, these tumours consisting of cells which, true, are all lipidic, but which differ morphologically, do not nonetheless constitute a single anatomo-clinical entity corresponding to a sub-group of the

endocrine mesenchymal tumours of the ovary.

Great strides have been made during the last few years in the experimental and descriptive *embryology* of the ovary. The common mesonephrotic origin of the interstitial gland of the male and female gonads and of the adrenal cortex is now considered a certainty. The "germinative" nature of the portion of the celomic mesothelium destined to become the germinal plate is not accepted by the majority of investigators. This celomic epithelium which undergoes stratification in order to form the germinal plate, releases only a single outflux of sex cords, deep in the embryonic mesenchyme in the direction of the mesonephrotic tracts which later they penetrate. This is true for either sex. In the ovary, these epithelial cords give birth exclusively to the cells of the granulosa. Thus the classic theory of two successive surges of sex cords is brought to naught. The primitive gonad is sexually bipotential and, while it possesses two antagonistic parts — the hilar and the cortical — which are preferentially male and female, nevertheless maintains this ambivalence within the cortex itself during infancy and adult life. WITSCHI, in 1963, wrote that "it seems probable that the entire steroid-producing organs, adrenal medulla, gonadal medulla and gonadal cortex are of mesonephric derivation, at least in an evolutionary sense. The production of the various steroids seems not to be distributed and restricted entirely to specific cell types". Thus for example, certain elements of mesonephrotic origin derived from the ovarian cortex probably retain their ability to secrete androgens.

The *histology* of the ovary helps us to locate those cells in the adult ovary that are susceptible of acquiring a lipidic endoplasm. Prior to ovulation, only the cells of the theca interna and those of the hilus are secretory. After ovulation, the transformation of the ruptured follicle into the corpus luteum is characterized by a lipidic vacuolization ("luteinization") of the cells of the theca interna and of the granulosa, and by a vascular penetration of the luteinized granulosa. Throughout the active phase of the corpus luteum the luteinized granulosa cells and thecal cells retain a morphologic and functional specificity. Little is known so far concerning the nature and physiological role of the "K cells".

The cells of the ovarian hilus have been successively termed "sympathicotropic cells", "extraglandular interstitial cells", and "cells of the hilus". They could easily be taken for the interstitial cells described by LEYDIG, so close is their resemblance. The different morphologic aspects they present, depending on the phase of their secretory activity, have recently been studied by R. and A. LOUBET (1961), who examined serial sections of 200 ovaries of children and adult women. In every case, they found cells of the hilus, even in the full-term and premature newborn. They hold that these cells are more frequent at the time of puberty, at the end of pregnancy, and especially during the menopause, when they remain abundant during the next 10 years. These investigators describe 4 cell types:

Type I: cell diameter of 14 to 12 microns. Cytoplasm with sharp contours, finely granular and eosinophilic;

Type II: narrow endoplasm, granular and eosinophilic, and extensive vacuolized exoplasm;

Type III: cytoplasm, entirely vacuolized, giving the cell a spongiocyte-like appearance;

Type IV: histiocyte-like aspect. Only the nucleolated vesicular nucleus is characteristic.

As in the case of the Leydig cells of the testis, separate enclaves are found in the cytoplasm of the hilar cells: these may be lipoidic bodies, a brownish lipochrome pigment, or crystalloids of Reinke (Fig. 5). The latter are not constantly present and are found in only a small proportion of cells.

Lastly, while the possibility of the existence of heterotopic adrenalcortical formations in the genital sphere is generally accepted, their site of predilection seems to be the broad ligament. The frequency of such heterotopic vestiges in the ovary itself (in the hilus and even in the cortex) is more difficult to appreciate.

Studies concerning the *hormonal biochemistry* of the steroids, a matter that has been constantly evolving during recent years, have brought to light a fact of cardinal importance. These hormones are all elaborated starting from a single precursor, the same derivative of cholesterol — progesterone. Progesterone is synthesized by the interstitial gland of the ovary and testis and by the adrenal cortex by means of an identical biosynthetic mechanism. "Aside from failure to demonstrate adrenal steroid formation by the normal ovary or placenta, all the steroid-producing glands can synthesize any of the major steroid hormones". (K. J. RYAN, 1963). Thus the ovary, for instance, can produce testosterone starting from progesterone. But as we stated previously, it would all be easy if, in pathological conditions, the functioning of the 17-ketosteroids would enable us to establish the adrenocortical or ovarian origin of the sex androgens excreted in the 24-hour urine determinations. Perhaps, in the future, the adrenocortical and ovary restraining-stimulating test will make it possible to pinpoint the cell family responsible for the elaboration of the 17-ketosteroids excreted. Present-day methods of urinary androgen determinations do not allow such precision.

From our study of these 11 new cases, the following points are worthy of comment:

1. *Clinical.* The hilar cell tumours were operated upon after the menopause, and the other lipidic tumours during the period of reproductive activity. The luteomas were not virilizing and were discovered in every instance at the end of a difficult pregnancy complicated by gravidic toxemia. The adrenal-like tumours bearing hilar cells were operated upon virilized in women, but none presented a Cushing's syndrome. Four out of the five masculinized patients in whom hormone determinations were obtained had raised levels of 17-ketosteroids; these were extremely elevated in the two cases of large-sized, clinically detectable tumours.

2. *Histologic.* The absence in the neoplastic cords of cells purely of the cellular types I, II and III described by R. and A. LOUBET is noteworthy. The predominance in each variety of tumour of one of these three types seems to confer on each tumour its characteristic physionomy but not pure specificity.

These reflections, together with the recently acquired data described above, seem to indicate an identical biological behavior on the part of all three tumour varieties and of all the cellular types which can predominate in the neoplastic cords with each one apparently secreting different substances. Thus, depending on the hormone content of their endoplasm, the same endocrine mesenchymal ovarian cells which, in proliferating, form the lipoidic tumours, can take on a new appearance, incarnating the three cytologic varieties: hilar, luteinic, and spongiocyte-like.

As the study of the 11 clinical reports shows, the "hilar" cells of type I are present in the tumours operated upon

during the menopause or postmenopause period. The "luteinic" cells of type II were found during the period of pregnancy in patients presenting a syndrome of gravidic toxemia. The "spongiocyte-like" cells of type III were operated upon in young women who were masculinized after an initial defeminization. These different physiological states — which, it seems, correspond to qualitative and quantitative differences in the secretion of the pituitary or placental stimulins — determine the morphology of the cells which make up lipoidic tumours.

The absence of a Cushing's syndrome in the virilized women seems to prove that the "adrenal-like" tumours are not truly adrenocortical, histogenetically speaking. For it is difficult to see why ovarian tumours, developing from hilar or adrenocortical vestiges, should not give rise to the Cushing's syndrome which eutopic adrenocortical adenomas so readily produce.

As regards the "luteomas", their personality seems to us to be more biological than morphologic. The lack of complete hormone counts[1] in the case reports to which we had access made it impossible for us to discover whether they are active during pregnancy, secreting or not secreting progesterone. Do these tumours represent hyperplastic reactional proliferations of certain areas of the ovarian mesenchyma that are particularly receptive to the L.H. hormones of pregnancy?

Conclusions. These considerations incite us to adopt for the histogenesis of hilar and adrenal-like cell tumours the concept of unity upheld in France by LAFFARGUE in 1955 and 1961 and by PAYAN in 1957. In their view, one cannot

---

[1] Determinations of F.S.H., L.H., and pregnandiol were not practised under satisfactory conditions in these patients.

set up a contradistinction between these two types of tumours, both of which are virilizing. "If at times they are more the Leydig type, or more the adrenal type, their origin is nevertheless the same, which explains why there are some intermediary aspects, between the two forms." Hence their appellation "lipidic cell endocrine arrhenomas".

The luteoma, with its endocrine architecture, and which is likewise composed of lipoidic cells, seems to have its own specific personality, as Sternberg hinted in 1963. The three cases we investigated were non-virilizing. They were discovered in a quite special physiological and pathological context. The rare cases of virilizing luteoma described in the literature could just as well have been considered as lipidic cell endocrine arrhenomas which had become functional and were discovered at the moment of pregnancy. The term "pregnancy luteoma" proposed by Sternberg thus seems the appropriate one.

From the viewpoint of nosology, endocrine lipidic cell arrhenoblastomas can be considered as the Leydig-like variety of Meyer's "arrhenoblastomas" or of Laffargue's "arrhenomas".

The "luteoma" should, in our opinion, be classified apart, in the generic group of ovarian tumours, on the same plane as the granuloso-thecal tumours and the arrhenoblastomas. Further studies will reveal whether these tumours are hormone secreting; provided, that is, that they can be operated upon several weeks after confinement and delivery. This delay is indispensable for appreciating whether, without the aid of the placenta, they secrete progesterone.

Summary

Under the heading "Lipoidic Cell Tumors" can be grouped various sexual endocrine tumours of the ovary, which are mesenchymal but bear no theca cell component, and which contain lipidic cells. All three varieties of hilar cell, luteinic cell, and adrenal-like cell tumours, already described in the literature under a diversity of appellations, were represented in the 11 cases on which we report. The histologic aspect and the clinical and endocrine features of the various neoplasms investigated indicate that the apparently generic group of lipoidic cell ovarian tumours in fact comprises two distinct anatomo-clinical entities: 1) the virilizing hilar cell and adrenal-like cell tumours, which seem clearly to be two morphologic expressions of one and the same type of neoplasm (the pure Leydig-type variety of Meyer's arrhenoblastomas), known in France since 1955 as "lipidic cell endocrine arrhenoma"; 2) the "pregnancy luteoma" described by Sternberg in 1963, with its own quite particular biological personality. It is not yet possible to establish the precise place of these two categories of mesenchymomas in what can at last be considered an acceptable classification for the sexual endocrine tumours of the ovary.

Résumé

On peut grouper sous le nom de «tumeurs à cellules lipoïdiques» diverses rares tumeurs endocrines sexuelles de l'ovaire, mésenchymateuses mais non thécomateuses, dont les cellules sont lipidiques. Parmi les onze cas rapportés dans ce travail, les trois variétés de tumeurs à cellules hilaires (Fig. 3, 5), lutéiniques (Fig. 4) et surrénaloïdes (Fig. 1, 2), déjà décrites dans la littérature sous des appellations diverses, étaient représentées. L'aspect histologique et le contexte clinique et endocrinien des différents néoplasmes étudiés permettent de penser que le groupe apparemment générique des tumeurs ovariennes à cellules

lipoïdiques comporte deux entités ana-
tomocliniques distinctes. D'une part, les
tumeurs à cellules hilaires et surrénaloïdes, virilisantes, qui semblent bien
être deux modalités morphologiques
d'un même type de néoplasme (variété
leydigienne pure des arrhénoblastomes
de MEYER), désigné en France depuis
1955 sous le nom «d'arrhénome endo-

crinien, à cellules lipidiques». D'autre
part, le «lutéome de grossesse», décrit
par STERNBERG en 1963, qui possède
une personnalité biologique très parti-
culière. La place exacte de ces deux caté-
gories de mésenchymomes, dans une
classification enfin acceptable des tumeurs
endocriniennes sexuelles de l'ovaire,
reste à préciser.

Discussion

SCULLY commented that to determine
the category in which a lipoidic cell
tumour belonged required the close cooperation of the clinician, the biochemist
and the pathologist. He cited, as an
example of the difficulties, a case report
he had read of a young patient who
became virilized. The testosterone level
in the urine was elevated and the patient
was given ACTH and dexamethasone
at various times; neither had any effect
on the urinary level of testosterone.
When she was given chorionic gonadotropin, the urinary level rose significantly. After the tumour was removed,
it was incubated with radioactive precursors and was found to form testosterone and other androgens which could
be attributed to gonadal tissue but it
did not produce corticoid or any of the
steroids that were thought to be more
characteristic of adrenal cortical tumour.
These tumours are occasionally malignant as shown in the case of an elderly
female who became virilized and who
had a level of 17-ketosteroids in the
range of 140 mg per 24 hours. She subsequently developed metastases and died
of her tumour; the 17-ketosteroid level
was 1,000 by that time.

SCULLY also gave a brief discussion
of pregnancy luteomas in which he presented experience with one patient that
indicated dependence of these tumours
on chorionic gonadotropin for their
structural, as well as their functional,

integrity. He also described a case history
of a patient with what he thought in
retrospect was a pregnancy luteoma
occuring in the first trimester, although
this tumour usually is found in the last
trimester of pregnancy. He added that
caution must be exercised during pregnancy, in diagnosing as malignant, tumours that have this cytological structure. He also made the point that some
authors have reported that these tumours
have a higher incidence in Negroes than
in Caucasians.

LUISI commented that some conflicting views had been expressed regarding the concept, described by GRICOU-
ROFF, that the adrenal-like tumours were
not actually adrenal cortical tumours.
Some patients with manifestations simu-
lating Cushing's syndrome or adrenal
virilism have been reported. In addition,
some adrenal-like morphologic aspects
have been observed. However, he added,
definite proof of the adrenal origin was
lacking. From his experience with two
patients, he agreed with GRICOUROFF and
SCULLY in considering the pregnancy
luteomas as probably chorionic dependent lesions. In one instance he observed
an intense theca lutein reaction in practically all the follicles, a reaction similar
to that seen in choriocarcinoma and
hydatidform mole.

TEILUM said that there was no morphological or embryological basis for
considering the lipoid cell tumours of

adrenal origin. Many investigators have reported adrenal-like or adrenal tumours differentiating from the stroma.

Scully agreed that there has been no proof that any of the lipoid cell tumours are of adrenal origin, but, he said, if the assumption is that they are all of Leydig or hilus cell origin, then there are difficulties, such as explaining the hormonal findings in certain cases. For example, the 17-ketosteroid levels are above 20 mg per 24 hours in only about one third of the patients with tumours that are known to contain Leydig cells such as the arrhenoblastomas or hilus cell tumours, but in the entire group of lipoid cell tumours, most patients have had high levels of 17 ketosteroids, sometimes as high as 100 or 300 mg per 24 hours. Therefore, the pattern of these tumours differs from those that are known to arise from hilus or Leydig cells.

Teilum replied that he agreed that there may be some difference in the hormone production but it is not constant and it is also known that typical hilus cell tumours in rare cases may be estrogen producing. There are also, he said, cases of "androblastoma tubular" associated with the constant production and excretion of corticosteroid, and that these disappeared after the tumour was removed.

In reply to a question from the floor, Scully said he did not believe there was any relation between the lipoid cell tumour and the so-called stromal cell hyperplasie in endometrial carcinoma that is sometimes associated with an increase in 17-ketosteroids. He did not think, he said, there was any real evidence that stromal hyperplasie was an estrogenic phenomenon; he thought it was common, and with careful search one could find these luteinized cells in areas of stromal hyperplasia. These cells, he thought, gave rise to the stroma luteomas and possibly to some of the larger lipoid cell tumours.

References

Barzilai, G., *Atlas of ovarian tumors.* New York: Grune & Stratton Inc. 1949.

Berger, L., La glande sympathicotrope du hile de l'ovaire; ses homologies avec la glande interstitielle du testicule. Les rapports nerveux des deux glandes. *Arch. Anat. (Strasbourg)* **2**, 255—267 (1923).

— Tumeur des cellules sympathicotropes de l'ovaire avec virilisation. *Rev. canad. Biol.* **1**, 539—566 (1942).

Brukhanov, N, Zur Kenntnis der primären Nebennierengeschwulste. *Z. Heilk.* **20**, 39—73 (1899).

Laffargue, P., Tumeurs mâles de l'ovaire. Etude anatomo-pathologique. *Presse méd.* **63**, 959—961 (1955).

—, Classification et diagnostic des tumeurs gonadiques spécifiques de l'ovaire. *Ann. Anat. path.* **6**, 305—322 (1961).

Meyer, R., Tubuläre (testikuläre) und solide Formen des Andreiblastoma ovarii. *Beitr. path. Anat.* **84**, 485—520 (1930).

Payan, H., Tumeurs des gonades. *Sud. méd. chir.* **90**, 6489—6493 (1957).

Peham, H., Aus akzessorischen Nebennieren-Anlagen entstandene Ovarial-Tumoren. *Wschr. Geburtsh. Gynäk.* **10**, 685—694 (1899).

Ryan, K., *The ovary,* p. 69—83. In: H. G. Grady, Internat. Acad. Path. Monograph. Baltimore: Williams & Wilkins Co. 1963.

Scully, R. E., *The ovary,* p. 143—174. Internat. Acad. Path. Monograph. Baltimore: Williams & Wilkins Co. 1963.

Serment, H., et Piana, L., *Tumeurs endocrines sexuelles de l'ovaire.* Marseille: Edit. Quo Vadis 1964.

Sternberg, W. H., The morphology, androgenic function, hyperplasia and tumors of the human ovarian hilus cells. *Amer. J. Path.* **25**, 493—521 (1949).

— *The ovary,* p. 209—254. Internat. Acad. Path. Monograph. Baltimore: Williams & Wilkins Co. 1963.

Witschi, E., *The ovary,* p. 1—10. Internat. Acad. Path. Monograph. Baltimore: Williams & Wilkins Co. 1963.

Zander, J., Steroids in the human ovary. *J. biol. Chem.* **232**, 117—123 (1958).

Metastatic Ovarian Tumours

Antonio Luisi, M. D.

Titular de Patologia, Instituto Central Hospital A.C. Camargo, São Paulo, Brasil

Introduction

In general pathology, a metastasis is considered as the reproduction of a tumour remote from the primary one and without anatomical connections with the latter. This definition excludes those tumours resulting from contiguous spread. Under such a view, the ovary can be reached via lymphatic or blood vessels or by superficial implantation. The latter alternative includes spread across the peritoneum or the tubes.

The study of the metastatic ovarian tumours has considerable practical and theoretical importance, affording, due to the numerous problems involved, a fertile research field.

It is never too much to recall Virchow's well-known pronouncement that the organs which show a great capacity for the production of tumours have a low tendency to be the site of metastases. In spite of the great controversy concerning the data presented, we can assert that the incidence of ovarian metastasis is significantly high, overpassing, indeed, in some statistical surveys, that of primary malignant tumours. Thus, while AHUMADA *et al.* (1953) reported that in 100 ovarian carcinomas, 14.5 per cent were metastatic, KITAIN had a figure of 61.5 per cent and JOHANSSON (1960) quoted LOCKYER and METZGER as authors stating that over 75 per cent of the malignant ovarian neoplasms are metastatic in nature. Another researcher,

GALLAGER (1962) also emphasized the frequency of such carcinomas in relation to the primary malignant ones.

The variability of the relative incidence presented in the literature depends on different factors. These include the type of material selected, the quality and the frequency with which the histological examination is performed. It is well known that many organs are not systematically submitted to histological examination when not showing gross lesions, and in the ovary, in a number of instances, the metastases are microscopic.

From a practical view, the difficulty found in recognizing the primary or secondary nature of ovarian neoplasm is remarkable in many cases. This recognition can even represent an unsurmountable difficulty, especially when based on morphological data only. The item concerning the so-called Krukenberg tumours, due to a mistake in the histogenetical interpretation, is at present based on morphological data not properly evaluated, although there is no doubt as to the accuracy of the descriptions made by KRUKENBERG.

As to the primary sites which are the source of ovarian metastasis, the following main groups are generally considered:

1. Tumours of digestive origin, particularly the gastrointestinal ones;

2. Tumours of genital origin;

3. Tumours of mammary origin.

To these basic groups, another one must be added: the reticulo-endothelial system neoplasms, for their frequency in ovary involvement and for the interesting information afforded by them in the momentous problem represented by the African Lymphoma (Burkitt's tumour).

Because of a shortage of time we had to limit the present review to the following aspects:

I. Frequency of the metastatic ovarian tumours in autopsies of cancer patients and in specimens from the Surgical Pathology Laboratory of an institution especially dedicated to the diagnosis and treatment of neoplastic diseases.
II. Age distribution.
III. Relation of the ovarian metastases to other metastases.
IV. Main primary sites:
   A. Digestive organs;
   B. Genitalia;
   C. Mammary gland;
   D. Reticuloendothelial System.
V. Pathways of ovarian involvement.
VI. Morphopathological aspects (the so-called Krukenberg tumour).

Material and Methods

The material studied was obtained at necropsies performed at the Instituto Central, Hospital A.C. Camargo, from 1953 to March 1966. During this time 1,000 necropsies with histological examinations were conducted. When males and those with different pathologic processes were excluded, 250 cases remained for investigation. Some further eliminations were necessary. These included cases which had undergone previous ovariectomy, usually in relation to hormonal deprivation in mammary carcinoma and cases presenting ovarian involvement by direct extension, as well as some other instances in which we could not arrive at a definite conclusion

as to their nature. Thus, a group of 90 cases remained for study. Clinicopathologic data were reviewed and all the histological preparations personally checked. In some, new sections were made and different staining methods were used in a search for or confirmation of the histological type of the primary tumour and its metastasis, as well as for the way in which the disease spread to the ovaries. Morphological evidence for lymphatic and cancerous emboli and for the existence of direct implantation on the ovary, was sought. Even those ovaries originally considered histologically negative, were re-examined for foci missed at the first survey.

The same method was used for all the specimens collected at the Laboratory of Surgical Oncological Pathology. These represented 560 cases of patients oophorectomized due to mammary carcinoma or to ovarian neoplasms which histological investigation proved to be metastatic.

Some of these cases represented patients who died later, but were not included in the necropsy series.

Routine techniques in histology were employed, mainly hematoxylin-eosin, P.A.S. and Meyer's mucicarmine, and the Fontana-Masson's method for the detection of argentaffin cells in some cases.

Because of time limitations, we could not perform semi-serial sections in the negative cases, a procedure which would be highly desirable in a review such as this.

Results

Tables I to V summarize the results obtained in the present review.

I. Frequency of the Ovarian Metastases

In the series of 90 cases studied (Table I), 27 instances of ovarian metastases were found, representing about

Table I. *Necropsy cases*

Primary tumour	No. of cases	Ovarian metastasis			Total
		R.Ov.	L.Ov.	Both	
Reticuloendothelial system	18			6	6 = 33.3%
Breast	15	1		5	6 = 40.0%
Uterus: Corpus	7			1	1 = 14.2% ⎫
Cervix	6			1	1 = 16.6% ⎬ = 15.3%
Stomach	7		1	5	6 = 85,7%
Skin	7	1			1
Intestine	5			1	1
Esophagus	5				0
Lung	4	1		1	2
Bone	4			1	1
Vulva	2				0
Gall bladder	3			1	1
Eye	2				0
Salivary glands	1			1	1
Tongue	1				0
Bladder	1				0
Lips	1				0
Kidney	1				0
Total	90	3	1	23	27 = 30.0%

Table II. *Surgical pathology cases*

Primary tumour	No. of cases	Ovarian metastasis			Total
		R.Ov.	L.Ov.	Both	
Breast	504	21	9	41	71 = 14%
Uterus *	29	8	3	3	14 = 48,2%
Intestine	9	2	1	6	9 = 100%
Stomach	9	1		8	9 = 100%
Reticuloendothelial system	2			2	2
Skin	3			1	1
Vulva	2			1	1
Thyroid gland	1			1	1
Total	559	32	13	63	108 = 19,3%

* *Corpus:* 8 cases, with 5 positives (62,5%). *Cervix:* 21 cases, with 9 positives (42,8%).

30%. This incidence is lower than that of 37 per cent verified by VIRIEUX (1963) but, nevertheless, more significant than the figures reported by other researchers — 11.7% by LEY; 5.0% by WARREN and MACOMBER (1935) and 8.5% by WILLIS (1952).

Table II refers to 559 ovarian specimens of which 108 contained metastases, which equals a rate of 19.3 per cent, lower than in the autopsy series. The nature of the specimens could well explain this reduced rate; necropsies were usually performed upon patients with neoplasms in a rather advanced stage of evolution, with a higher chance of metastic development. In the specimens collected surgically, most were removed

Table III. *Distribution of ovarian metastases by age groups (necropsy cases)*

Age	Cases	Ovarian metastasis		Frequency
		negative	positive	
Minus of one year	1	1		
1—10	7	4	3	*21 in 63 = 33.3%*
11—20	5	4	1 (20%)	
21—30	10	7	3 (30%)	
31—40	21	13	8 (38%)	
41—50	19	13	6 (31.5%)	
51—60	16	13	3 (18.7%)	*6 in 27 = 22.2%*
61—70	6	4	2	
71—80	4	3	1	
81—90	1	1		
Total	90	63	27	*27 = 30%*

Table IV. *Distribution of ovarian metastases by age groups (surgical pathology cases)*

Age	Cases	Ovarian metastasis		Frequency
		negative	positive	
11—20	1	1		*88 in 413 = 21.3%*
21—30	23	19	4 (17.3%)	
31—40	164	121	43 (26.2%)	
41—50	225	184	41 (18.2%)	
51—60	109	92	17 (15.6%)	*18 in 136 = 13.3%*
61—70	23	22	1 (4.3%)	
71—80	3	3		
81—90	1	1		
Age not known	10	8	2	
Total	559	451	108	*108 = 19.3%*

because of breast cancer and with no clinical manifestations of ovarian involvement.

As to the side affected, with the exception of 4 cases, all the autopsy specimens had bilateral ovarian involvement. Among the surgical specimens were observed the following points: Over one-half of the 71 cases of ovarian metastases plus breast carcinomas (41) were bilateral; 9 were in the left and 21 in the right ovary. This higher incidence in the right ovary when metastasis was unilateral, was also noted in the 14 cases metastasing from the uterus. Eight of these presented metastases involving the right ovary alone while the remaining 6 had metastases either to the left ovary or to both of them. Such bilateral disease also prevailed in the cases with gastric and intestinal disease.

The data assembled in the present investigation allow us to conclude that in the greater number of instances the metastases are bilateral, and that the unilateral processes affect, preferentially, the right ovary.

II. Age Distribution

The figures shown in Tables III and IV, show the prevalence of metastases in the age group 31—40 years, with a maximum rate both in necropsies (38 per cent) and in cases provided by the Surgical Pathology (26.2 per cent).

When the proportion of ovarian metastases is analyzed up to the age of 50 years, the rate turns out to be 33.3 per cent, decreasing to 22.2 per cent thereafter. In the surgical specimens the corresponding values amount to 21.3 and 13.3 per cent, respectively. These rates show a higher susceptibility of ovaries physiologically active to the implantation of metastasis.

The same fact is recorded in the literature. VIRIEUX (1963) reported, in necropsies, 51.7 per cent of ovarian metastasis taking place before the fiftieth year of age, as opposed to a rate of 30.9 per cent thereafter. The same author, for ovaries extirpated for hormonal dependency in cases of mammary carcinomas, found a rate of 44.4 per cent against 33.3 per cent respectively.

Authors such as WARREN and MACOMBER (1935) and KASILAG jr. and RUTLEDGE (1957), also found that the ovarian metastases are proportionally more frequent before the menopause.

JOHANSSON (1960), on the contrary, found a higher incidence of metastasis in patients over 50 years of age, attributing this finding to the particular conditions brought about by the high standard of living in Sweden.

III. Relation of the ovarian Metastases to Other Metastases

When there are metastases present in the ovaries, they are to be found in other organs as well. As a matter of fact, in the 27 necropsies studied by us, we did not find exclusive involvement of the ovaries in any instance.

Table V shows the frequency of metastases occurring in other organs, simultaneously; the pathway and extent of in-volvement evidently depend on the primary site of the process.

WARREN and MACOMBER (1935), in their 40 positive cases reported, mention the restriction of metastases to the ovaries alone or to ovaries and regional nodes, in 5 cases only.

IV. Main Primary Sites

In Table I, a variety of primary sites are listed, notice should be taken of the importance assumed especially by the tumours of the stomach, breast, reticulo-endothelial system and uterus, which have metastasized to the ovary, in percentages of 85.7, 40.0, 33.3 and 15.3 respectively, in the autopsy series. In the material provided by the Surgical Pathology Laboratory (Table II), 100 per cent of the gastrointestinal tumours 48.2 per cent of uterine and 14 per cent of mammarian tumours, metastasized to the ovary.

A. Digestive System

The importance of the digestive site, particularly of the gastrointestinal tumours, as a source of ovarian metastases, is emphasized practically by every researcher in this field.

POJARISSKY (cited by AHUMADA et al., 1953), collecting 681 ovarian carcinomas, verified that 503 were derived from organs of the digestive system.

GAUTHIER-VILLARS (1928), in a series of 365 ovarian metastases of digestive origin, found out that most of them, namely 247, were related to the stomach.

JOHANSSON (1963), pointed out the gastrointestinal site as responsible for 84.0 per cent of his recorded ovarian metastases, the stomach being the source of 39.0 per cent and the intestine of 45.0 per cent of the cases.

AHUMADA et al. (1953), in a sample of 15 metastatic ovarian carcinomas, were able to establish the gastroenteric

Table V. *Relation of the O.M. with other metastases. Necropsy cases*

Primary tumour	No. of cases with O.M.	Fre-quency	Localization of the other metastases
Reticuloendo-thelial system	7	5	Liver, kidney, ganglionar generalization
		4	Spleen
		3	Heart, fallopian tubes, pancreas
		2	Lung, bones, uterine corpus, cervix, adrenal, tonsils
		1	Brain, intestine, skin, estomach, periaortic, iliac lymph nodes, spinal cord.
Stomach	6	2	Liver, intestine, peritoneum
		1	Lung, uterine corpus, kidney, adrenal, thyroid gland, gall bladder, pancreas, esophagus, breast, cecal appendix, muscles, periaortic, suprapancreatic, perigastric, mesenteric lymph nodes and lymph nodes of the greater and lesser curvatures
Breast	6	5	Lung, liver, bones
		3	Adrenal, brain
		2	Uterine corpus, axillary lamph nodes
		1	Spleen, heart, thyroid gland, intestine, gall bladder, esophagus, muscles, inguinal, periaortic, peritraqueal, iliac, mediastinal lymph nodes
Lung	2	2	Liver
		1	Bones, uterine corpus, vulva, kidney, adrenal, brain, thyroid gland, intestine, skin, ganglionar generalization
Uterus: Corpus	1	1	Lung, liver, spleen, thyroid gland, periaortic, retro-peritoneal, mesenteric and mediastinic lymph nodes
Cervix	1	1	Lung, adrenal
Skin	1	1	Lung, liver, bones, kidney, spleen, adrenal, brain, heart, thyroid gland, intestine, inguinal, periaortic, peri-tracheal and suprapancreatic lymph nodes
Intestine	1	1	Kidney, adrenal, retroperitoneal lymph nodes
Gall bladder	1	1	Liver, bones, kidney, spleen, periaortic lymph nodes
Salivary glands	1	1	Lung, liver, kidney, brain, thyroid gland

tract as the primary site of 8 cases. In 17 cases of ovarian metastases studied by WILLIS (1952), 6 had their primary site in the stomach.

ABRAMS *et al.* (1950), pointed out a rate of 15 per cent of ovarian metastases in cases of gastric carcinoma.

B. Genitalia

Among ovarian metastases from tumours of the reproductive system, the most interesting ones are those originat-ing from the uterus, from the endo-metrium in particular, which can be mistaken for primary endometrial tu-mours of the ovary. MILLER (quoted by AHUMADA *et al.*, 1953), reported that in 403 cases of endometrial carcinoma, col-lected in the literature, 7.2 per cent gave rise to ovarian metastases, whereas a rate of only 0.65 per cent in 924 cases was due to cervical carcinomas. AHUMADA (1953) observed 0.69 per cent of metas-tases in a group of 542 cases of cervical carcinomas, and none in 124 cases of corporeal carcinomas. NOVAK (1927), reported an incidence of 4.8 per cent of ovarian metastasis in a series of 147 carcinomas of the uterine body studied.

As to the simultaneous involvement of the ovary and endometrium, it is particularly difficult in some instances to determine which is the primary tumour or whether both neoplasms have developed simultaneously and independently.

FINN (1951), in a group of 292 cases of endometrial carcinoma, detected 25 cases of ovarian metastases, namely 7.5 per cent. Of this group, not less than 5 were first considered to be primary tumours of the ovary, since the clinical picture suggested an ovarian tumour and the endometrial neoplasms were of a rather smaller size.

In the specimens studied by us, we found in 31 cervical carcinomas, 9 cases with ovarian metastases, which amounts to a rate of 42.8 per cent, and 5 cases in 8 corporeal tumours, corresponding to 62.5 per cent.

Altogether, the cases of uterine tumours supplied by the Surgical Pathology Laboratory represented 48.2 per cent of the ovarian metastases; in necropsies, the corresponding rate was 15.3 per cent.

C. Mammary Gland

The breast is one of the most important primary sites for neoplasms. Recently, some studies have been undertaken regarding the effectiveness of the ovary resection in cases of mammary carcinomas. Compared to our findings — 33.3 per cent in autopsies and 15.3 per cent in surgical specimens — the pertinent literature shows a great variability in its incidence, as follows:

WARREN and WITHAM (1953) recorded 15 instances of ovarian metastases (about 9.1 per cent) in 162 cases of mamary carcinoma.

VIRIEUX (1963) points out that 18.9 per cent of all the ovarian metastases studied by him in necropsies are due to the mammary carcinoma which, in turn, has shown metastases in 41.7 per cent of the cases. In surgically excised material, the author reports an approximate rate of 21.2 per cent. KARSH (1951) refers to 12.2 per cent of ovarian metastases in autopsies of mammary carcinomas, such an incidence being equivalent to that of the tumours of the gastrointestinal tract. KASILAG Jr. and RUDLEDGE (1957) established a frequency of 25.0 per cent.

SIRTORI et al. (1958) reported 26.1 per cent, 15.9 per cent of which were bilateral. LUMB and MACKENZIE (1959) refer to 29.4 per cent, stressing that in 63.3 per cent of the affected ovaries there was no gross evidence of metastasis. This observation emphasizes the value and the need for the microscopic investigation. JOHANSSON (1960), however, presented a rate of 14 per cent, similar to that observed by us in surgical specimens.

D. Reticuloendothelial System

The study of ovarian involvement in cases of neoplastic lesions of the reticuloendothelial system is particularly important because of its frequency. In the present investigation 6 of 18 necropsies of cases with reticuloendothelial tumours have shown lesions of the ovaries, which means a rate of 33.3 per cent. Of these 6 cases, 5 were of leukemic with intense dissemination; the uterus and the Fallopian tubes were also affected. The remaining case was a reticulosarcoma of the oral cavity with involvement of the mandible and deep nodes, mainly the periaortic and iliac nodes, and of the brain, medulla and pancreas as well. Both ovaries were affected, but only the left presented gross evidence of metastasis, being largely increased in volume. Karsh (1951) has reported, in his review of the subject, the bilateral and diffuse involvement of the ovaries in 4 lymphosarcomas and 1 reticulosarcoma.

One of the most up-to-date aspects of the present subject is the ovarian involvement in cases of African lymphoma

12 cases; the lesions were mostly bilateral, symmetrical, with diffuse infiltration of the ovaries; O'Conor et al. (1965) found the same alteration in 2, of an additional 5 cases. Dorfman (1965), in 6 of a group of 7 cases of lymphosarcoma studied in female children from St. Louis, verified the bilateral involvement of the ovaries, detecting as well

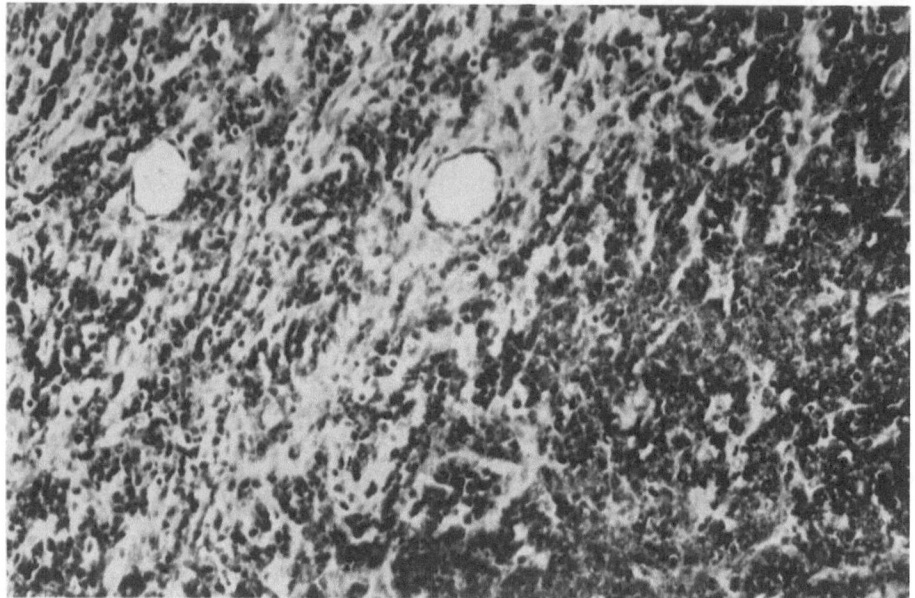

Fig. 1. Ovarian involvement in a case of malignant lymphoma (Burkitt's tumour). H.E.

(Burkitt's tumour). Cases similar to those observed in Africa were studied by us, Luisi (1965), in Brasil. Our 9 cases of Burkitt's tumour were from the States of São Paulo and Paraná; 2 were females but nothing could be ascertained in relation to their ovarian condition, because no autopsy was performed. In 2 additional cases of African lymphoma the bilateral involvement of the ovaries was noticed by us (unpublished data). Figs. 1, 2 and 3 are from one of these cases.

The importance of the subject can be evaluated from the following literature data: O'Conor (1961) has observed large tumour growths on the ovaries in 7 of his

bulky tumorous growths measuring up to $21 \times 12 \times 6$ cm. Of these 7, 2 cases presented oral manifestation of the disease. In St. Louis also, a similar case was identified and reported in 1928 by Brown and O'Keef (1928). A later review of this case, has shown it to be identical to the Burkitt tumour — the patient had a lymphoma-like tumour in the four maxillary quadrants, in both breasts and ovaries.

V. Pattern of Ovary Involvement

As to metastasis, the ovary may be reached via the following paths:

A. Lymphatic vessels;

B. Blood vessels;

C. Transperitoneal and transtubal implantation.

A. Lymphatic Vessels. Lymphatic permeation and mainly the retrograde embolism are considered possible pathways

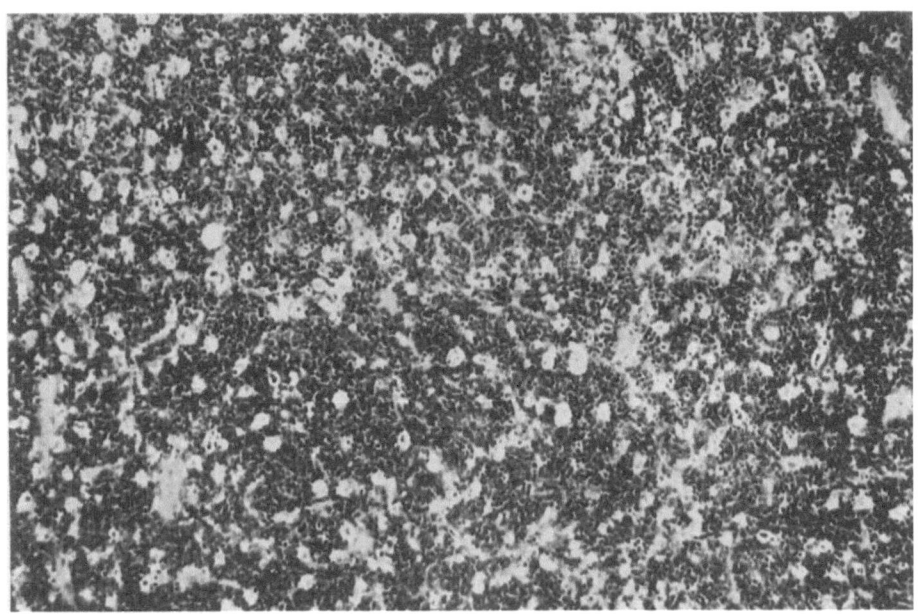

Fig. 2. The same case showing lymphoid anaplastic cells intermixed with numerous reticular cells. This aspect is considered characteristic of the "African Lymphoma" by some authors. H.E.

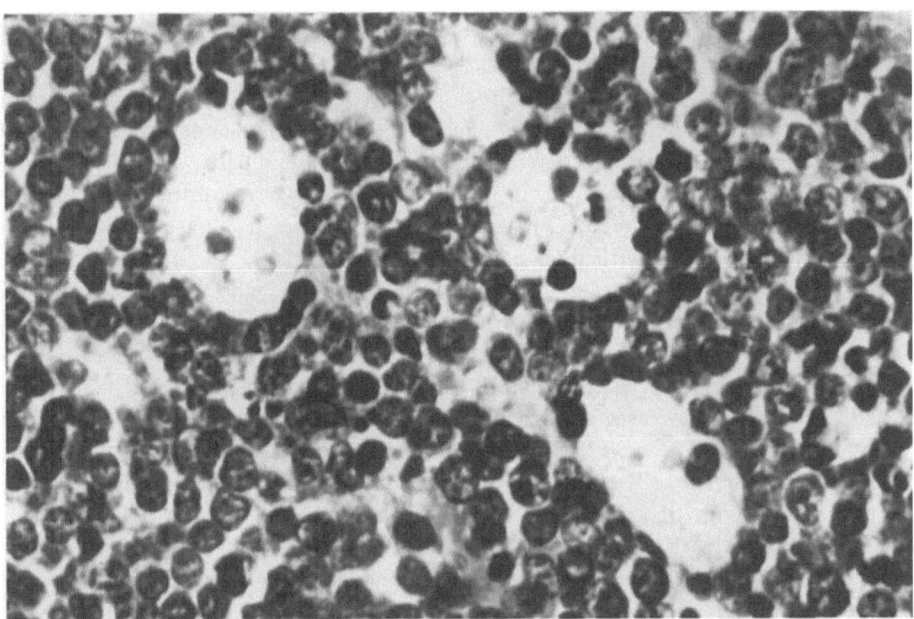

Fig. 3. Same case, showing the reticular cells with macrophagic activity. H.E.

of spread. By the last process, in cases of blockage of lymphatic vessels responsible for the ovary drainage — namely the latero-aortocava and right inter-aortocava, and the latero- and preaortica lymph-nodes to the left (ROUVIERE) — a reflux of the lymphatic flow towards the ovary would take place. VIRIEUX (1963) criticizes the reasoning behind this attempt to explain this reflux; according to him, the reflux would be prevented by the existance of valves in the lymphatic vessels. However, VIRIEUX (1963) recalls that the direction of the flow is immaterial, since the lymphatic vessels are ducts offering a minimal intrinsic resistence.

In cases of Krukenberg tumours, some authors have demonstrated a striking and generalized endolymphatic carcinosis. Thus FANFANI (1950) accepts, in gastric tumours, the invasion of the lymphatic submucous network spreading up to the perigastric, nodes, the mediastinum and tracheobronchial nodes being reached via transdiaphrammatic lymphatics. The dissemination towards the small pelvis would lead to the involvement of the pre- and para-aortic nodes, and henceforth the ovaries would be involved.

If the lymphatic path is accepted in objective cases, the existence of neoplastic emboli in the lymphatic vessels of the ovaries has to be verified, as well as the integrity of the ovarian surface which must be maintained apart from the metastasis by normal tissue. VIRIEUX (1963) pointed to this path as responsible for 8.7 per cent of the cases studied by him.

B. Hematogenic Route. The presence of neoplastic emboli in blood vessels, the widespread dissemination by the hematogenic houte to different organs and the integrity of the ovarian cortex, sum up arguments supporting spread by this path.

VIRIEUX (1963) stated such a dissemination in 26.5 per cent of his cases.

C. Surface Cellular Implantation. The presence of extrinsically originated small cellular lumps must be corroborated. That superficial cellular implantation can occur through the peritoneal via, is well accepted by some authors. VIRIEUX (1963), for instance, accepts this mode of spread in 64.8 per cent of his cases and WILLIS (1953) is another author who regards this means as highly important.

In cases of mammary carcinoma, the following explanation is put forth by HANDLEY (cited by VIRIEUX, 1963): lymphatic cells spread through the superficial *fascia* up to the *linea alba*, beneath the xiphoid appendix, to invade the connective and reaching the subserous fat; from there such cells reach the peritoneum, affecting abdominal or pelvic organs.

In intra-abdominal tumours the emergence of neoplastic cells to the external surface of the organ affected, before spreading as far as the ovary via the peritoneum, is necessary.

WARREN and MACOMBER (1935) noted superficial ovarian implantation in 3 cases of mammary carcinomas, which have also shown evidence of transmission by the lymphatic path; 3 of their reported cases of gastrointestinal carcinomas produced ovarian metastasis by implantation.

KASILAG Jr. and RUTLEDGE (1957), in 23 positive cases of ovarian metastases from breast carcinoma, observed implantation in 7 cases, in which other serous implants were noted as well. In the remaining cases, these authors report the following: arterial emboli in 5, lymphatic emboli in 4 and diffuse propagation in 4.

The seeding of tumour cells over the ovarian surface can take place in cases of uterine or Fallopian tube carcinoma, via the ductal lumen. Opinions differ in the literature about this mode of spread. NOVAK (1927), who has studied the problem, considers it of little importance, putting stress essentially on the lymphatic embolism.

From a practical point of view, it is very difficult to establish clearly the precise route by which the ovarian invasion by the neoplastic cells is brought about; the bulky tumours, due to the extension of the lesions, afford little information on the subject. The smaller tumours, the microscopic ones in particular, represent the most adequate substrate for proper study and even in these, with rare exceptions, it is quite difficult to point at one definite mechanism to the exclusion of others.

We have found the occurrence of tumour lymphatic embolism in 21 cases, exhibiting different patterns, moderate or intense, but in 18 the presence of nodules and a variable degree of ovary infiltration were also well marked.

In some cases the nodules were separated from the surface by a normal cortical layer, which could not be detected in other instances. In 2 such cases, we also noticed the presence of neoplastic plugs in the blood vessels.

Neoplastic embolism only was established by us in 3 cases, one of which is described as follows:

A 32-year-old patient was operated upon for a mammary carcinoma, and three years later had a recurrence of the process. A tumourous nodule was detected in the axilla. Bilateral oophorectomy was performed and the patient died five months later at home. In the right ovary, measuring $3.5 \times 2.5 \times 0.5$ cms, nothing was observed grossly. Histological sections disclosed only the presence of carcinomatous plugs in the lymphatic vessels, with no other alterations.

In approximately four cases, which had mammary carcinoma, morphological evidence of direct implantations with the simultaneous presence of discrete nodules was found; in one of the cases a lymphatic embolism suggested also a secondary involvement following external penetration. Figs. 4, 5 and 6 are demonstrative of carcinomatous superficial ovarian implantation.

In all the remaining instances, it was impossible to establish and explain on morphological grounds, the path responsible for the metastatic progress.

VI. Morphological Aspects. The Problem of the so-called Krukenberg Tumour

The aspect of ovaries affected by metastases is evidently very variable, depending upon a series of factors. It is important to stress that, in most of the cases, the gross examination affords no information, thus emphasizing the importance of a systematic histological study.

Of the 135 instances of ovarian metastases considered in the present paper, 30 showed largely normal ovaries. Bulky tumours, often bilateral, measuring up to $29 \times 12 \times 8$ cms, were observed in about 25 cases. In the remaining cases, the ovaries presented small or moderate volume increase, homogeneous or not, attaining up to 7 cm in its larger diameter; in such instances, tumour nodules of reduced size — quite evident at sectioning — or a combination of nodules and irregular areas, generally moderately firm or whitish, were observed.

In the large tumours we observed some firm, solid bodies and others with myxomatous degeneration in various degrees, as well as cystic and solid forms with regressive hemorrhagic alterations.

In the material supplied us by the Surgical Pathology Laboratory, 10 cases had the characteristics described by Krukenberg. Six originated from the stomach and the remainder from the sigmoid colon, rectum and breast, the primary tumour in the latter instance measured only 3 cm in diameter. In all these cases, the tumours were bulky, bilateral, and clinically evident. The external surface was smooth or bulging with infection and of homogeneous and steady con-

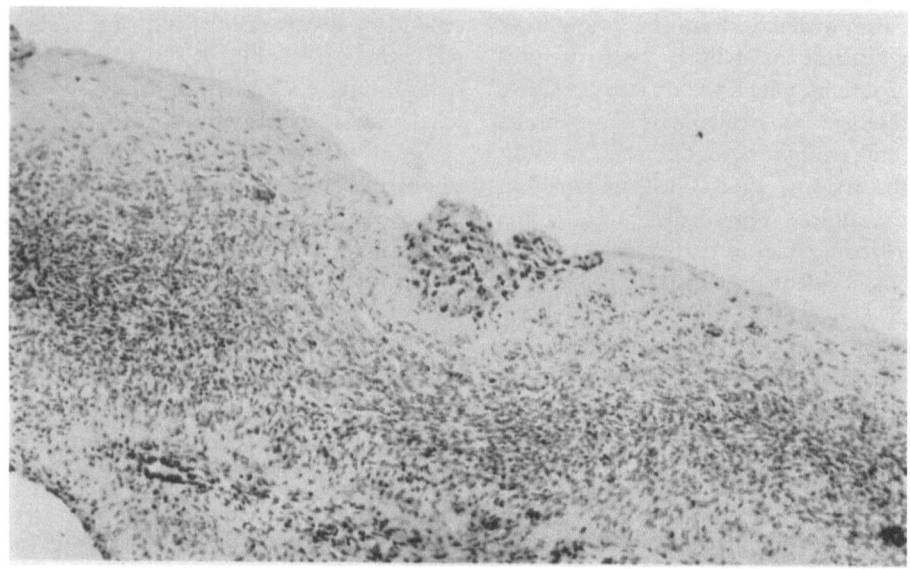

Fig. 4. Superficial ovarian implantation of carcinomatous cells originating in a Mammary Carcinoma. The oophorectomy was made one year after the radical Mammary operation. H.E.

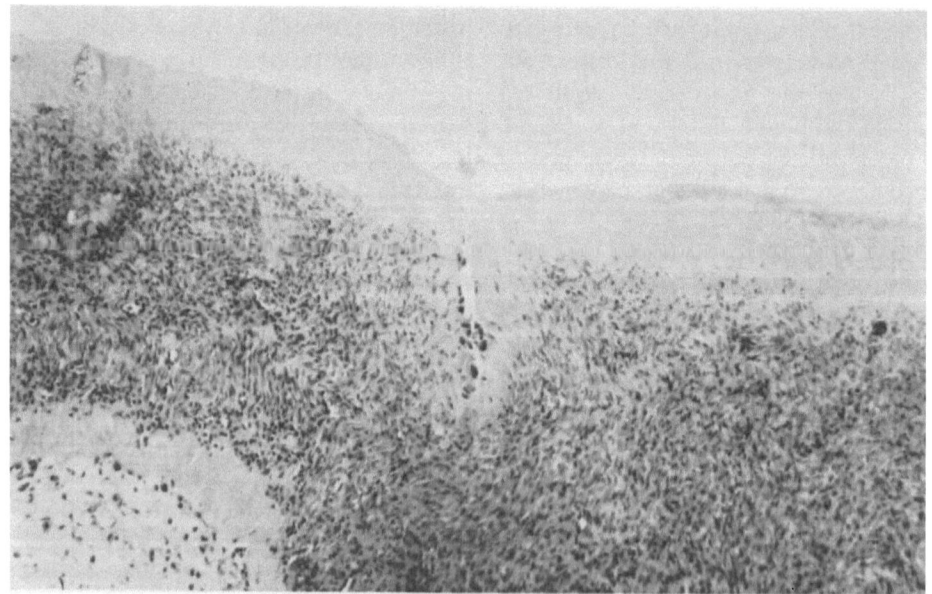

Fig. 5. Same case, showing discret carcinomatous cells in the ovarian surface. H.E.

sistence, with the exception of one of the cases of a Krukenberg-type in which the ovaries in their largest length attained only 5.5 × 4 × 3 cms, with discrete nodules. In the remainder, the involvement was diffuse. The largest sized ovary measured 18 × 10 × 8.5 cms; the other one was comparatively smaller. The of the Krukenberg type were observed.

One of the interesting cases in our series is the following:

The patient, 44 years of age, presenting a gelatinous mammary carcinoma had the ovaries removed, the right one measuring 3 × 3 × 1,5 cms, the left one 5 × 3 × 2.5 cms; both showed an elastic

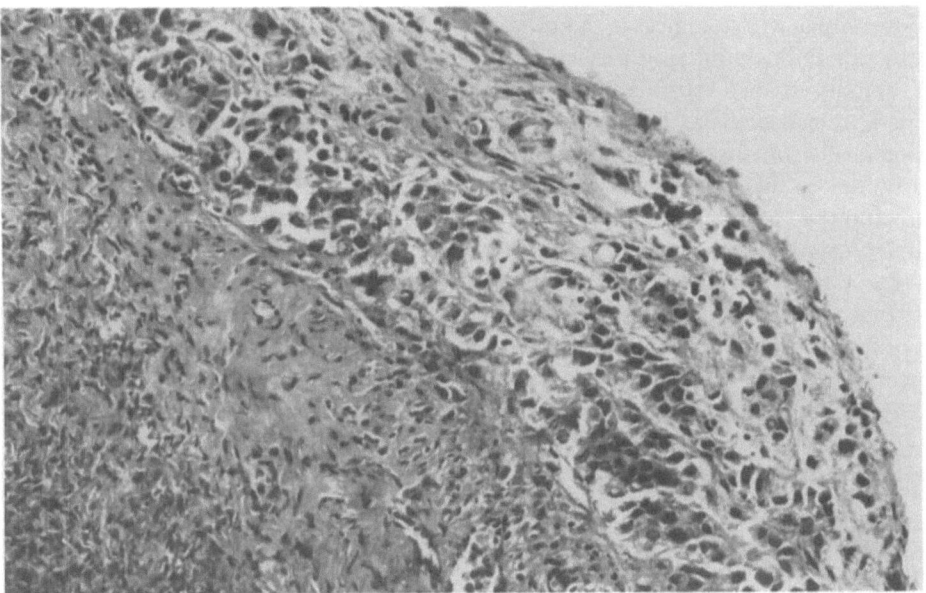

Fig. 6. Detailed aspect of the superficial carcinomatous implantation. H.E. (Same case)

average age of the patients was around 37.7 years.

The existence of a primary gelatinous tumour is not essential to the subsequent development of Krukenberg-like metastases; on the contrary, these can be found in the absence of mucus-secreting activity in the primary tumour. Of the 7 cases of gastric adenocarcinomas necropsied by us, 6 had given to ovarian metastases, 5 of which were bilateral, but were not of the Krukenberg type. In the case of metastatic carcinoma originating from the intestine, the metastases were not of that kind either. Forms that could possibly be considered evolutionary stages

consistency. The microscopic examination disclosed intense embolism in the lymphatic vessels, veins and arteries, with mucous-secreting epithelial cells, including some signet-ring cells; the ovarian stroma showed a discrete involvement, with similar cells present. Such features would probably evolve, in due time, to the classic type described by KRUKENBERG, since the proliferative reaction of the stroma was the only element missing.

In view of the disagreement in literature as to what concerns the actual concept of Krukenberg tumour, it is impossible to establish a comparison within a series of correlated and pertinent observations. In the original description by KRUKENBERG, the following aspects were emphasized: These were bilateral tumour growths of slow development, with the ovaries morphologically more or less torus-molded. The transverse-section was generally consistent and dense, especially in its outer surface, alternating with firm, or myxomatous areas towards the deeper inner portion of the organ. Histologically, KRUKEN-BERG describes the intense proliferation of spindle shaped stromal cells and round, tumefied cells, frequently with some mucin contents. Although impressed by the epithelial aspect of this neo-formation — as the mucocellular and carcinomatous designations demonstrate — the author, nevertheless, interpreted the cases studied as an uncommon kind of primary fibrosarcoma with mucin producing areas.

In the literature, the following viewpoints as to what constitutes a Krukenberg tumour, can be found:

a) metastatic tumours of any nature;

b) metastatic tumours originating from the gastrointestinal tract;

c) metastatic tumours with mucin-producing cells;

d) primary tumours of KRUKENBERG.

MASSON (1956) states that this designation is universally accepted as describing the ovarian metastases of digestive origin, describing among the microscopical characteristics even the existence of tubuli and acini.

Furthermore, the eminent French pathologist stresses another special feature of the metastases: the presence of argentaffin cells, even when the primary neoplasm does not show them.

The artificiality of all these conceptions is self-evident, even if we consider the limitation of the eponym to those cases where mucus secreting cells are present in association with an outstand-ing proliferation of the ovarian stoma, as we did in our 10 observations. When bulky tumours — partially studied in the histological features — are considered, the possibility of glandular structures settled in other areas cannot be excluded. This is even more of a possibility when transitional forms are present; these vary from the metastatic adenocarcinomas producing mucus to instances of complete loss of glandular structure. As NOVAK (1962) puts it: It would be solely the final result of a mucoid adenocarcinoma that, in the ovary, is considered characteristic of the Krukenberg tumour.

As to the primary Krukenberg tumours, only a few cases with necroscopic and histopathological studies for which the existence of a possible primary site could not be ascertained are found in the literature.

In a recent investigation, WOODRUFF and NOVAK (1960) said that of their 48 cases of Krukenberg tumours, about 10 seem to be of a primary nature; these authors also reported one case of unilateral tumour with a 10-year survival.

Primary tumours are not considered here in relation to the originally established pattern of fibrosarcoma mucocellulare carcinomatodes, but as primary mucus-secreting adenocarcinomas of the ovary which can, eventually, take over the characteristics already discussed.

Summary

In the present review 90 autopsies of cancer patients and 560 surgical specimens, removed either because of breast cancer or because of tumours which were later identified as metastatic, were analyzed.

The following results were obtained:

1. The frequency of ovarian metastasis was 30 per cent in the autopsy series and 19.9 per cent in the surgical specimens with maximum incidence rates

of 38 and 26.2 per cent in the group aged between 31 to 40 years.

2. In all the cases with ovarian metastases submitted to necropsy, metastases were also found in other locations.

3. The main primary sites were in the mammary gland, and the digestive, reproductive, and reticuloendothelial systems.

4. The pathways of spread were by the lymphatic vessels, the blood vessels and by direct implantation. In 21 cases a marked lymphatic embolism was observed, and in 18, nodules and a variable degree of ovarian infiltration were also present. Three other cases were considered highly interesting because lymphatic tumour embolism only was detected without other alterations. Direct implantation was ascertained in 4 cases, where the surface penetration and subsequent ovarian infiltration were found, the lymphatics being only secondarily involved. In the majority of the cases, however, it was almost impossible to state that the process spread by any one path.

5. The so-called Krukenberg tumours — characterized by a striking proliferation of the stroma and the presence of mucus secreting cells, signet ring-like and of different sources — was observed in 10 cases, 6 of which had the primary focus of the disease in the stomach.

The artificiality of the conception on the Krukenberg tumours was discussed and the discarding of the eponymic term was suggested.

Discussion

TEILUM remarked that LUISI's paper and two similar ones, by VILLIER and by KASILAG and RUTLEDGE, indicated that the incidence of metastases to the ovary apparently is higher than generally believed. The 30 to 37 per cent reported by LUISI is similar to the incidence reported by KASILAG and RUTLEDGE. LUISI's studies also show that the lymphatic spread is more common than was generally believed in spite of the difficulties of determining how the disease metastasized. Another point of interest is the association with proliferation of functioning cells in some cases. This has been reported by other investigators, but the reason is not known. In LUISI's series, as reported also by KASILAG and RUTLEDGE, no evidence of ovarian dysfunction was noted in premenopausal patients. The course of stromal proliferation in the typical Krukenberg tumour is difficult to explain. It is known that some of the primary gastric cancers are often associated with fibrous proliferation of the stroma and possibly the stimulus is from the tumour cells themselves. There is generally agreement that the usual site of the primary neoplasm is in the stomach or in the intestine, with the breast and the reticuloendothelial system next in that order.

Although the concept of the "Krukenberg" tumour is not valid for considering the histologic metastatic changes in the ovary, the term was useful for clinicopathological reasons, and he thought it should be retained.

SCULLY commented that the question of practical interest was how often the tumour was metastatic when the preoperative diagnosis was probable ovarian tumour. His own estimate was similar to that of KOTTMEIER's, about four per cent. He thought that the eponymic designation had glamorized the tumour so that when one thought of a metastatic tumour, one thought of a tumour that had metastasized from a mucous carcinoma of the stomach. In his own experience, he said, cancer metastatic from the large intestine was more common than cancer that had metastasized from the stomach. He did not think that those tumours which metastasized from the large intestine should be called "Krukenberg tumours" because they had different clinicopathologic connotations. Tumours with the microscopic appearance that KRUKENBERG described have a characteristic gross appearance. They are almost always solid, show degenerative changes but usually not cyst formation, and are often bilateral. The adenocarcinomas that metastasize from the large intestine are less often bilateral and usually are extensively necrotic, hemorrhagic, and show cystic degeneration so that at operation they are easily confused with papillary cystadenocarcinomas, primary in the ovary.

In his own series, metastases were relatively more frequent in premenopausal women than in postmenopausal women, when the lesser frequency of primary cancer in the stomach and intestine in these women is considered. This may mean only that the ovary is more vascular in this age group or it may be because these women are ovulating and opening up little holes in the surface of the ovary in which the tumour cells can implant.

As for treatment, SCULLY said, he believed that menopausal or postmenopausal patients who have cancer of the large intestine and probably those who have gastric cancer should have both ovaries removed at operation because some will return later with ovarian masses.

R. GRAHAM said that at her institution, every patient who died came to autopsy and ten per cent of the cases

which were classified clinically and histologically as primary ovarian carcinoma were shown to be metastatic at postmortem. In no instance had the primary site been the stomach; in two cases, the primary site was the pancreas, and the remainder were in the large intestine.

DAVIDSOHN inquired if LUISI had seen any examples of involvement of the ovary in leukemia. He had personally known one patient, an old lady, who died of causes unrelated to either ovarian disease or leukemia. At autopsy, an enlarged ovary was found to be the site of a chronic granulocytic leukemic lesion; only at autopsy were there found to be changes in the bone marrow suggesting chronic granulocytic leukemia. She had never received any irradiation. This was interesting, he said, because although chronic lymphocytic leukemia is known to have a mild course in elderly people, chronic granulocytic leukemia does not behave in that way.

KOTTMEIER asked the question of what should be done if an ovarian tumour is removed and at examination is diagnosed as metastatic ovarian cancer. Should a second operation be performed if the patient had a primary lesion in the stomach or the intestine? Patients have been reported for whom the primary lesions had been removed with subsequent cure. In his own experience, he said, he had seen patients for whom both ovaries had been removed and for whom no other metastatic site was detected at the time of operation.

KOTTMEIER also said that in the Radiumhemmet series several postmenopausal patients, who were treated with heavy doses of estrogen for extensive carcinoma of the breast, developed an ovarian tumour one to three years after treatment for the breast carcinoma. In several instances, the ovarian tumour was removed, but the pathologist could not tell whether the tumours were primary ovarian lesions or metastases from the breast carcinoma.

GENTIL commented that it was routine in his institution to perform oophorectomy for a female patient who had any type of intestinal resection, but he and his colleagues had been hesitant to follow this routine when the lesion was in the stomach because of the lower incidence of metastases. Another point of interest, he said, was that lesions of the large intestine arising below the peritoneal reflexion seldom metastasize to the ovaries. This point indicates that the most likely route of this particular type of metastasis is the lymphatic one.

GENTIL cited experience with a patient who, at the age of 54 years, had undergone surgical treatment for a large gastric cancer. She had not returned for examination for eleven years, and when she did, she had vaginal bleeding, weight loss, and an extensive cystic mass in the abdomen. Although she was not in good general condition, a laparotomy was performed and a solitary metastatic tumour of the left ovary was removed. LUISI, who saw the specimen but did not know the clinical history of the patient, made a diagnosis of metastatic Krukenberg tumour. This was an example of an estrogen producing metastatic tumour of the stomach with a long evolution and supported the contention that females undergoing surgical intervention for cancer of the stomach or colon should also have bilateral oophorectomy.

As to KOTTMEIER's question about the patient with a pelvic mass which was diagnosed as metastatic tumour, he recommended a carefuly inventory before any surgical procedure is performed. In many instances, a second operation can be avoided. He cited as examples two cases in which ovarian tumours, believed to be primary, were removed and found to be metastatic. He performed a second operation in both instances despite negative radiological studies of the stomach and large intestine. In both instances, he found a tumour in the right colon.

GRICOUROFF agreed with the difficulties of the morphological diagnosis of primary and metastatic tumours, mainly in the endometrioid ovarian tumours. The co-existence of ovarian and uterine cancer is not exceptional, he said, but they are seldom simultaneously arising tumours, except possibly when the ovarian tumour is a granulosa cell tumour. It is always difficult, however, to tell which is the primary site, although usually it is the uterus. The propagation of an ovarian cancer to the uterus by the lymphatic route, with secondary serous myometrial or endometrial sites, is not rare. The endometrial lesion can resemble a superficial deposit, which naturally suggests a type of direct implantation from the tube, but the presence of neoplastic particles in the lymph vessels favors the vascular route. In the endometrioid tumour, the second ovary is involved in over one half of the cases. The explanation is in the transit from one ovary to another through the lymphatic drainage. Even when the second ovary appears to be intact, microscopic examination will often show cancer cells present in the lymphatic vessels of the hilus.

References

ABRAMS, H. L., SPIRO, R., and GOLDSTEIN, N., Metastases in carcinoma; analysis of 1.000 autopsied cases. *Cancer (Philad.)* **3**, 74—85 (1950).

AHUMADA, J. C., and COLAB., *El cancer ginecológico*, tomo II. Buenos Aires: Librería El Ateneo 1953.

Brown, J. B., and O'Keef, C. D., Sarcoma of the ovary with unusual oral metastases. *Ann. Surg.* **87**, 467—471 (1928).

Dorfman, R. F., Childhood lymphosarcoma in St. Louis, Missouri, clinically and histologically resembling Burkitt's tumor. *Cancer (Philad.)* **18**, 418—430 (1965).

Fanfani, M., La carcinosi endolinfatica toraco-abdominale e il suo contributo al significato della "sindrome di Krukenberg". *Arch. De Vecchi Anat. pat.* **15**, 1279—1294 (1950).

Finn, W. F., Diagnostic confusion of ovarian metastases from endometrial carcinoma with primary ovarian cancer. *Amer. J. Obstet. Gynec.* **62**, 403—408 (1951).

Gallager, H. S., Differential diagnosis of primary and metastatic ovarian cancer. In: *Carcinoma of the uterine cervix, endometrium and ovary*, p. 299—303. Chicago: Year Book Med. Publ. Inc. 1962.

Gauthier-Villars, P., Étude des métastases ovariennes des epitheliomas digestifs. *Ann. Anat. path.* **5**, 1 (1928).

Handley, Cit. by C. Virieux, p. 476.

Johansson, H., Clinical aspects of metastatic ovarian cancer of extragenital origin. *Acta obstet. gynec. scand.* **39**, 681—697 (1960).

Karsh, J., Secondary malignant disease of the ovary. Study of 72 autopsies. *Amer. J. Obstet. Gynec.* **61**, 154—160 (1951).

Kasilag jr., F. B., and Rutledge, F. N., Metastatic breast carcinoma in ovary. *Amer. J. Obstet. Gynec.* **74**, 989—992 (1957).

Kitain: Cit. by J. C. Ahumada, p. 261.

Ley: Cit. by R. A. Willis, The spread of tumour in the human body, p. 220.

Luisi, A., Bertelli, A. P., Machado, J. C., and Freitas, J. P. A., "Linfoma Africano" em crianças brasileiras. *Rev. bras. Chirurg* **49**, 280—295 (1965).

Lumb, G., and Mackenzie, D. H., The incidence of metastases in adrenal glands and ovaries removed for carcinoma of the breast. *Cancer (Philad.)* **12**, 521—526 (1959).

Masson, P., *Tumeurs humaines,* 2e. ed., p. 754—755. Paris: Librarie Maloine, S. A. 1956.

Miller: Cit. by J. C. Ahumada, p. 261.

Novak, E., Ovarian metastases with cancer of uterine body; is transtubal implantation an important factor? *Amer. J. Obstet. Gynec.* **14**, 470—486 (1927).

Novak, E. R., and Woodruff, J. D., *Novak's gynecologic and obstetric pathology.* Philadelphia and London: W. B. Saunders Co. 1962.

O'Conor, G. T., Malignant lymphoma in African children, II. A pathological entity. *Cancer (Philad.)* **14**, 270—283 (1961).

— Rappaport, H., and Smith, E. B., Childhood lymphoma resembling Burkitt tumor in the United States. *Cancer (Philad.)* **18**, 411—417 (1965).

Pojarissky: Cit. by J. C. Ahumada et al., p. 253.

Sirtori, C., Pizzetti, F. e Catania, V. C., Studio istologico ed istochimico dei surreni e delle ovaie in pazienti portatrici di carcinoma mamario. *Tumori* **44**, 263—282 (1958).

Virieux, C., Untersuchungen über Häufigkeit und Entstehungsweise von Krebsmetastasen in den Eierstöcken. *Gynaecologia (Basel)* **153**, 209—224 (1962). In: Progresos de obstetricia y ginecologia, vol. VI/3, p. 470—479. Barcelona: Editorial Praxis 1963.

Warren, S., and Macomber, W. B., Tumor metastasis, VI. Ovarian metastasis of carcinoma. *Arch. Path.* **19**, 75—82 (1935).

—, and Witham, E. M., Studies on tumor metastases: Distribution of metastases in cancer of breast. *Surg. Gynec. Obstet.* **57**, 81—85 (1933).

Willis, R. A., The spread of tumors in the human body, 2nd ed. London: Butterworth & Co. Ltd. 1952.

— Pathology of Tumors, 2nd ed. London: Butterworth & Co. Ltd. 1953.

Woodruff, J. D., and Novak, E. R., Krukenberg tumors of the ovary. *Obstet. and Gynec.* **15**, 351—360 (1960).

Ovarian Cancer: Immunological Aspects.
Influence on Prognosis and Treatment*

Israel Davidsohn, M. D.

*Professor and Chairman, Department of Pathology, The Chicago Medical School
Director, Department of Experimental Pathology
Mount Sinai Hospital Medical Center, Chicago, Illinois, U.S.A.*

Stanislav Kovarik, M. D.

*Research Associate, Department of Pathology
The Chicago Medical School and Department of Experimental Pathology
Mount Sinai Hospital Medical Center, Chicago, Illinois, U.S.A.*

Rudolf Stejskal, D. D. S.

*Research Assistant, Department of Experimental Pathology
Mount Sinai Hospital Medical Center, Chicago, Illinois, U.S.A.*

Introduction

The literature on immunological aspects of ovarian cancer is meager, and even more so when it comes to the consideration of the immunological aspects of ovarian neoplasms in relation to prognosis and treatment. Similar limitations of our knowledge regarding immunologic aspects of human cancer apply to most other organs with the possible exception of the colon, thyroid and stomach. These three will be discussed later.

Considerably more is known about cancer in some experimental animals, as would be expected. Transplantation, carcinogenesis and other experimental designs have contributed to this knowledge.

It is in the nature of immunologic phenomena that an antigen-antibody reaction is taken for granted, but in human cancer it has not been established that there is a specific cancer antigen, although such claims have been made. Somewhat better founded is the claim that normal tissues have antigenic properties that are lacking in cancer.

Carcinogens may behave as haptens and initiate an "autoimmune" reaction directed against the tissues of the host. Under such circumstances, absence of normal tissue antigen or antigens gives the cancer cells a selective survival advantage (Goudie, 1963).

There is experimental evidence in support of the hypothesis that cancer cells are deprived of certain antigenic properties. Loss of a tissue-specific antigen has been demonstrated in cells of experimental tumours of hamster kidney and rat liver (Weiler, 1959) and of spontaneous tumours of human skin (Nairn et al., 1960) and gastrointestinal tract (Nairn et al., 1961) by the use of heterologous antibodies.

* This study was supported in part by Public Health Service Grant GM-1109 of the Institute of General Medical Sciences and a grant of the American Cancer Society, Illinois Division.

In the present state of the meager knowledge of immunologic aspects of human ovarian cancer, the best we can do is to gather scattered bits of information that may have at least some bearing on the subject. This will be done in the hope that such seemingly unrelated parts of the jigsaw puzzle of immunology of ovarian cancer may eventually add up to something more meaningful (Davidsohn, 1965).

With these reservations, we may now address ourselves to the question: what are the immunologic aspects of ovarian cancer?

We may get some help by applying the question to other organs.

Established Immunologic Aspects of Human Cancer

A good example of established immunologic aspects of human cancer is found in the thyroid. Autoantibodies against thyroid tissue are frequently present in chronic thyroiditis. They are reacting with thyroid tissue and can be readily detected. It was noted that such autoantibodies were significantly less frequent in cancer of the thyroid. The explanation is based on the assumption that in a situation where autoantibodies are developed in the course of chronic inflammation, non-neoplastic cells would be at a disadvantage and growth and proliferation of neoplastic cells would be favored. This point was demonstrated by the toxicity of thyroid-specific autoantibody present in chronic thyroiditis for normal thyroid cells but not for neoplastic cells (Pulvertaft et al., 1959). If this concept of enhanced survival of neoplastic cells resulting from greater susceptibility of normal cells is correct, then an increased incidence of neoplasia would be expected in so-called autoimmune diseases. This conclusion is supported by an increased incidence of

thyroid carcinoma in chronic thyroiditis (Lindsay et al., 1952; Roitt and Doniach, 1958; Stuart and Allen, 1958; Doniach et al., 1958; Belyavin and Trotter, 1959).

A similar situation exists in cancer of the colon in patients with chronic ulcerative colitis. Here too, autoantibodies against normal colonic epithelium can be demonstrated (Broberger and Perlmann, 1962), and cancer of the colon is much more frequent in patients with ulcerative colitis than it is in persons without this condition (Slaney and Brooke, 1959). Also, the age of onset of cancer is significantly earlier in patients with chronic ulcerative colitis.

Another example is pernicious anemia where autoantibodies reacting with epithelial cells of the gastric mucosa have been demonstrated (Irvine et al., 1962; Taylor et al., 1962). As in the two preceding examples, cancer of the stomach is presumed to be more frequent in patients with pernicious anemia than in those without it (Mosbeck and Videbaek, 1950).

Immunologic Aspects of Benign Cystic Teratoma of Ovary

In general, when one considers immunologic aspects of an organ or of a specific lesion in the organ, one has to demonstrate an antigen-antibody relationship between the organ and/or its lesion and the host as a whole. In such a situation the organ or the lesion may contain an antigen capable of stimulating the production in the host of an antibody reacting with the host's own tissues, or conceivably the host could produce an antibody against the lesion (Davidsohn, 1964).

There are a few examples that are indicative of such relationship in the case of the ovary. One of these examples is hemolytic anemia in patients with dermoid cysts or other teratomas of the ovary.

A sufficiently large number of instances of this type of lesion have been reported to permit certain generalizations. The natural history of this condition is about as follows:

The patients present the usual manifestations of progressive anemia, such as tiredness, shortness of breath on effort, buzzing of the ears, and moderate tachycardia. The anemia ranges from moderate to severe. There is significant increase of reticulocytes, spherocytes, and of osmotic fragility of erythrocytes. The indirect serum bilirubin is elevated. Normoblastemia may be present. Autoantibodies reacting with the patient's erythrocytes may be demonstrated with the direct antiglobulin test (Coombs Test). If the test is negative, more than one batch of antiglobulin serum should be used. The detection of autoantibodies is facilitated if one tests trypsinized erythrocytes in an albumin rich medium (ANDRÉ et al., 1955). Platelets are not decreased in number. The spleen may be palpable, but is only rarely significantly enlarged. Steroids, the drug of choice in the treatment of autoimmune hemolytic anemia, are usually only transiently effective (McANDREW, 1964). Splenectomy does not help.

A substantial number of cases have been reported with this clinical picture, in which an examination or operation revealed the presence of an ovarian cyst and after its removal the hemolytic anemia was cured (BARRY and CROSBY, 1957). One of the earliest was reported in 1938 (WEST-WATSON and YOUNG, 1938). In most instances the ovarian lesion was a dermoid cyst, less frequently a malignant teratoma and occasionally a carcinoma. One of the reported cases was a pseudomucinous cystadenocarcinoma (JONES and TILLMANN, 1945). Of inter-

est in this connection is the opinion that a pseudomucinous cystadenoma may be the result of a one-sided development of a teratoma.

The cause-and-effect relationship between the teratoma and the anemia was demonstrated after the teratomectomy was followed by the cessation of hemolysis as manifested by reticulocytosis, spherocytosis and bilirubinemia, and by the reduction and later complete and permanent disappearance of the anemia.

There are several possible explanations of the pathogenesis of the anemia:

1. A substance generated in the cyst and secreted into the circulation coats the erythrocytes and is responsible for their hemolysis. This substance may be an autoantibody, or it may be an abnormal protein lacking the characteristics of a true antibody.

2. The cyst may contain an antigen which stimulates the antibody producing cells in the host to elaborate an autoantibody. This hypothesis is especially attractive.

The validity of these hypothetical explanations remains to be established. Association of hemolytic anemia with dermoid cysts is rare, but consideration of such a possibility may reveal more cases that are less obvious. This is a distinct possibility since about 11 per cent of all ovarian tumours are teratomas.

Based on these observations, pelvic examination for the possible presence of an ovarian cyst is indicated before one resorts to splenectomy in cases of hemolytic anemia that do not respond to steroids, and even in cases with a slight or moderate splenomegaly. Interestingly, there have been reports of removal in a patient with hemolytic anemia of a simple cyst not followed by cure and, conversely, of removal of a dermoid cyst from the mediastinum with consequent cure. X-ray examination of the pelvis may reveal the presence of a dermoid cyst by demonstrating teeth or bone or even large masses of hair.

In the cases reported, the ages of most of the patients were between 30 and 50, though occasionally patients were in the first decade of life and the age range extended to the eighth decade.

Other Suggestive Immunologic Implications of Ovarian Neoplasms

Dales reported subsidence of purpura following removal of a pseudomucinous cystadenoma in a 51-year-old woman with a 10-year history of a bleeding tendency, a normal platelet count and no other detectable abnormalities of blood coagulation (Dales, 1965).

In a recent carefully controlled study of 97 cases of ovarian malignant neoplasms compared with a similar number of benign growths, a history of mumps parotitis seemed to decrease the incidence of malignancy (West, 1966). This observation can be interpreted to imply that mumps in childhood may have a protective value against development of an ovarian malignancy in later years or that resistance against mumps decreases resistance to development of ovarian malignancy.

The lower incidence of cancer of the ovary in Japan and in Japanese in the U.S. (Segi *et al.*, 1957; Smith, 1956) is more likely to have a hormonal basis. These findings are possibly related to the lower incidence of cancer of the breast in Japanese women.

A Hypothetical Immune Reaction in Man Against Dysgerminomas, Seminomas, Pinealomas, and So-Called "Germinal Tumours" of the Mediastinum

A hypothesis of a common immunologic reaction by the host against seminomas, dysgerminomas, pinealomas (atypical teratoma of the pineal) and the so-called "germinal tumours of the mediastinum" (Oberman and Libcke, 1964) was suggested (Marshall and Dayan, 1964). This hypothesis was based on similar histologic appearances, frequently granulomatous infiltrates and certain similarities in clinical behavior (Friedman, 1951).

Clinical and histopathologic similarities of the four neoplasms have been reported. The former include: age incidence and sex dependence, with more frequent occurrence in males (except for dysgerminomas). The latter neoplasm is characterized by the appearance of the neoplastic cells, infiltration with lymphocytes and plasma cells and association with teratomas. The basis for the immunologic implication is provided by the cellular reaction in the stroma.

Histology. The predominant cell is large, round, with a narrow clear or eosinophilic cytoplasm, and dark nuclei with one or more nucleoli. In biopsies, mitoses are abundant. Focal necrosis can be seen, though rarely. Accumulations of tumour cells are separated by bands of connective tissue carrying blood vessels, and infiltrated with large numbers of lymphocytes, plasma cells and some eosinophils (Figs. 1—6). Also present are epithelioid cell granulomas, multinucleated giant cells, occasionally with included asteroids and Schaumann's bodies, and lymph follicles with germinal centers. There are quantitative and qualitative variations in these infiltrations. Some of the cellular and reactive infiltrates are so dense that they may even mask the neoplastic cells. The abundance and extent of the inflammatory reaction may obscure the neoplastic character of the lesion. The reactive inflammatory changes are not related to the areas of focal necrosis. In pinealomas perivascular infiltrates may be the only finding without neoplastic cells.

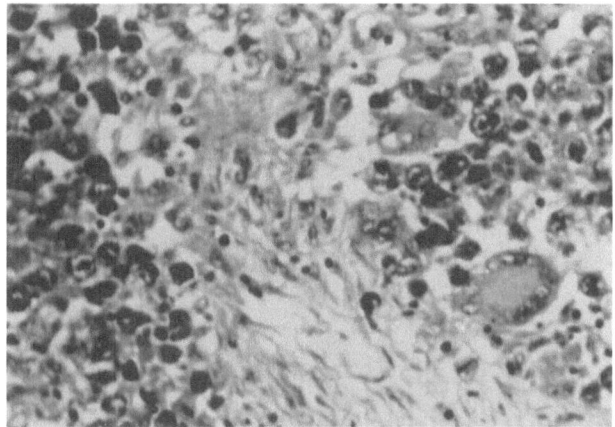

Fig. 1. Dysgerminoma. Two islands of tumour cells are separated by a broad band of loose connective tissue which is infiltrated with lymphocytes and plasma cells. A giant cell containing a large number of vesicular peripherally arranged nuclei is seen in the right lower corner (hematoxylin and eosin, ×400)

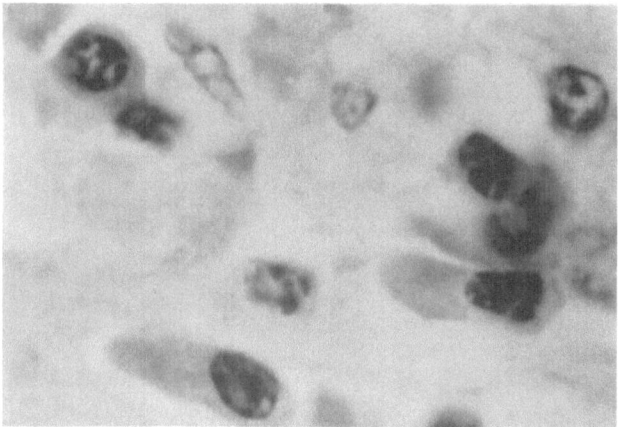

Fig. 2. A segment of Fig. 1 with a group of plasma cells (hematoxylin and eosin, ×2,500)

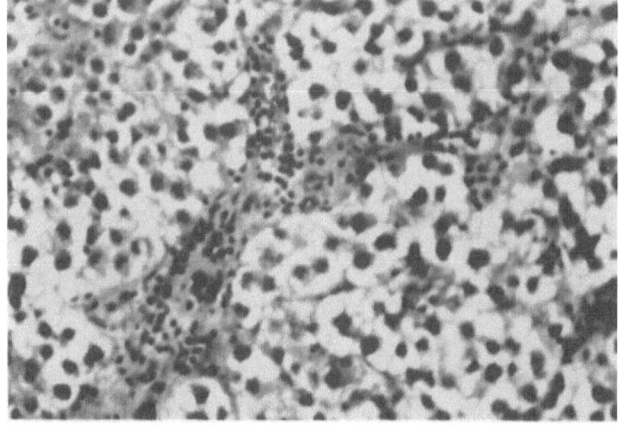

Fig. 3. Seminoma. Connective tissue bands infiltrated with lymphocytes and plasma cells, separate islands of tumour cells very much like in the dysgerminoma (Fig. 1) (hematoxylin and eosin, ×400)

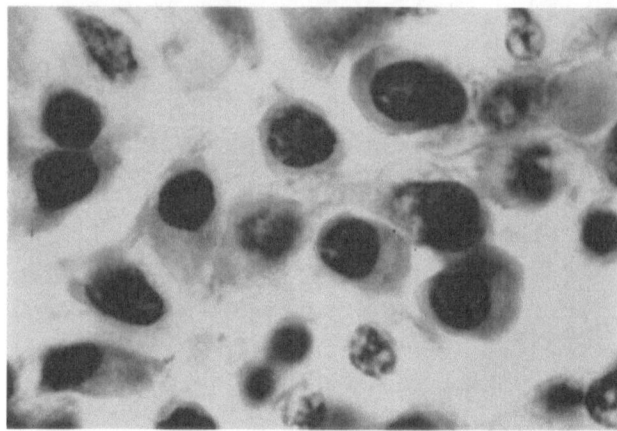

Fig. 4. A detail of Fig. 3 with a group of plasma cells (hematoxylin and eosin, ×2,500)

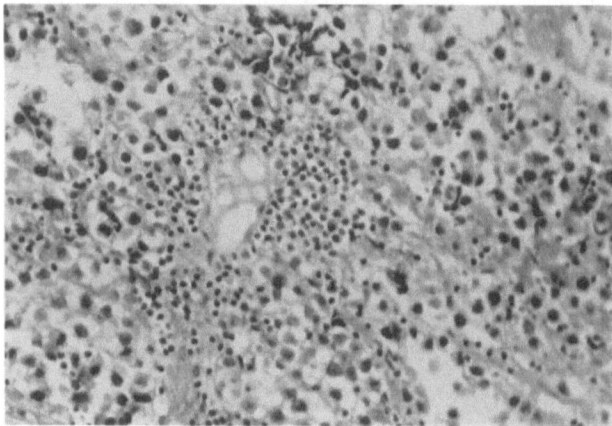

Fig. 5. Pinealoma. Essentially the same general pattern as in Figs. 1 and 3 (hematoxylin and eosin, ×300)

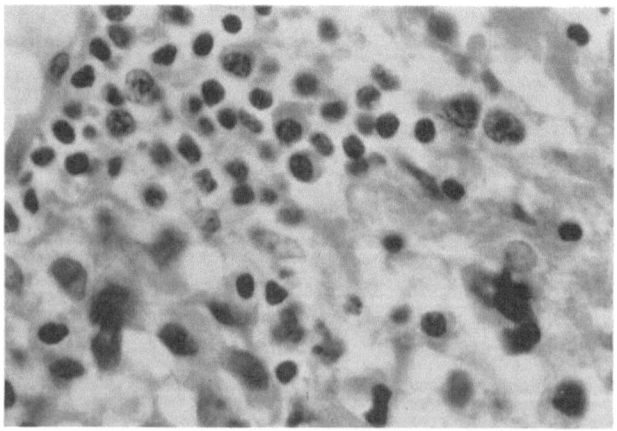

Fig. 6. An enlarged detail of Fig. 5. Here too, plasma cells are conspicuous in an area of lymphocytc infiltration (hematoxylin and eosin, ×1,100)

There are only few reports about the appearance of lymphoid tissue elsewhere, especially in regional lymph nodes and spleen. There are no reports about regional lymph nodes and spleen in dysgerminomas.

The infiltration of the stroma is interpreted as an immune reaction against an antigen or antigens in neoplastic cells. The epithelioid-cell granulomas may be a reaction to lipids of the neoplasms, as reported in response to injections of complete Freund's adjuvant (WHITE and MARSHALL, 1958).

Another possible explanation is a response to breakdown products of the neoplasms. However, there is no relation between quantity and quality of infiltrates and necrosis in the tumour. Occasionally, only isolated neoplastic cells may be present in a sea of the lymphocytic or granulomatous infiltrate. Reports of systematic studies of lipids in the four neoplasms are lacking. Lipids have been studied in seminomas. The reported findings have not been confirmed in a study of three cases of pinealomas (MARSHALL and DAYAN, 1964).

The hypothesis of an immunologic reaction against the tumour presupposes: (1) A special antigen in the neoplasm not present in the host, as was reported in a renal cortical carcinoma (NAIRN et al., 1963). (2) Variations in the antigenic potency of the neoplastic cells and variations in antibody producing ability of host, which would account for the variability of the cytologic composition and of the intensity of the infiltrates. (3) The assumption that the immune reaction is not destructive to the neoplasm, but only growth retarding, which is supported by the lack of correlation between necrosis of tumour cells and the stromal infiltrate. There is no evidence as yet that the inflammatory infiltrates are the result of an antibody response.

It may be that evidence in support of the hypothesis could be furnished with the help of modern sensitive methods of antibody demonstration.

Association of Ovarian Neoplasms with other Diseases

Peutz-Jeghers' syndrome, said to be hereditary, is characterized by the presence of intestinal polyps and intra-oral melanin spots. Ovarian neoplasms have been found in 9 of approximately 180 cases in women, reported till now. In the most recent publication, the ovarian lesion was a papillary cystadenoma. Numerous polyps were present from the mouth to the anus. One of them in the transverse colon was an infiltrating adenocarcinoma. According to the authors the frequency of ovarian tumours, approximately in 5 percent of females with the syndrome, suggests that they are related to the same mutant gene (HUMPHRIES et al., 1966).

The association is mentioned here not because of an evident immunologic implication but because the present lack of knowledge of immunology of ovarian neoplasms makes it necessary to record even single observations for future correlation.

Non-Immunologic Systemic Effects of Ovarian Neoplasms

Some non-immunologic systemic effects are of biochemical nature. Here belongs migratory thrombophlebitis in a patient with thrombophlebitis of arms and legs, not responding to antibiotics. The removal of a papillary cystadenoacanthoma of the right ovary and of a Brenner tumour of the left ovary was followed by complete recovery without any additional therapy (WOMACK and CASTELLANO, 1952).

Blood Group Antigens in the Ovary

Blood group specific substances (BGS), considered to be the same as in the blood, are present in various tissues including the ovaries. In ovarian cyst fluids they may be present in large amounts. The first to demonstrate it was YOSIDA (YOSIDA, 1928). MORGAN demonstrated chemical properties of factors A and Le[a] in ovarian cyst fluid (AMINOFF *et al.*, 1950). Large amounts of one or the other were found in the cyst fluid.

By chemical extraction with saline or ethanol, different amounts of BGS were obtained from different tissues and secretions. Aqueous extracts of saliva contained 12 units[1] of BGS. Whereas no detectable water soluble BGS could be demonstrated in blood, up to 5 units were present in alcoholic extracts.

Large amounts of water soluble BGS are present in mucus producing epithelial cells. Alcohol soluble BGS are present in various tissues but only in small amounts. The formerly available extraction technique did not permit to demonstrate the exact localization of BGS in various tissues. This became possible with two recently introduced techniques: immunofluorescence and mixed cell agglutination. Specific fluorescent antisera permit to detect water soluble A, B, and O (H) BGS in mucus containing epithelial cells and secretions. Alcohol soluble BGS are found in endothelial cells and in many epithelial cells, e.g., in the skin, mouth, esophagus, ureters, urinary bladder, etc. The principle of the mixed cell agglutination reaction (COOMBS *et al.*, 1956) is that bivalent or multivalent antibodies can combine with the antigen on the surface of the cells under investigation and at the same time with the erythrocytes of known antigenic composition. The following procedure is followed in our laboratory: the section is treated with specific antiserum for several minutes,

washed in saline and then covered with the erythrocyte suspension. The erythrocytes settle. The slide is inverted. The erythrocytes containing the same ABO antigen as the cells in the histologic section remain attached, the other cells fall off. With this technique water soluble and alcohol soluble BGS are demonstrated in paraffin sections (KOVARIK *et al.*, 1967). Immunofluorescent conjugated antisera detect only water soluble substances.

The ability of mixed cell agglutination to demonstrate alcohol soluble substances is probably due to higher sensitivity of the technique that is capable of detecting small amounts of alcohol soluble BGS left behind by alcohol extraction during the dehydration of paraffin sections.

We have used both techniques (immunofluorescence and mixed cell agglutination) for detection of BGS A and B in various tissues.

Much has been written on the effect of cancer on the blood group substances in tissues. The consensus has been that these substances are not affected by the cancerous transformation. All these reports dealt with alcohol soluble substances demonstrable with immunofluorescence exclusively in fresh frozen sections. We investigated the effect of malignant transformation on water soluble group substances A and B and we found that, in some cancers, production

---

[1] The amounts of BGS in a tissue are determined with the hemagglutination inhibition test. One unit is the amount of antibody present at the titration endpoint. "If the titer of a serum is 100, and the quantity of antiserum used in the hemagglutination test is 0.1 ml, this volume is said to contain one hemagglutinating unit." (KABAT, E. A., Blood Group Substances. Academic Press, New York, 1956, p. 105.) A 1:10 dilution of such serum would contain 10 units in 0.1 ml, and similarly there are 20 units in 0.1 ml of a 1:5 dilution.

of BGS is reduced or absent. These observations were made first in mucinous adenocarcinomas of the gastrointestinal tract (DAVIDSOHN *et al.*, 1966a) and later in some neoplasms of the ovary (DAVIDSOHN *et al.*, 1967b).

The following results were obtained with the two methods: (1) with immunofluorescence by conjugating appropriately selected anti-A and anti-B sera of human or animal origin with fluorescein isothiocyanate; (2) with the mixed cell agglutination technique.

Our studies on neoplasms of the gastrointestinal tract can be summarized as follows: the presence of water soluble blood group substances A and B was investigated with fluorescence technique in formalin-fixed, paraffin-embedded tissues of the gastrointestinal tract, including the stomach, small intestine, ascending and transverse colon, and proximal portion of the descending colon in 81 adenomatous polyps and adenocarcinomas, and in controls.

In the absence of cancer, the blood group substances were present abundantly in the epithelial cells and in secreted mucus. In cancer, the antigenic substances were absent in the secreted mucus. The failure to secrete the blood group antigens is interpreted as a manifestation of dedifferentiation resulting from the cancerous process (DAVIDSOHN *et al.*, 1966a).

Our studies of neoplasms of the ovary included the following five groups:

1. Normal ovarian tissue.
2. Serous cystadenomas.
3. Serous cystadenocarcinomas.
4. Pseudomucinous cystadenomas.
5. Pseudomucinous cystadenocarcinomas.

In sections from pseudomucinous cystadenomas, abundant BGS were present in the epithelial cells with both techniques (Figs. 7, 8).

In pseudomucinous cystadenocarcinomas the presence of BGS was related to the degree of differentiation of the epithelial cells. In poorly differentiated neoplasms, BGS were demonstrated by immunofluorescence only in the form of extracellular accumulations in small cystic areas. In similar areas the more sensi-

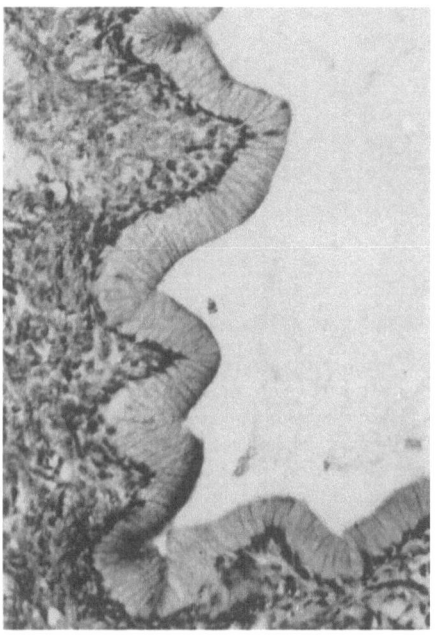

Fig. 7. Ovary. Blood Group A. Pseudomucinous cystadenoma. High columnar epithelial cells are filled with abundant mucus. Some of it is also present in the lumen (hematoxylin and eosin, ×350)

tive mixed cell agglutination revealed small amounts of BGS in extracellular accumulations of secretions and in some irregularly distributed patches of epithelial cells.

With the mixed cell agglutination technique the BGS were found in paraffin sections of normal ovarian tissue only in erythrocytes and in endothelial cells (Figs. 9, 10). Immunofluorescence was entirely negative.

In serous cystadenoma the epithelial cell lining the cysts and the papillary

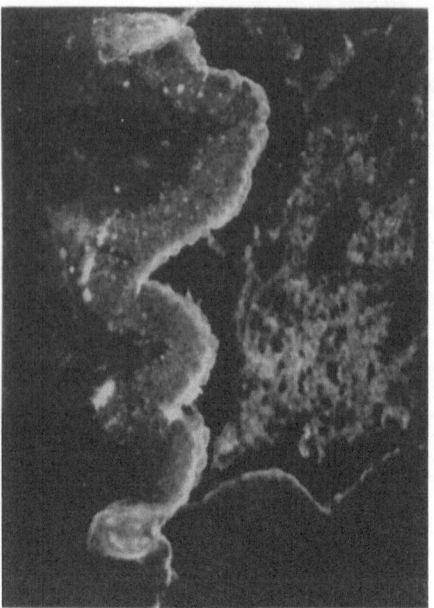

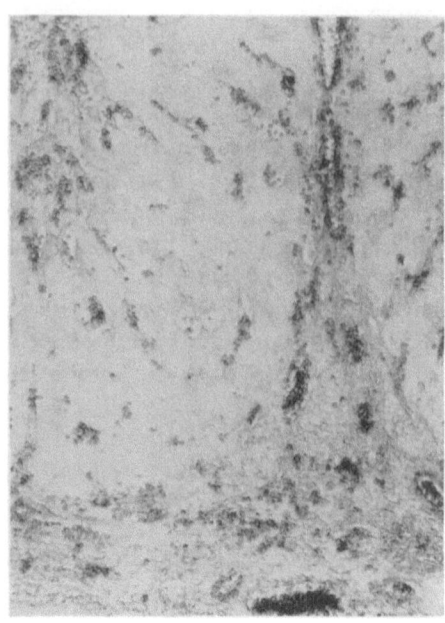

Fig. 8. Same section and same field as Fig. 7. Section was treated with anti-A fluorescent conjugate. The brilliant white material in the cells and in the lumen is group substance A. In the actual stained preparation, the A antigen has a brilliant green color (hematoxylin and eosin, ×350)

Fig. 10. Same section and same field as in Fig. 9. Mixed cell agglutination technique. The presence of blood group A antigen is indicated by the aggregates of red cells. It is demonstrable only in endothelial cells lining vascular spaces and in the erythrocytes left in the lumina (×180)

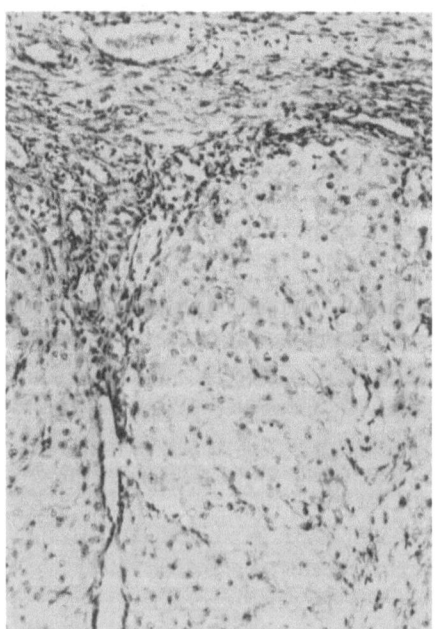

Fig. 9. Ovary. Blood Group A. Corpus luteum and adjacent normal ovarian tissue (hematoxylin and eosin, ×180)

projections reacted positively with both techniques. This finding indicates that water soluble BGS are not limited to mucus.

In serous cystadenocarcinomas the presence of BGS was related to the degree of differentiation of the neoplasm.

In areas where the neoplastic cells were well differentiated, both reactions were positive. In less well differentiated areas and in metastases both were negative (Figs. 11, 12). In highly anaplastic carcinomas, sections taken from various areas were all negative with the immunofluorescence technique. In a few highly anaplastic papillary carcinomas the mixed cell agglutination technique was positive. The significance of this finding is being investigated further.

These results have added to our understanding of the process of dedifferentiation as it occurs in the course of malignant transformation.

Other Aspects of a Possible Relation between Blood Groups and Cancer of the Ovary

HELMBOLD (1961) and more recently OSBORNE and DE GEORGE reported pos-

sible association of blood group A with certain neoplasms of the ovary (OSBORNE and DE GEORGE, 1963). In the latter publication, of a total of 453 malignant and of 260 benign neoplasms of various

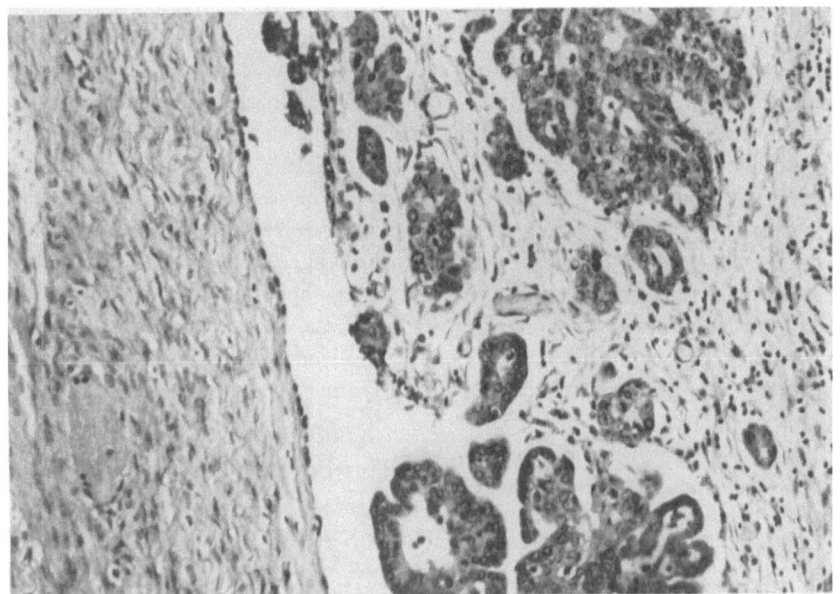

Fig. 11. Ovary. Blood Group A. Poorly differentiated papillary serous cystadenocarcinoma; metastasis in omentum (hematoxylin and eosin, ×250)

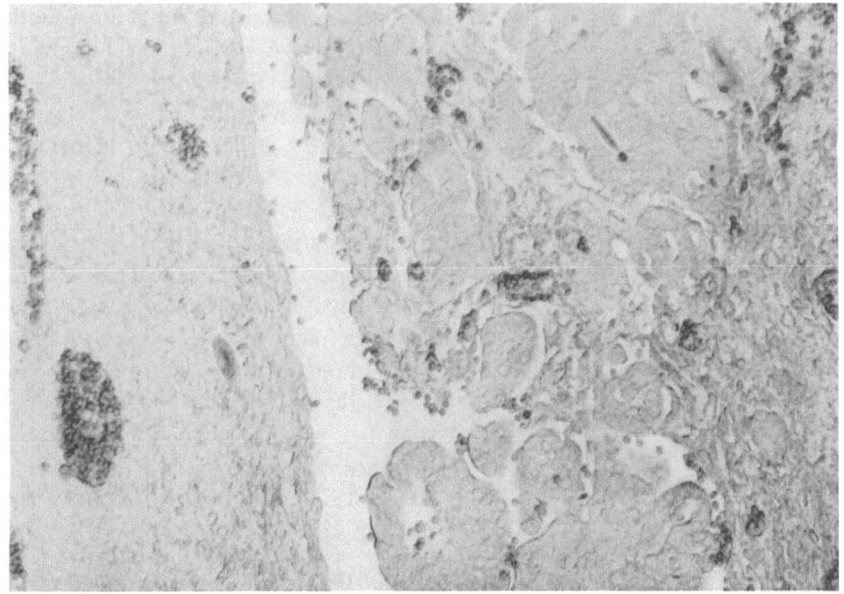

Fig. 12. Same section and area as in Fig. 9. Mixed cell agglutination technique. Blood Group A antigen demonstrated only in the lining endothelial cells and lumina of vascular spaces (×250)

8*

types, the incidence of group A was compared with group O. In both groups the relative incidence of group A was greater than that of group O. In the benign group the difference was more marked than in the malignant. The excess in the benign neoplasms was contributed by only four of the ten categories: pseudomucinous cysts, simple cysts, endometriosis, and dermoid cysts. The increase in the dermoid cyst group was the only one statistically significant. The excess in malignant neoplasms was contributed only by two of the nine categories, both of them statistically significant: papillary adenocarcinoma and metastatic carcinoma. The primary sites were mainly gastrointestinal tract, breast, and cervix.

The ovarian neoplasms which associate with blood group A are of a glandular type of epithelium. They contain an atypical or extra-ovarian type of epithelium. The ovarian neoplasms which do not appear to associate with group A are solid rather than cystic, and if of epithelial origin, the epithelial cells are entirely of ovarian type. The authors conclude that an association of blood group A with a precancerous process may be the responsible factor.

Interesting, though difficult to correlate, is the well-known fact that very large amounts of BGS, even larger than in saliva, are found in the pseudomucinous cystadenomas (FREIESLEBEN et al., 1961).

Immunotherapy of Cancer of the Ovary

Intravenous or intraperitoneal injections of immunocompetent cells given to eight patients with advanced cancer who had previously received cytotoxic drugs were reported to be followed by objective evidence of improvement, though temporary, in most patients. A graft-versus-tumour reaction was claimed to be responsible. The cells were obtained from spleens removed from patients with idiopathic thrombocytopenic purpura, hemolytic anemia, portal hypertension or gastric cancer (WOODRUFF and NOLAN, 1963).

All the patients treated with splenic cells were in advanced stages of cancer; three had ovarian carcinoma with peritoneal dissemination and ascites. In every patient some changes had occurred either in the patient's symptoms, the physical signs, or the findings on serial biopsies. The impression was gained that some of the changes were due to a direct action by the transplanted cells on the tumour. In all three ovarian cancers, the ascites was abolished during periods of observation from two to four months.

Resistance to Cancer of the Ovary

This problem is considered in a report (CUTLER et al., 1960) of a survival analysis of cancer of the ovary between 1935 and 1954.

The outlook for younger women, relative to general population mortality, was better than for older women. The five-year survival rate for women under 35 years of age was 74 per cent. For the age groups 35—44, 45—54, 55—64, 65—74, 75—84, the five-year survival rates were 34, 28, 20, 15 and 15 per cent, respectively.

This is a confirmation of previous studies analyzing survival rates. There is no reason to assume that these differences have an immunologic basis. The data are included merely because differences in resistance to disease require consideration of immunity. In this connection the greater frequency of chronic lymphocytic leukemia and the lower titers of iso-agglutinins anti-A and anti-B in advanced age come to mind.

The Problem of Metastases to the Ovary

A reference to metastases is natural when immunologic aspects of cancer are discussed. What happens when a local cancer begins to metastasize?

There has been no lack of attempts to answer this question, but none prevailed. In recent years there has been increasing interest in the possible role of immunologic mechanisms. In a report of a symposium sponsored by the U.I.C.C. on the topic "The Mechanism of Invasion in Cancer", STRÄULI, the referee, emphasized the increasing importance of immunology in cancer research as reflected in several papers dealing with possible connections between immune processes and formation of metastases (STRÄULI, 1966). The reports included evidence of decreased activity of lymphocytes in advanced cancer, suggesting a loss of immunological defense. Partial immunologic tolerance towards cancer antigens was another hypothesis based on an experimental study of sarcomas induced by carcinogenic hydrocarbons. Several other possible immunologic mechanisms have been suggested at the meeting.

The frequency of metastases of mammary carcinoma to the ovaries has been investigated by various authors. Figures quoted varied, probably depending on the stage of the involvement of the breast. In KASILAG and RUTLEDGE's (1957) series of 91 cases of oophorectomy done for breast carcinoma, metastases were found in 25 per cent. Histologic study revealed multiple mechanisms of metastases. The breast carcinoma entered the ovaries from the surface and through the hilar vessels. Bilateral involvement was common. In previous reports the frequency of mammary carcinoma metastases to the ovary was considerably lower.

Summary

Our knowledge of immunologic aspects of cancer of the ovary is still in its very early stages. Isolated items have been accumulated, and more are being added at a rapidly increasing rate. Some have already matured to find clinical application through a better understanding of ovarian cancer, and a few have become useful in early diagnosis, prognosis and even therapy. This applies mainly to autoimmune hemolytic anemia when it occurs in women having dermoid cysts of the ovary. Other observations pointing to a possible role of immunologic phenomena in ovarian neoplasms have been reported. There is good reason to hope that some of these observations eventually will prove to be equally applicable. Experience has taught us that this is the natural history of scientific progress.

Recently published results of our studies on the effect of cancerous transformation on the production, secretion or storage of A, B blood group substances in epithelial cells of neoplasms of the gastrointestinal tract are reviewed. Also included is a summary of results of our recent similar studies on ovarian neoplasms. These studies are being prepared for publication.

We interpret the impairment of ability to produce, secrete or store the A, B blood group substances to be the result of functional dedifferentiation in cancer, analogous to the better known morphologic dedifferentiation.

Résumé

Nos connaissances des aspects immunologiques du cancer ovarien sont très récentes. Des faits isolés ont été amassés et leur nombre s'accroît constamment. Quelques-uns de ces faits ont déjà trouvé une application clinique par une meilleure compréhension du cancer; certains d'entre eux aident le diagnostique, la prognose et même la thérapeutique. Ceci s'applique surtout à l'anémie hémolitique-autoimmune, quand elle s'associe avec le kyste dermoïde de l'ovaire. D'autres observations récentes nous laissent croire que des phénomènes immunologiques jouent un rôle dans le cancer ovarien. On peut s'attendre à ce que quelques-unes de ces observations puissent avoir également une application pratique. L'expérience nous enseigne que c'est-là le train naturel du progrès scientifique.

Dans un compte-rendu qui vient de paraître et que nous résumons ici, nous avons présenté les résultats de nos études sur l'effet de la transformation cancéreuse sur la production, sécrétion ou accumulation des substances des groupes sanguins A et B dans les cellules épithéliales des tumeurs du système gastro-intestinal. Egalement inclus est un résumé des résultats obtenus au cours d'études pareilles dans le cancer ovarien. Ces résultats seront publiés.

C'est notre avis que la diminution de pouvoir produire, sécréter ou accumuler les substances des groupes sanguins A et B suit la dédifférentiation fonctionnelle dans le cancer, comparable à la dédifférentiation morphologique mieux connue.

Discussion

Brunschwig described investigations which he and Southam had conducted in advanced ovarian cancer patients by injecting into the thigh suspensions of tumour cells in dilutions of from 1,000 to 100,000,000. If there was a "take", an artificial metastasis, a nodule developed and, in about a month, grew to a firm mass which could be measured. These investigators found that as the patients' condition deteriorated, the number of cells required to induce an artificial metastasis diminished. They found also that when cultivated tumour cells obtained from cell lines grown in the laboratory were injected, the speed with which they were rejected was related to the patient's general condition: as the disease progressed, the rejection was delayed. This evidence, he said, could be interpreted as a measurable something that could be called host resistance. Davidsohn inquired as to whether the changes in advanced cancer which were attributed to diminished host resistance could not be explained partly by an alteration in the transplant that was used. Brunschwig replied that, as yet, a method to measure the aggressiveness of cancer had not been developed.

J. Graham described studies with an autogenous vaccine prepared with Freund's adjuvant. Not much success had been achieved, he said, although there was one long-term survivor in a group of four patients with pseudomyxomas. Recently, Graham said, he and his colleagues had been using a vaccine prepared with killed pertussis organisms, and the impression, based on limited experience, was that more benefits were being achieved.

Graham remarked that antibodies to cancer had been demonstrated by several groups of investigators and there was little doubt that antibodies and characteristic antigens of tumours existed. How important these observations are in the control of cancer is not known, however. Of equal importance is the observation of impaired resistance in patients with cancer. If this resistance is examined closely, he said, it will be found that it is the ability to react to a new antigen that is impaired. Apparently, there is no impairment of the ability to react to a previously encountered antigen. It was his impression, said Graham, that at least part of this impairment is a function of production of substances by the tumour that acts on the body.

The response of dysgerminomas to relatively small doses of radiation is significant, because this tumour is heavily infiltrated by lymphocytes and plasma cells, cells of defense mechanism. This response supports the dictum that radiation achieves its benefit by stimulation of the local defense mechanism. In contrast to the paralyzing effect of whole body irradiation on the immune mechanisms, study of the effect of the local irradiation will demonstrate that the immune response in the local area that was irradiated was stimulated. In his own studies, he had injected an antigen into the extremity of an animal, irradiated the area immediately, and observed an increased production of antibodies in the area, as well as an increase in the circulating antibodies in these animals in comparison with control animals.

LUISI inquired as to the significance of the granulomatous reaction observed in dysgerminomas and asked if asteroids and Sherman bodies had been observed in the giant cells in dysgerminomas.

MULLER said that the response of seminoma to relatively small doses of irraditation might well be due to the presence of many lymphocytes in the tissue. However, he said, when localized exteriorized loops of lymphatic nodes on the spleen were irradiated, apparently an antimitotic factor was released into the blood and had a general effect. His particular interest was because he used colloidal radioactive isotopes in large interstitial injections; in these circumstances, the center of the nodes would receive a rather high dose, which would mean that such antimitotic factors were released.

BRULÉ inquired as to whether DAVIDSOHN's findings meant that chemotherapy might be harmful, because a chemo-

therapeutic agent which was active against tumour cells would destroy the immunological cells and there would be little chance that the tumour cell with a low mitotic index would be destroyed.

SCULLY inquired as to whether DAVIDSOHN's work would be helpful in determining the histogenesis of some of the tumours. If the antigens were present in all mucous-secreting cells throughout the body or if all parts of the intestinal tract contained these substances, would this point be significant, since there was the question of whether the mucinous tumours of the ovary are related to the Müllerian or enteric epithelium. In regard to DAVIDSOHN's statement that the presence or absence of the cells might be useful in determining the metastatic potential, he also asked if any study had been made of the borderline tumours that cytologically are benign but that implant on the peritoneum.

TEILUM said that he had not observed the SHERMAN or asteroid bodies in dysgerminoma; he thought that these structures were typical of sarcoidosis. He was aware that the SHERMAN bodies are considered an expression of a high degree of immunity, but he had never observed them.

DAVIDSOHN, in closing, said that the only claim that could be made for his work is that he and his colleagues had demonstrated loss of isoantigens, particularly A and B, in the material that he had studied. O has not been studied, because of the difficulties of obtaining a potent anti-H serum, but this work is now in progress.

There are two schools of thought, DAVIDSOHN said, as to whether there is a specific cancer antigen or whether there is a loss of antigen. His own work supported the latter theory because it demonstrated that the isoantigen is lost, although this is not an autoantigen. This may indicate that this biochemical change takes place before metastasis develops.

As to BRULÉ's question, he could offer no conclusion, he said; the benefit or harm seemed to be a matter of dosage at times, and from the immunological viewpoint, it was interesting that one dose stimulated antigenic or antibody-producing ability, whereas another might decrease this ability.

As to LUISI's question, he had, of course, observed the granulomatous reaction in dysgerminoma, seminoma, pinealoma, and in certain teratomas of the mediastinum. He had not seen the SHERMAN bodies or asteroid bodies in the cases he had studied.

References

AMINOFF, D., MORGAN, W. T. J., and WATKINS, W. M., Studies in immunochemistry: Isolation and properties of human blood group A substance. *Biochem. J.* **46**, 426—438 (1950).

ANDRÉ, R., DREYFUS, B., et SALMON, C., Anémie hémolytique et kyste dermoïde de l'ovaire. *Bull. Soc. med. Hôp. Paris* **71**, 1062—1069 (1955).

BARRY, K. G., and CROSBY, W. H., Auto-immune hemolytic anemia arrested by removal of an ovarian teratoma: Review of the literature and report of a case. *Ann. intern. Med.* **47**, 1002—1007 (1957).

BELYAVIN, G., and TROTTER, W. R., Investigations of thyroid antigens reacting with Hashimoto sera: Evidence for an antigen other than thyroglobulin. *Lancet* **1959** I, 648—652.

BROBERGER, O., and PERLMANN, P., Demonstration of an epithelial antigen in colon by means of fluorescent antibodies from children with ulcerative colitis. *J. exp. Med.* **115**, 13—26 (1962).

COOMBS, R. R. A., BEDFORD, D., and ROUILLARD, I. M., A and B blood group antigens on human epidermal cells demonstrated by mixed agglutination. *Lancet* **1956** I, 461—463.

CUTLER, S. J., EDERER, F. C., and GREENBERG, K. A., Survival of patients with ovarian cancer. *J. nat. Cancer Inst.* **24**, 541—549 (1960).

DALES, M., Purpura associated with ovarian tumour. *Brit. med. J.* **1965** I, 127.

DAVIDSOHN, I., Recent advances in immunopathology. *New Phycn* **13**, 233—237 (1964).

— Immunohematologic aspects of cancer of clinical significance. *Proceedings of Fifth Nat. Cancer Conference*, Philadelphia, Penn., Sept. 17—19, 1964, p. 705—712 (1965).

— KOVARIK, S., and LEE, C. L., A, B, and 0 substances in gastrointestinal carcinoma. *Arch. Path.* **81**, 381—390 (1966a).

— —, and STEJSKAL, R., Blood group specific substances in ovarian neoplasms (in preparation, 1967).

DONIACH, D., ROITT, I. M., and HUDSON, R. V., Auto-antibodies in thyroid carcinoma: letter to the editor. *Lancet* **1958** II, 265—266.

FREIESLEBEN, E., KISSMEYER-NIELSEN, F., CHRISTENSES, J., JENSEN, K. G., and KNUDSEN, E. E., Excessive content of blood-group substances in serum from patients with ovarian cysts. *Vox Sang. (Basel)* **6**, 304—311 (1961).

FRIEDMAN, N. B., The comparative morphogenesis of extragenital and gonadal teratoid tumours. *Cancer (Philad.)* **4**, 265—276 (1951).

GOUDIE, R. B., Auto-immune selection of carcinoma cells in man. *Nature (Lond.)* **197**, 1020 (1963).

HELMBOLD, W. v., Sammelstatistik zur Prüfung auf Korrelationen zwischen dem weiblichen Genitalcarcinom und dem ABO und Rhesus System. *Acta genet. (Basel)* **11**, 29—51 (1961).

HUMPHRIES jr., A. L., SHEPHERD, M. H., and PETERS, H. J., Peutz-Jeghers syndrome with colonic adenocarcinoma and ovarian tumour. *J. Amer. med. Ass.* **197**, 296—298 (1966).

IRVINE, W. J., DAVIES, S. H., DELAMORE, I. W., and WILLIAMS, A. W., Immunological relationship between pernicious anaemia and thyroid disease. *Brit. med. J.* **1962** II, 454—456.

JONES, E., and TILLMAN, C., A case of hemolytic anemia relieved by removal of an ovarian tumour. *J. Amer. med. Ass.* **128**, 1225—1227 (1945).

KASILAG jr., F. B., and RUTLEDGE, F. N., Metastatic breast carcinoma in ovary. *Amer. J. Obstet. Gynec.* **74**, 989—992 (1957).

KOVARIK, S., DAVIDSOHN, I., and STEJSKAL, R., Detection of ABO antigens in cancer with the mixed cell agglutination reaction. Submitted for publication (1967).

LINDSAY, S., DAILEY, M. E., FRIEDLANDER, J., YEE, G., and SOLEY, M. H., Chronic thyroiditis: A clinical and pathologic study of 354 patients. *J. clin. Endocr.* **12**, 1578—1600 (1952).

McANDREW, G. M., Haemolytic anemia associated with ovarian teratoma. *Brit. med. J.* 1964 II, 1307—1309.

MARSHALL, A. H. E., and DAYAN, A. D., An immune reaction in man against seminomas, dysgerminomas, pinealomas, and the mediastinal tumours of similar histological appearance? *Lancet* 1964 II, 1102—1104.

MOSBECK, J., and VIDEBAEK, A., Mortality from and risk of gastric carcinoma among patients with pernicious anemia. *Brit. med. J.* 1950 II, 390—394.

NAIRN, R. C., FOTHERGILL, J. E., McENTEGART, M. G., and RICHMOND, H. G., Specific antibody against gastrointestinal mucosa. *Lancet* 1961 II, 109.

— PHILIP, J., GHOSE, T., PORTEOUS, I. B., and FOTHERGILL, J. E., Production of a precipitin against renal cancer. *Brit. med. J.* 1963 I, 1702—1704.

— RICHMOND, H. G., McENTEGART, M. G., and FOTHERGILL, J. E., Immunological differences between normal and malignant cells. *Brit. Med. J.* 1960 II, 1335—1340.

OBERMAN, H. A., and LIBCKE, J. H., Malignant germinal neoplasms of the mediastinum. *Cancer (Philad.)* 17, 498—507 (1964).

OSBORNE, R. H., and DE GEORGE, F. V., The ABO blood groups in neoplastic disease of the ovary. *Amer. J. hum. Genet.* 15, 380—388 (1963).

PULVERTAFT, R. J. V., DONIACH, D., ROITT, I. M., and HUDSON, R. V., Cytotoxic effects of Hashimoto serum on human thyroid cells in tissue culture. *Lancet* 1959 II, 214—216.

ROITT, I. M., and DONIACH, D., Human autoimmune thyroiditis: Serological studies. *Lancet* 1958 II, 1027—1033.

SEGI, M., FUKUSHIMA, I., FUJISAKU, S., KURIHARA, M., SAITO, S., ASANO, K., and NAGAIKE, H., Cancer morbidity in Miyaji prefecture, Japan, and a comparison with morbidity in the U. S. *J. nat. Cancer Inst.* 18, 373—383 (1957).

SLANEY, G., and BROOKE, B. N., Cancer in ulcerative colitis. *Lancet* 1959 II, 694—698.

SMITH, R. L., Recorded and expected mortality among the Japanese of the United States and Hawaii with special reference to cancer. *J. nat. Cancer Inst.* 17, 459—473 (1956).

STRÄULI, P., The mechanism of invasion in cancer. Un. int. *Cancer* 4, 3—5 (1966).

STUART, A. E., and ALLEN, W. S. A., Autoantibodies in thyroid carcinoma. *Lancet* 1958 II, 47.

TAYLOR, K. B., ROITT, I. M., DONIACH, D., COUCHMAN, K. G., and SHAPLAND, C., Autoimmune phenomena in pernicious anemia: Gastric antibodies. *Brit. med. J.* 1962 II, 1347—1352.

WEILER, E., *Carcinogenesis*. In: WOLSTENHOLME and O'CONNOR (eds.), Ciba Foundation Symposium. London: Churchill 1959, p. 165.

WEST, R. O., Epidemiologic study of malignancies of the ovaries. *Cancer (Philad.)* 19, 1001—1007 (1966).

WEST-WATSON, W. N., and YOUNG, C. J., Failed splenectomy in acholuric jaundice, and the relation of toxaemia of the haemolytic crisis. *Brit. med. J.* 1938 I, 1305—1309.

WHITE, R. G., and MARSHALL, A. H. E., The role of various chemical fractions of *M. tuberculosis* and other mycobacteria in the production of allergic encephalomyelitis. Immunology 1, 111—122 (1958).

WOMACK, W. S., and CASTELLANO, C. J., Migratory thrombophlebitis associated with ovarian carcinoma. *Amer. J. Obstet. Gynec.* 63, 467—469 (1952).

WOODRUFF, M. F. A., and NOLAN, B., Preliminary observations on treatment of advanced cancer by injection of allogenic spleen cells. *Lancet* 1963 II, 426—429.

YOSIDA, K. I., Über die gruppenspezifischen Unterschiede der Transsudate, Exsudate, Sekrete, Exkrete, Organextrakte und Organzellen des Menschen und ihre rechtsmedizinischen Anwendungen. *Z. ges. exp. Med.* 63, 331—339 (1928).

Diagnosis of Ovarian Carcinoma by Cul-de-sac Aspiration

Ruth M. Graham, Sc. D.

Roswell Park Memorial Institute, Buffalo, New York, U.S.A.

The need for earlier diagnosis of ovarian carcinoma is obvious. The same statement was being made for cancer of the cervix twenty years ago. Yet today the mortality rate from cancer of the cervix has decreased by fifty per cent, largely because cytologic examinations have detected the disease at an earlier stage.

In our attempt to apply the cytology of cul-de-sac aspirations to the earlier diagnosis of ovarian cancer we have applied the same principles we used in confirming Papanicolaou's thesis that carcinoma of the cervix could be diagnosed by identifying malignant cells in the vaginal smear (Meigs *et al.*, 1943).

These principles are embodied in the following questions:

1. Can malignant cells in unknown samples from clinical cancer be identified with accuracy?

2. Can malignant cells be identified in less advanced cases?

3. How often are cells erroneously called malignant in patients with no demonstrable malignancy.

This paper is a report of our findings.

Advanced carcinoma of the ovary often produces ascitic fluid. If the diagnosis of malignancy can be made with accuracy on fluid obtained by paracentesis, it would suggest that diagnosis by cul-de-sac aspiration would be profitable. In a previous series (Graham, 1963) the accuracy of diagnosis in ascitic fluid in 84 patients with metastases to the peritoneum was 92%. However, this series included all cases of peritoneal involvement and was not confined to ovarian carcinoma.

In the past six years we have examined ascitic fluid from seventy-eight cases of carcinoma of the ovary. Seventy of these were diagnosed as positive on the *first* examination or 90% (Table I). There was a 4% false negative error. One patient whose tumour was considered a cystadenoma had cells in the fluid, which were considered malignant. Since seventy fluids were correctly diagnosed, this represents a false positive figure of 2%. From this experience it is apparent that malignant cells desquamating from far advanced ovarian cancer can be accurately identified.

A question of technique must be considered in the use of material obtained by cul-de-sac aspiration. Is the small amount of fluid obtained a representative sample? A large volume of fluid is often obtained at paracentesis. A cul-de-sac aspiration may obtain only a fraction of a milliliter of fluid. Cul-de-sac aspiration was done in fourteen cases of ovarian carcinoma that either had ascitic fluid at the time or developed fluid within three months. Twelve of the fourteen were called positive, or 86%; one negative and one doubtful. We concluded that the cul-de-sac aspiration contains a representative sample of the cells in the abdominal cavity, even though the fluid examined is much smaller in quantity.

Cul-de-sac aspirations have been done on three hundred and forty-three patients at the Roswell Park Memorial Institute. Since for a patient to be referred to the

Table II indicates the results in seventy-three cases of primary ovarian carcinoma. Eighty-one per cent were diagnosed as positive on the *first* cul-de-

Table I. *Accuracy of cytologic examinations of ascitic fluid*

Final diagnosis	Cytologic diagnosis			
	positive	doubtful	negative	unsatis-factory
Carcinoma of ovary	68	4	3	1
Adenocarcinoma of pelvis (primary not determined)	2			
Dysgerminoma			1	
Cystadenoma of ovary	1		1	

Table II

Primary ovarian carcinoma	Cul-de-sac aspiration		
	+	±	−
Papillary adenocarcinoma	23	3	1
Serous cyst adenocarcinoma	3	1	1
Adenocarcinoma	11		4
Anaplastic carcinoma of ovary	3		1
Carcinoma of ovary	8	2	1
Clinical — no path — dead	2		
Microinvasive of ovary	3 *		
Breast carcinoma — adenocarcinoma of ovary	1 *		
Carcinoma in situ of Cx microinvasive Adenocarcinoma of ovary	1 *		
	1		
Treat Cx — adenocarcinoma of ovary	1		
Corpus I$_1$ — papillary adenocarcinoma	1 *		
Corpus II — adenocarcinoma of ovary	1 *		
	59/73	6/73	8/73
	81%	8%	11%

* Unsuspected clinically 7/73 — 10%.

Institute, the diagnosis of cancer or a question of cancer is necessary, this series is heavily weighted with symptomatic patients, and those with established malignant disease. The use of cul-de-sac aspirations as a screening procedure has been reported elsewhere (GRAHAM and GRAHAM, 1966).

sac aspiration. There was an erroneous negative report in 11%. Eight per cent of the aspirations were considered doubtful, but not repeated. It is of interest that four cases of ovarian carcinoma were found in patients with other malignancies (three of the cervix and one of the breast) and that two of these were not suspected clinically. The two cases of carcinoma of the corpus were originally thought to be primary at that site, but were subsequently shown to be primary

The diagnosis of unusual ovarian malignancies by cul-de-sac aspiration is not good as shown in Table III. Of the six cases, only two were recognized as

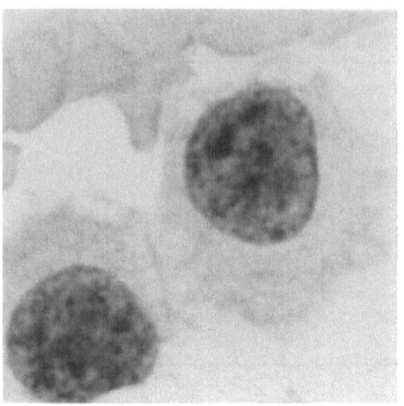 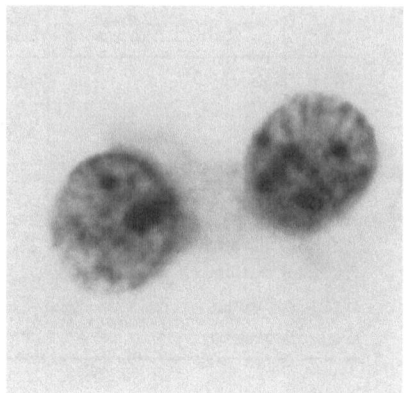

Fig. 1. The two malignant cells on the left were found in ascitic fluid from a far advanced ovarian cancer. Those on the right were in a cul-de-sac aspiration of a 49 year old woman with no gynecologic symptoms and normal appearing ovaries. On histologic examination a micro-invasive carcinoma of the ovary was found

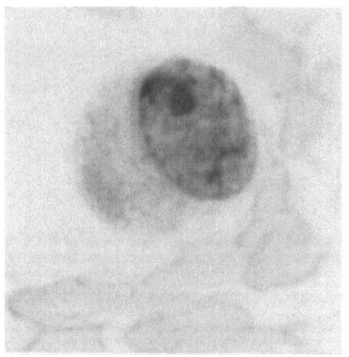 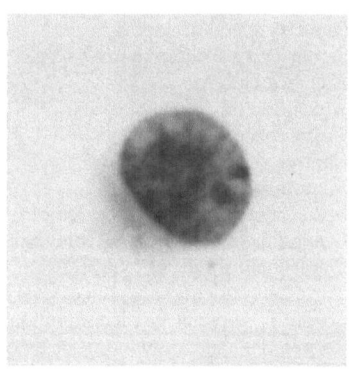

Fig. 2. Two more examples from the two cases described in Fig. 1. Note abnormal nucleoli and distinctly abnormal distribution of chromatin in the cell seen in ascitic fluid (left) and the cell seen in the cul-de-sac aspiration (right)

carcinoma of the ovary with metastases to the corpus.

The four cases of microinvasive detected cytologically are gratifying. The malignant cells desquamating from these early lesions were indistinguishable from those desquamating from an advanced ovarian carcinoma (Figs. 1, 2).

Table III. *Rare ovarian neoplasms*

	+	±	−
Malignant teratoma			1
Granulosa cell carcinoma	1		1
Fibro sarcoma of ovary			1
Carcino sarcoma of ovary	1		
Leimyosarcoma of ovary			1
	2		4

malignant. This is also seen in the ascitic fluids in which a case of dysgerminoma was considered negative. These poor results may be due to our inexperience in recognizing these tumours. In the sarcoma, it is more likely that the malignant cells are not desquamating in appreciable numbers. Sarcomas tend to have malignant cells, which are tightly adherent to one another. The only sarcoma recognized as malignant had carcinoma elements.

An occasional case of carcinoma of the ovary is referred to the Institute for question of further therapy after the cancer is thought to have been removed completely. The use of cul-de-sac aspirations in this small group has been worthwhile (Table IV). Eleven such patients

Table IV

Carcinoma of ovary 100% removal	+	−
Well 3—15 years	10	
Recurrence	1	

were seen. Ten had no malignant cells in the cul-de-sac aspiration and all are well without evidence of disease from 3 to 15 years. One patient had malignant cells in the aspiration and promptly developed recurrence.

There were seven primary cases with disease in the abdominal cavity but not classified as ovary. One was a carcinoma of the Fallopian tube. Four were classified as carcinoma of the pelvis since it was impossible to determine whether the adenocarcinoma originated in the cervix, corpus or ovary. Two cases were classified as carcinoma of the corpus, Stage III, indicating that clinically the disease was considered to be beyond the confines of the uterus. All these seven cases had malignant cells in the cul-de-sac aspirations (Table V).

Table V

Primary cases — not ovary but disease in pelvis	Cul-de-sac aspiration		
	+	±	−
Carcinoma of the pelvis	4		
Carcinoma of Fallopian tube	1		
Corpus Stage III	2		
	7	0	0

Recurrent disease in the abdominal cavity from a carcinoma other than ovary ocurred in twenty-one patients (Table VI).

Table VI

Recurrent — metastatic in abdominal cavity	Cul-de-sac aspiration		
	+	±	−
Recurrent corpus	7		3
Recurrent cervix	7*		1
Recurrent sarcoma of uterus	1		1
Recurrent carcinoma of vagina	1		
	16		5

* 1 case unsuspected clinically.

One case of recurrent cancer of the cervix was detected by cul-de-sac aspiration in a patient thought to be free of disease and has been reported elsewhere (GRAHAM et al., 1964). Fourteen patients, diagnosed as having carcinoma of the breast, had cul-de-sac aspirations. One adenocarcinoma of the ovary and one metastatic lesion in the ovary from the breast were discovered (Table VII).

Table VII

Carcinoma of breast	Cul-de-sac aspiration		
	+	±	−
Normal ovaries			2
Cystadenoma			1
No pelvic exploration		4	5
Adenocarcinoma of ovary	1		
Metastatic breast carcinoma	1		

There were ninety-eight cases of benign gynecologic disease in this series. A considerable number had palpable masses (Table VIII). The cases of leiomy-

an erroneous positive diagnosis. It was in a patient with carcinoma of the cervix with severe radiation damage to the bowel (Table IX).

Table VIII. *Benign gynecologic pathology*

	+	±	−
Consultation — no gyn disease			20
Pathology — cervitis			12
Pathology — hyperplasia of endometrium		2	13
polyps of endo-cervix of endo-metrium		1	8
Benign palpable masses			
Leiomyoma	.	1	16
Pelvic inflammatory disease			
Chronic			5
Acute			1
Cystadenoma of ovary			6
Endometriosis	1*	1	2
Dermoid		1	1
Thecoma			1
Stein Leventhal			1
Fibroma of ovary		2	1
Fibro adenoma of ovary			1
No disease in ovary	2**		
	3	8	88

* Borderline lesion — composite papillae with malignant epithelium biopsy only.

** Considered false positive reports.

Table IX. *Primary gynecologic malignancy other than ovary*

	+	±	−
Carcinoma in situ of cervix	2	1	24
Invasive carcinoma of cervix		1	17
Carcinoma of vulva			5
Carcinoma of vagina			1
Carcinoma of corpus Stage 1	2	4	21
Carcinoma of corpus Stage II	2	1	5
Treated Cx	2		5
	8	7	78

Of the 8 positives: 5 were ovarian carcinoma, 1 false positive, 2 corpus carcinoma.

The other two positive reports were in carcinoma of the corpus, one Stage I and one Stage II. No disease was demonstrated in the abdominal cavity. Whether this represents retrograde passage of malignant cells from the endometrial cavity, through the tube to the abdominal cavity is a matter of conjecture. More cases will be needed to determine the source of the cells. Careful step sections of the tube would be helpful.

oma, pelvic inflammatory disease and cystadenoma were correctly diagnosed as benign cytologically. In this series there were two cases in which the source of the malignant cells could not be found. On review the cul-de-sac aspirations are still considered positive but these cases are classified as false positive reports.

Cul-de-sac aspiration was performed on ninety-three cases of primary gynecologic malignancy other than ovary. There were eight positive cul-de-sac aspirations — five of these were proven to have carcinoma of the ovary and three of these were discovered by cul-de-sac aspiration. One must be considered as

The most interesting group of patients in this series are nineteen in whom pelvic examination under anesthesia was negative, yet the cul-de-sac aspiration contained malignant cells (Table X).

Table X. *Borderline lesions of the ovary*

Being followed without exploration	7
Borderline lesions — oophorectomy	8
Borderline lesions — biopsy only	2
In situ of tube	1
Borderline, but blood vessel invasion	1

Seven of these patients are being followed at three month intervals and these seven patients have not had a laparotomy.

Two patients, in their early forties, have been explored and had biopsies of both ovaries. Ten patients, all postmenopausal, have had bilateral salpingo-oophorectomy.

One of these twelve patients had a carcinoma in situ of the fimbriated end

desquamating from an advanced clinical carcinoma (Figs. 6 and 7).

2. Such histologic lesions are present on the edge of clinical invasive carcinoma (Figs. 8, 9 and 10).

Summary

The examination of fluid obtained by cul-de-sac aspiration is an accurate

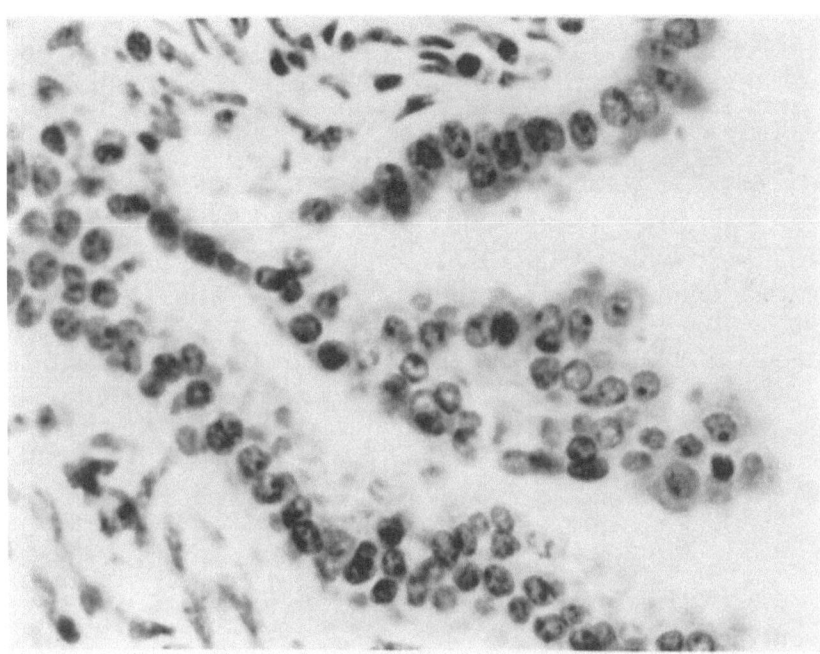

Fig. 3. Multilayering of the germinal epithelium. Nuclei have abnormal structure. Borderline lesion

of the Fallopian tube. The remaining eleven had lesions of the surface of the ovary, which we regard as borderline and pre-malignant. The histologic picture was either that of multilayering of the germinal epithelium or extensive papillary processes of the surface, or transition of normal germinal epithelium to single layer of typical malignant cells (Figs. 3, 4, and 5).

The basis for considering these lesions borderline and pre-malignant are:

1. The cells desquamating from these cells are indistinguishable from the cells

method in diagnosed carcinoma of the ovary. The false negative error is 12%. Three cases were called positive in whom no source for the abnormal cells could be found, a false positive error of 5%.

Four microinvasive carcinomas of the ovary have been discovered by cul-de-sac aspiration and one carcinoma in situ of the tubal epithelium. Eleven cases have been detected in whom the germinal epithelium is distinctly abnormal. These are regarded as borderline and pre-malignant.

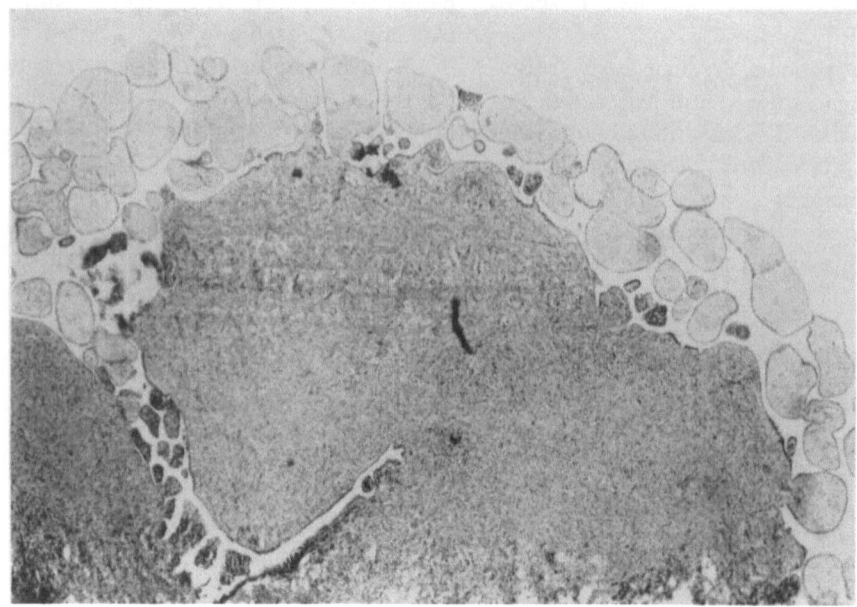

Fig. 4. Extensive papillary process on surface of ovary, and in crypts. Considered borderline lesion

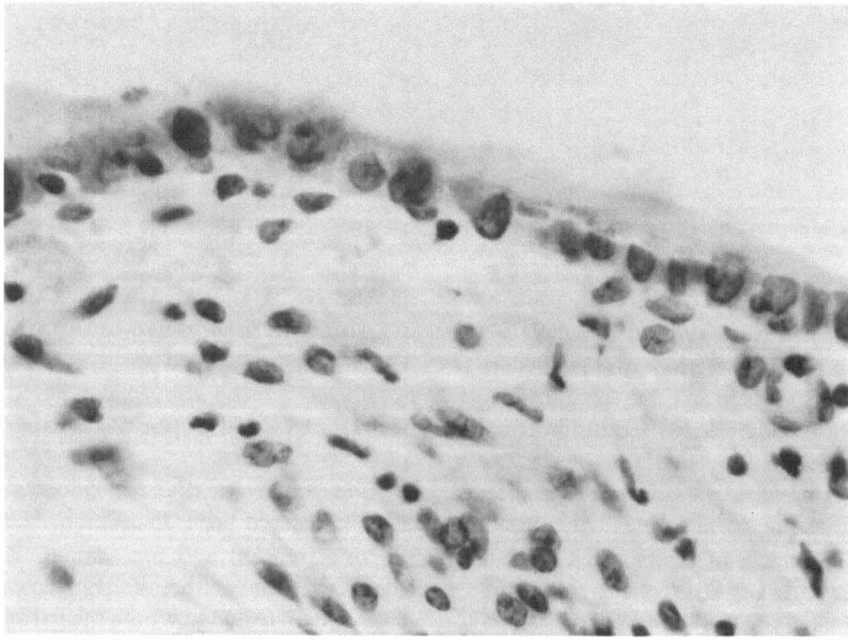

Fig. 5. Single layer of malignant cells on surface of ovary. Borderline lesion. Note abnormal nuclear configuration

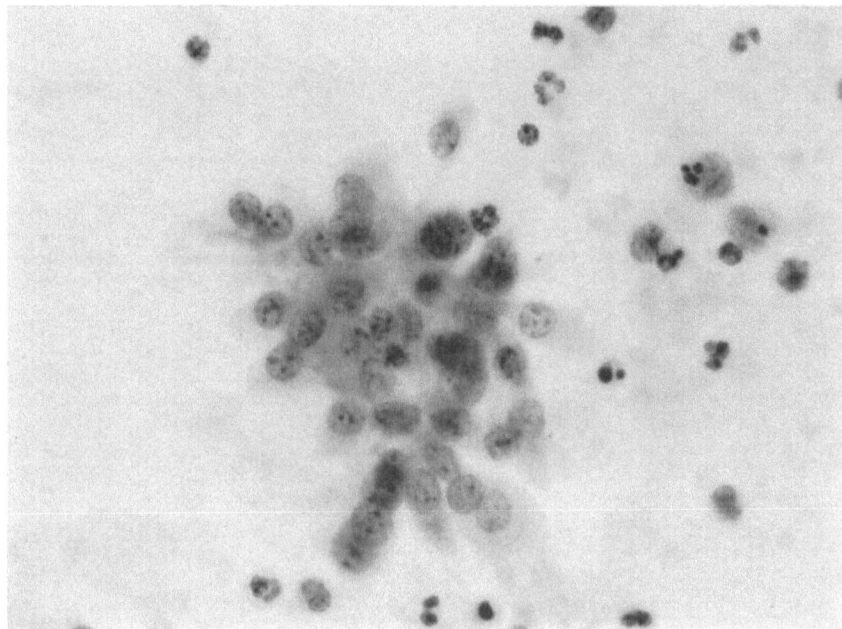

Fig. 6. Cells found in cul-de-sac aspiration of a 75 year old patient. Histologic diagnosis-borderline lesion

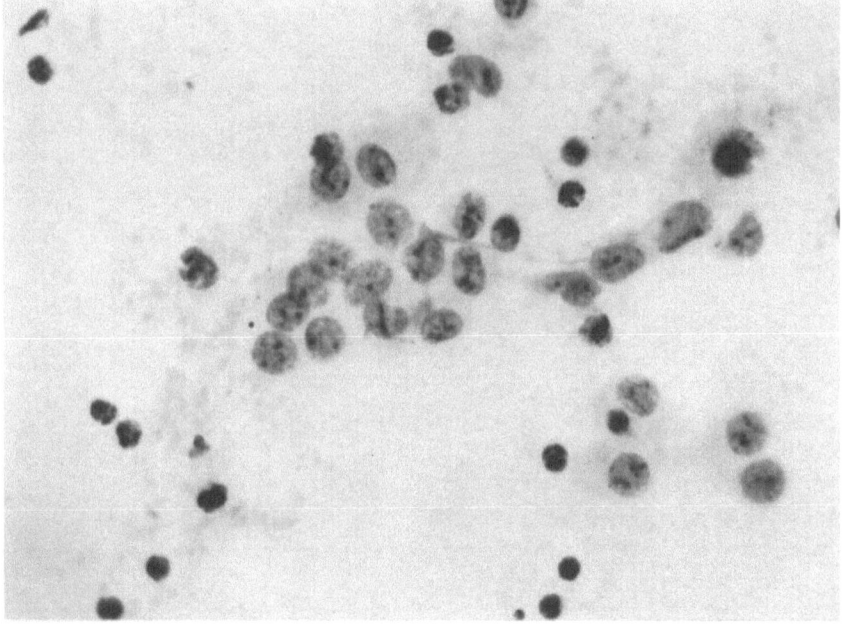

Fig. 7. Cells in the ascitic fluid of a 33 year old patient who has since died of her disease. Compare with Fig. 6

9 Ovarian Cancer

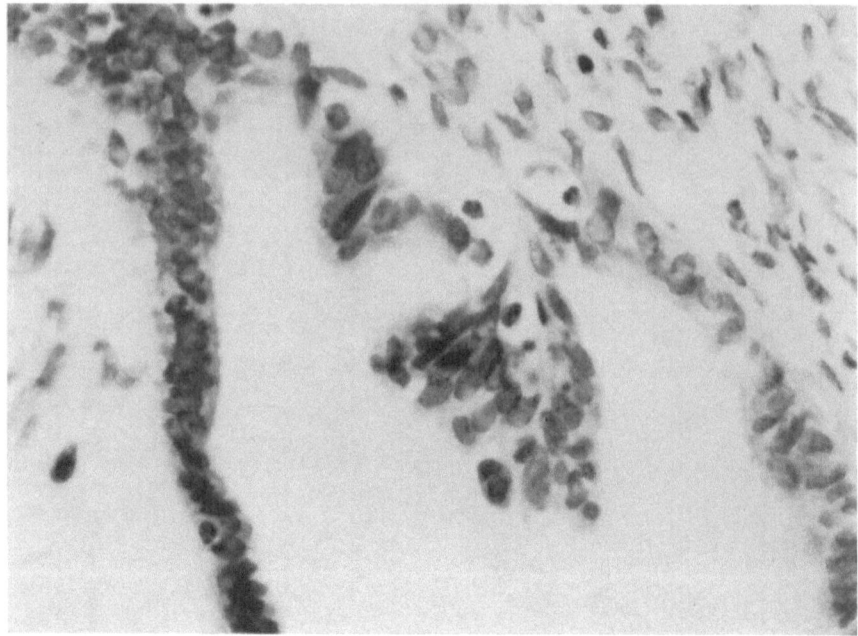

Fig. 8. Surface near an invasive carcinoma of the ovary. Cancer cells were found in lymphatics in wall of hernial sac. Compare with Fig. 3

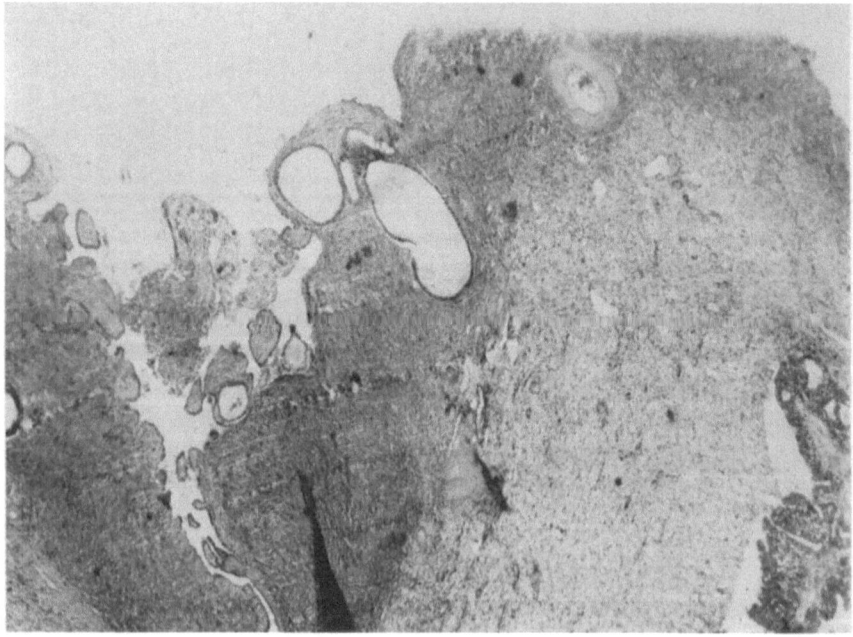

Fig. 9. Ovarian surface in Stage IIb ovarian carcinoma. Notice papillary projections on surface and in crypts. Invasive tumour in right hand corner. Compare with Fig. 4

Routine use of cul-de-sac aspirations particularly in symptomatic women may result in the detection of early occult ovarian carcinoma.

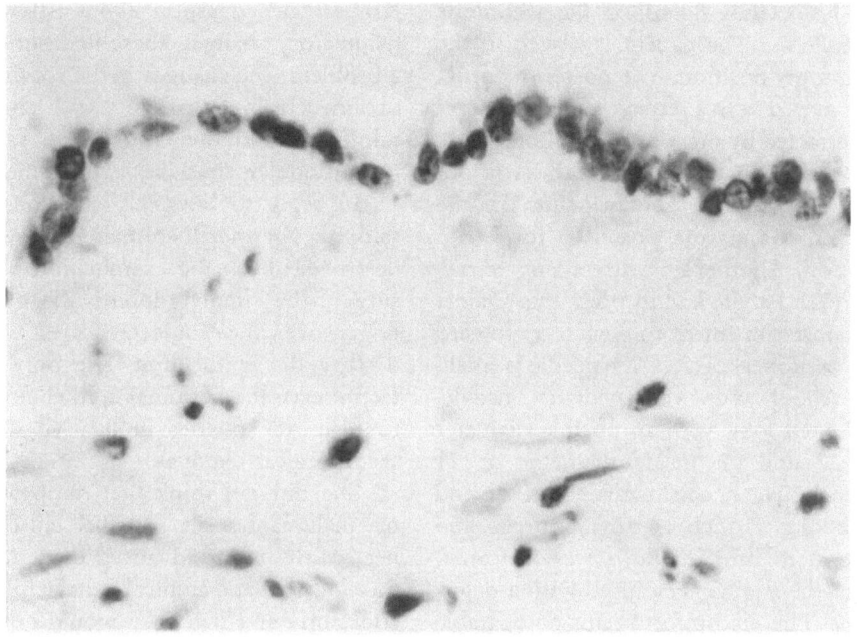

Fig. 10. Single cell layer composed of malignant cells near an invasive cancer of the ovary. Patient died of her disease. Compare with Fig. 5

Discussion

KOTTMEIER remarked that at the Radiumhemmet, cul-de-sac aspirations had been done in 127 patients and in only nine instances were abnormal cells found. He inquired as to the technique of cul-de-sac aspiration, the size of the needle if no ascites or fluid were present, and if fluid should be obtained by aspiration only or by lavage also. He also asked if inflammatory changes are found in patients who have had salpingitis.

SCULLY remarked that perhaps this type of study would stimulate a more careful examination of the germinal epithelium of the ovary. Unfortunately, he said, most specimens have been examined so much by the time they are received for sectioning that, except in the cer-

vices, no epithelium was left. Although there was no proof, he said, it was the impression that many cystadenocarcinomas of the ovary arose from the germinal epithelium after it dipped into the ovarian stroma to form germinal inclusion cells. If this was true, cells would probably not be found in the cul-de-sac washings. Another question, he said, was whether it was too late for effective therapy when cells were already present in the cul-de-sac washings. Theoretically, the cells are already exposed to the peritoneal cavity, and implantation can take place.

RUTLEDGE inquired about the relationship of these cells with ovulation. He also asked if anything was known about the time lag between detection and invasion such as occurs in cervical carcinoma in situ, for example.

J. GRAHAM described the technique as follows: The patient is placed in the lithotomy position. The posterior fornix is exposed with a retractor and the cervix is retracted by one of two methods. One method is to use a tenaculum, without actually putting the tenaculum in the cervix, to put the posterior fornix on tension. Another is to use a ring retractor on a handle and to press this against the posterior fornix to push it up toward the peritoneal cavity. The needle is small, an Abbot scalp vein pediatric needle, one inch long with an outside diameter of 22 and an inside diameter of 21 French. The needle is carried on the end of a long, 11-inch, Hartmann forcep, and is passed through the posterior fornix, after the vagina is cleansed with a detergent. The discomfort seems comparable to that caused by a venipuncture. When aspiration is done in the operating room under anesthesia, an ordinary one and one-half inch No. 20 needle and a 5 or 10 cc. syringe is used; this method is really more satisfactory. He had only aspirated material as yet, but he had considered the possibility of injecting saline or Ringer's solution into the peritoneal cavity through the anterior abdominal wall, and then attempting to recover it through the cul de sac. Better techniques are needed because satisfactory specimens are obtained in only about 70 per cent of cases.

In only one instance in several thousand specimens had there been any complication; one patient had a large pelvic mass which was aspirated, proved to be cancerous, and became infected. When there were no abnormalities in the pelvis, no complications occurred, although occasionally bowel content is obtained.

R. GRAHAM said that it was particularly difficult to get good cul-de-sac aspirations after hysterectomy. As to KOTTMEIER's question about pelvic inflammatory changes, these had not been a problem; the changes in the specimens obtained from six patients with chronic salpingitis and one with acute salpingitis (done by mistake) were different.

In reply to SCULLY's question, she said, the germinal epithelium is easily destroyed; even the examination of the surgeon by simply rubbing the gloved finger over the single cell layer would destroy the epithelium. The only way to preserve the germinal epithelium was to place the ovaries in fixative within seconds after removal.

She did not think that the presence of malignant cells in the cul-de-sac necessarily meant advanced disease. She thought that the atypical cells exfoliated constantly and that they would not implant on the peritoneal surface as long as it was healthy. As to the time lag, she thought possibly that there was a time interval between the development of cancer and invasion although she had only one case to support this belief. This was a patient from whom exfoliated cancer cells in the vaginal smear had been obtained for three years. Although she was examined under anesthesia twice, seen in the clinic every three months for a long period of time, had a dilatation and curettage, and cervical biopsies, the source of the malignant cells could not be located. She had a severe viral infection and encephalitis, after which she discovered her clothes were too tight. She consulted a physician and was found to have inoperable carcinoma of the ovary with both ascites and pleural effusion. A smear obtained 11 years before treatment showed the same type of malignant cells that were present in the tumour.

References

GRAHAM, J. B., and GRAHAM, R. M., Cul-de-sac puncture in the diagnosis of early ovarian carcinoma. In press 1966.

— —, and SCHUELLER, E. F., Preclinical detection of ovarian cancer. *Cancer (Philad.)* **17**, 1414—1432 (1964).

GRAHAM, R. M., The cytologic diagnosis of cancer. Philadelphia: W. B. Saunders & Co. 1963.

MEIGS, J. V., GRAHAM, R. M., FREMONT-SMITH, M., KAPNICK, I., and RAWSON, R., The value of the vaginal smear in the diagnosis of uterine cancer. *Surg. Gynec. Obstet.* **77**, 449—461 (1943).

Cancer Cells in the Blood: Incidence and Importance to Prognosis and Treatment

STUART S. ROBERTS, M. D.

Attending Surgeon Markle Scholar in Academic Medicine, University of Illinois Research and Eductional Hospitals and Associate Professor of Surgery and Acting Head of Department, University of Illinois College of Medicine, Chicago, Illinois, U.S.A.

ELIZABETH E. McGREW, M. D.

Associate Pathologist, University of Illinois Research and Educational Hospitals, and Professor of Pathology, University of Illinois College of Medicine, Chicago, Illinois, U.S A.

JONAS VALAITIS, M. D.

Pathologist, Lutheran General Hospital, Park Ridge, Illinois and Clinical Associate Professor of Pathology, University of Illinois College of Medicine, Chicago, Illinois, U.S.A.

WARREN H. COLE, M. D.

Professor of Surgery Emeritus, University of Illinois College of Medicine, Chicago, Illinois, U.S.A.

Introduction

One of the most devastating events to take place in the natural history (or altered natural history) of many types of malignant tumours is the development of hematogenous metastases. This type of dissemination places cancer cells beyond the confines of primary surgical resection. Although it is true that the vast majority of cancer cells in the circulating blood are probable destroyed *within* vascular channels, the frequent occurrence of hematogenous metastases following resection of "favorable" lesions is ample proof that *some* cancer cells in the bloodstream are quite viable and capable of forming distant metastases. Although surgical excision, radiation therapy, and/or chemotherapy have resulted in apparent long-term control of disseminated disease in some cases, the occurrence of blood-borne metastases is still a factor that is usually lethal. Accordingly, this route of dissemination deserves intensive study.

The subject of cancer cells in the circulating blood (ROBERTS, 1961) is one phase, i.e., transportation, in the mechanism of vascular dissemination which can be thought of as occuring in a sequence of four phases including:

1. *entrance* of cancer cells into vascular channels,

2. *transportation* in the blood stream,

3. *lodgment* of the embolic cancer cells in arterioles and capillaries, followed by the

4. *fate*, which is either death or survival of the embolic cancer cells.

The *transportation* phase can be better understood by considering how cancer cells *enter* blood vessels, and what happens to them in the blood stream, i.e., lodgment and fate.

There are three routes by which cancer cells may gain entrance into vascular channels. Two of these routes are the direct result of the invasive growth of the malignant tumour, including:

1. invasion of blood vessels, and
2. invasion of lymphatics, some of which have direct communications to veins.

Pathologists and surgeons have long recognized the grave prognosis associated with the demonstration of vein invasion in a resected tumour, including lung, kidney, colon, breast, etc.

Contrary to any assumption that invasive growth by the primary tumour provides the only routes of entry of cancer cells, there is mounting evidence that on some occasions cancer cells may gain entrance into vascular channels in the same manner as do bone marrow emboli. This route of entrance, termed intravasation (YOUNG and GRIFFITH, 1950), is the passage of adjacent disrupted tissue cells (normal or neoplastic) into blood vessels through anatomic defects in the walls of the vessels. Thus, intravasation is the reverse of extravasation of formed elements of blood out of blood vessels into adjacent tissue. Intravasation may occur under certain circumstances when the extravascular (tissue) pressure rises even momentarily above the intravascular pressure. The fact that the normal counterpart of cancer cells, i.e., tissue cells, such as fat, bone marrow, liver, and brain can be demonstrated as blood-borne emboli in the pulmonary blood vessels of accident victims is strong evidence that invasion

is not the only route of entry. If normal tissue cells, which do not possess invasive qualities of their own, can and do on occasion enter blood vessels, perhaps cancer cells might also gain entrance by the route of intravasation. Therefore, the tendency of some malignant tumours to spread by vascular channels may be the result not only of invasion, but also the result of certain iatrogenic procedures such as incision biopsy which may set the stage for intravasation of cancer cells (ROBERTS, 1961). Intravasation of cancer cells may also help to explain how a clump of cancer cells (Fig. 1) can be detected in the blood stream immediately after accidental rupture of an ovarian tumour during pelvic examination (Fig. 2) and yet no evidence of vascular invasion subsequently be found in the resected specimen.

The demonstration of a large clump of cancer cells in the peripheral blood from an ovarian tumour as illustrated in Fig. 1 indicates that embolic cancer cells may not lodge in predicted arteriolar or capillary beds. Such a finding can be explained by certain by-pass routes, i.e., paravertebral veins of Batson which by-pass the lungs or liver. Also, there may be transorgan passage through arteriovenous shunts, or by actual transcapillary passage by distortion of the embolic cancer cells. The prompt appearance of cancer cells in the antecubital venous blood after manipulation of a malignancy within the abdominal cavity, e.g., carcinoma of the ovary, indicates that transorgan or transtissue passage has occurred *twice* — through the lungs and then through the tissues of the arm, distal to the antecubital fossa. On rare occasions, the pulmonary vasculature may be filled with cancer cells lodged in the arterioles and capillaries to such an extent as to obstruct the pulmonary blood flow with resultant strain on the

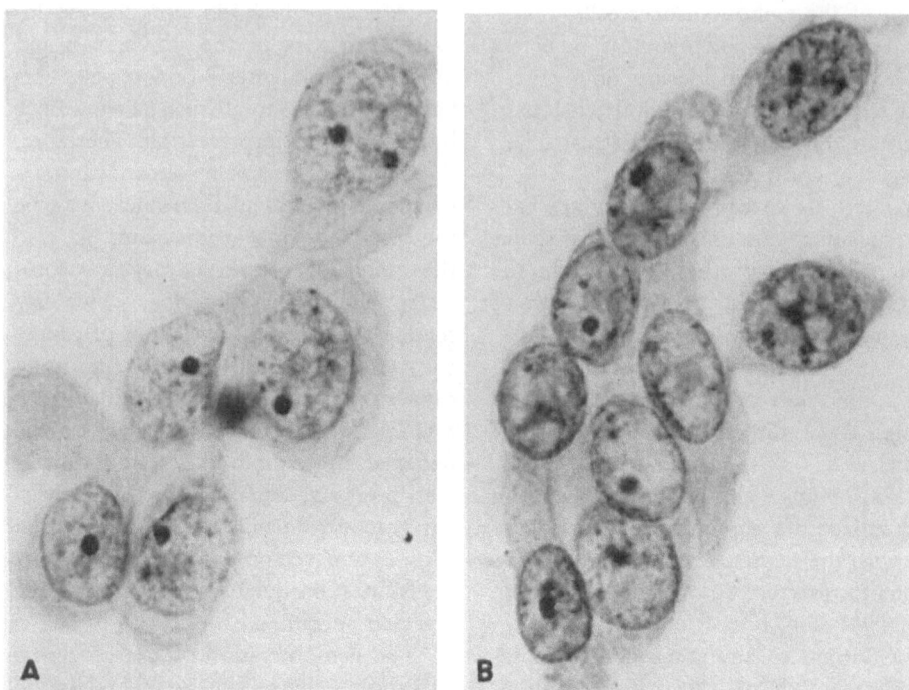

Fig. 1 A and B. Carcinoma of the ovary, Papanicolaou stain, × 1,100. A. Clump of cancer cells isolated from peripheral blood after accidental rupture of the tumour during pelvic examination. B. Direct smear of resected tumour. [From ROBERTS, S. S., *et al.*, *Cancer (Philad.)* *15*, 232—000 (1962)]

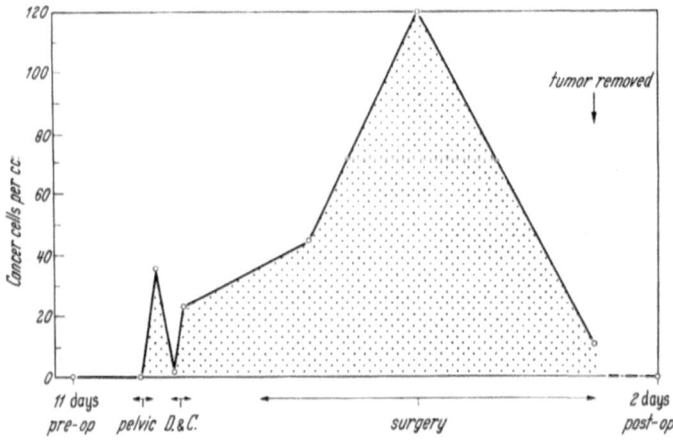

Fig. 2. Cancer cells in the peripheral blood during operation for carcinoma of the ovary. [After ROBERTS, S. S., *et al.*, *Arch. Surg. 76*, 334—000 (1958)]

right heart, that eventually subacute cor pulmonale occurs in a patient without antecedent cardiorespiratory disease.

The fate of blood-borne cancer cells is not predictable in any given patient. As previously emphasized, only a small portion of cancer cells found in the bloodstream will survive because of host resistance and other factors, i.e., tumour embolism is not necessarily equivalent to metastases formation. The sequence leading to the death or survival of cancer cell emboli at the point of lodgment has been clearly shown by the in vivo observations of SUMNER WOOD (1958) who utilized serial cinephotomicrographic records of the vascularized ear chamber in rabbits. These observations suggest that the ability of the cancer cells to evoke the formation of a surrounding intravascular thrombus at the point of lodgment is an important, but not invariable, step in the evolution of blood-borne metastases.

Materials and Methods

Patients. During the past ten years in our laboratory, more than 1,700 patients have been studied for the presence or absence of cancer cells in the circulating blood. Almost one half, 767 of these patients, were studied more than five years, and many as long as ten years ago. The patients were classified as "curable" or "incurable" at the time the blood samples were obtained. The term "curable" implies only a theoretical possibility based upon radiographic, gross, and microscopic exclusion of all evidence of tumour extension beyond the confines of surgical resection. Of the 767 patients studied five to ten years ago, 242 were classified as "curable". A total of 205 patients were studied before, during, and after operation. The 767 patients represent a cross-section of all types of tumours, although it should be emphasiz-

ed that the patient material does not represent the consecutive admissions to the hospital. A total of 22 patients of this group had ovarian carcinoma.

Collection of Blood Samples. An aloquit of 10 cc heparinized blood samples were collected from a variety of sites including 1) the antecubical vein, 2) local venous blood samples from veins draining the tumour, 3) by a catheter (cardiac or polyethelene) which was inserted into the superior or inferior vena cava depending on the tumour area. As few as one and as many as 55 blood samples were collected from each patient.

Methods of Isolation of Cancer Cells from Whole Blood. Blood samples from the patients in this study were processed by one of three methods of isolation of cancer cells (reported in detail elsewhere) including:

1. Albumin floatation (ROBERTS and Associates, 1958).

2. Streptolysin Method (LONG and Associates, 1960).

3. Dextran Sedamentation Method (RAMSDAHL and Associates, 1962).

Cytologic Identification. All slides were prepared by means of PAPANICOLAOU's technique of preservation and staining. Eight to twelve slides were made for each 10 cc blood sample. In this series of patients, the final interpretation of all slides scanned and marked as suspicious by technicians has been made by one of us (E.A.M.) cyto-pathologist. The original diagnosis of blood sample was reviewed recently by two cyto-pathologists (E. M. and J. V.). Whenever possible a direct smear of the resected tumour was prepared to allow comparison with abnormal cells isolated from the blood stream (Fig. 1).

Incidence of Cancer Cells in the Blood

Results of Blood Studies. Only those cancer cases that were studied more than five years ago, and were available for follow up were included under this heading, i.e., 767 patients. Not included are 23 cancer patients lost to follow up. The patients have been categorized under three headings including:

only one of 50 blood samples was positive.

The original cytologic diagnosis was positive for cancer cells in 279 of 767 (36%) cancer patients. However, in the recent review, only 52 (7%) of the 767

Table I. *All cancer patients*

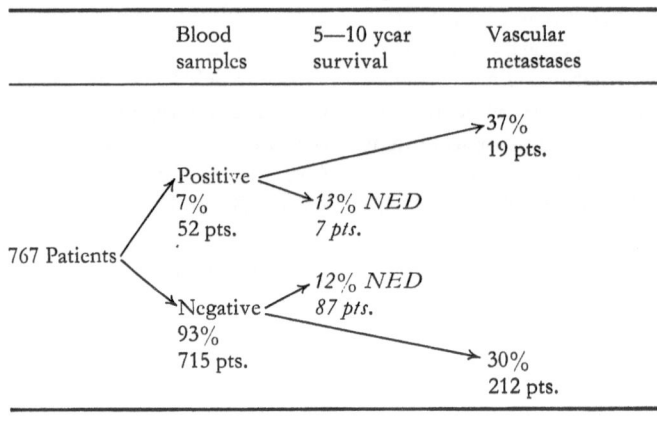

Table II. *All "curable" patients*

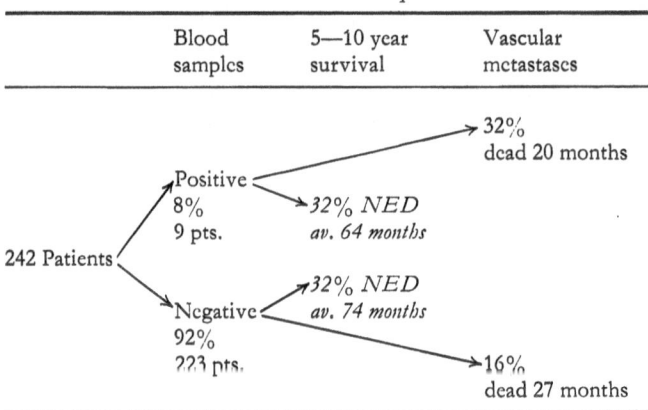

1. All Cancer Patients (Table 1).
2. All "Curable" Patients (Table 2).
3. All Patients During Operation (Table 3).

No distinction is made with regard to the *source* or *number* of blood samples. In other words, a patient is recorded as positive only once, regardless of whether the blood sample was obtained from the vena cava or antecubital vein, or whether

cancer patients had blood samples which were upheld as positive for cancer cells. All cases with only suspicious findings are included in the negative classification. Therefore, with the review of the original positive cases, only one in twenty had a diagnosis which was upheld as positive. This same reduction rate resulting from the review of the positive cases held true when considering the "curable" patients or the patients studied during operation. Hereafter, all results in this report will refer to data resulting from the recent review. As seen in Tables 1, 2 and 3, there was no apparent difference in the incidence of positive blood samples in the various categories, including 7% of all cancer patients, 8% of all "curable" patients, and 9% of all patients studied before, during, and after operation. A positive

and NADELL (1965), there is no doubt that cancer cells *have* been demonstrated in blood samples from cancer patients, including approximately 20% of "curable" and 30% "incurable" cases in the literature. In recent reports, the frequency of positive blood samples tends to be lower than ten years ago. The wide variation in the frequency of positive blood samples reported in the literature is to be expected when one considers

Table III. *All patients during operation*

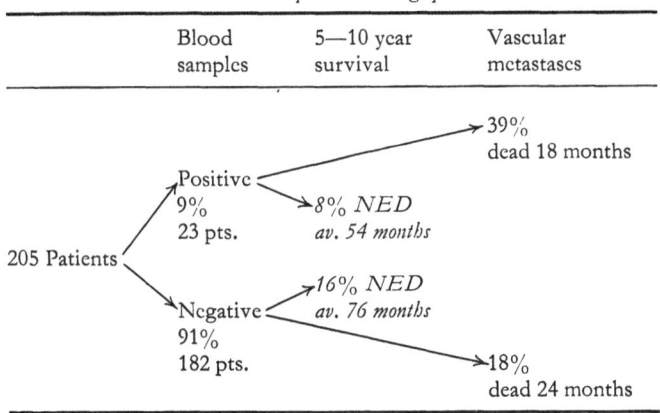

case in this latter category refers only to those patients who had a negative blood sample prior to operation, but developed a positive blood sample either during or following operation. Of the 22 cases with carcinoma of the ovary, only one (5%) had a positive blood sample (Fig. 2). Only one case of the entire group of 22 cases of carcinoma of the ovary was considered to be "curable" and this patient had negative blood samples.

Discussion. The incidence of positive blood samples in the literature has varied widely in the more than 5,000 patients reported during the past ten years by more than forty different investigative teams in various parts of the world. Although many of the reported frequencies of positive blood samples are conflicting, as summarized by GOLDBLATT

the widely different approaches to the methods of isolation, collection of blood samples, and cytologic criteria of malignancy. In spite of these variations, there are several areas of agreement with regard to the many factors which govern the frequency of positive blood samples:

The site of the blood samples appears to be of great importance. A greater percentage (approximately three-fold) of blood samples are positive when they are obtained from the local venous blood draining the tumour area, compared to the peripheral blood samples from the antecubical vein. Clumps of cancer cells are far more common in local venous blood samples then in peripheral blood samples where they are rare indeed (Fig. 1 A). The timing of these blood samples is of equal importance; blood samples must be drawn at frequent intervals before, during, and after the various forms of any manipulation of the primary tumour in order to detect an isolated shower of cancer cells in the blood stream which may be undetectable in a matter of minutes after a positive blood sample is obtained.

Although cancer cells have occasionally been seen on routine blood smears, such a chance finding is so rare that some method must be utilized to isolate or concentrate the relatively few cancer cells from the numerous formed elements of whole blood. The 20 different methods that have been reported in the literature reflect the situation that there is no current perfect method in terms of ease of performance, quantitative recovery, good cytologic quality of nucleated elements, etc. Most methods are either too complicated or time-consuming for general usage. Some of the methods preserve the quality of the cytologic preparation of the isolated cancer cells at the expense of the quantitative recovery, e.g., albumin floatation and dextran sedimentation. Other methods preserve the quantitative recovery at the expense of quality of the cytologic preparation, i.e., streptolysin.

Probably the most important single factor which influences the incidence of cancer cells in the blood stream is the cytologic criteria used for identifying a cell in a peripheral blood as actually malignant. During the past ten years in our laboratory (Cole et al., 1954) (Roberts et al., 1966), more than 40,000 slides have been scanned for the presence of abnormal nucleated cells in blood. With our recent review of the original positive cytologic diagnosis rendered five to ten years ago, the reduction rate in positive cases is 81% (from 279 cases to only 52 cases). During the first two to three years of our study, the mega-

karyocytes and immature cells of the blood series were the major problem areas of differential diagnosis. With a refined technique of double filtration (McGrath et al., in preparation), during the past two years, endothelial cells singly or in sheets have been a problem area of differential diagnosis. Experience in our laboratory and others has clearly shown that, in the blood studies, the problems are different from other areas of diagnostic cancer cytology. In 1961 the Diagnostic Research Branch of the National Cancer Institute initiated correspondence with senior investigators in this country who were active in the study of circulating tumour cells, and who were willing to meet in order to exchange information. In early 1962 a circulating cancer cell cooperative (CCCC) was formed. Those senior investigators with the authority to sign out diagnostic cancer cytology in their respective laboratories focused attention on the nature of the criteria used, and to be used, for identifying cells in peripheral blood as malignant. In a report of this cooperative, attention is brought to "those cells that have or could provide pitfalls in diagnosis, particularly magakaryocptes, endothelial cells, and young cells of the blood series" (Nadel et al., 1965).

Importance of Cancer Cells in the Blood to Prognosis and Treatment

Five- to Ten-Year Survival Studies. When all 767 cancer patients were considered, a total of 94 patients were alive five to ten years later. Only seven per cent of these patients had positive blood samples, while 93% had negative blood samples. Again, in all patients, there was no difference in the five- to ten-years survival when considered by positive or negative blood samples, i.e., 13% versus 12% (Table 1). Likewise, the 242 patients classified as "curable" showed no difference in the five- to ten-year survival according to the positive or negative blood samples, being 32% for both categories (Table 2). In the 205 patients studied before, during, and after operation, the survival rate for those patients with blood samples which became positive during or after operation was 8% compared to a 16% survival rate for those patients with a negative blood samples. The survival rate for patients with ovarian carcinoma was 9% for the 21 with negative blood samples; the one patient with positive blood samples did not survive.

The development of vascular metastases made no statistical difference in the total cancer patients by comparing positive and negative blood samples (Table 1). However, in the "curable" patients and the patients studied during operation, the development of blood-borne metastases was more than doubled in those patients with positive blood samples compared to those with negative blood samples (Tables 2 and 3).

Discussion. Although considerable data concerning cancer cells in the blood has accumulated in the past ten years, there have been very few reports concerning clinical survival studies. ENGELL, in 1959, reported the five- to nine-year follow-up of 125 cancer patients. Cancer cells were found in either the peripheral or regional blood samples in 61% of these patients, most of whom had an operation for an intestional-tract cancer. Of the 55 patients who survived more than five years, one half (51%) had cancer cells in the blood samples at the time of operation. ENGELL, therefore, concluded that the demonstration of cancer cells in the blood had very little prognostic significance. WATNE and associates (1960) reported an 18-month follow-up study of 817 patients with

various stages of cancer after palliative or curative types of surgery. The survival rate was 54% for the 57 patients who had cancer cells in the circulating blood compared to 71% for those patients with negative blood samples. This decreased survival rate was most apparent in patients with carcinoma of the stomach, rectum, urinary tract, reproductive organs, sarcoma and melanoma. The decreased survival rate was apparent in patients with carcinoma of the esophagus, breast or lung.

There are several possible explanations for the similar survival rates of the 767 cancer patients with positive or negative blood samples reported from our laboratory. As mentioned previously, this patient material does not represent consecutive admissions to the hospital, but rather a highly selected group. Because of the time and personnel required to process completely each blood sample (four to six hours), the study was initially limited to those patients who were thought to have a possibility of circulating cancer cells. The high degree of selection of patients in this series is reflected in the very low over-all five- to ten-year survival rate of 12—13%. Although 242 patients were classified as having so called "curable" lesions, very few of these patients had a small early tumour. It is also quite probable that many patients with blood samples interpretated as negative did in fact have cancer cells in the blood stream which were either too few to be isolated or were lost during processing of the blood sample. The fact that 212 (30%) patients with *negative blood samples* in the entire group of 767 patients developed vascular metastatic disease supports this hypothesis.

The decreased survival rate of patients with previously negative blood samples which became positive during or after operation is to be expected from experimental data. The number of "tumour" takes in the lungs of animals has been shown to be directly proportional to the number of cancer cells injected intravenously. Also, there is good experimental evidence that animals subjected to celiotomy will have increased "tumour" takes compared to normal control animals subjected only to anesthesia. Accordingly, a shower of cancer cells during operation may well occur at a time when the natural "host resistance" of the patient may be reduced because of operative stress. Of particular interest in this regard is the patient with ovarian carcinoma illustrated in Figs. 1 and 2 who had a shower of cancer cells detectable in the peripheral blood within minutes after inadvertent rupture of the tumour during pelvic examination under anesthesia. When this patient died eleven months after operation of locally recurrent ovarian carcinoma, there was no clinical evidence of blood-borne metastases in the liver or lungs, although no autopsy was performed.

Summary

Dissemination of cancer by vascular channels has been presented in sequence of four phases including 1) entrance, 2) transportation, 3) lodgment and 4) fate, which is either death or survival of the embolic cells. Seven per cent of 767 cancer patients, studied more than five and many as long as ten years ago in our laboratory, had positive blood samples. A similar frequency of positive blood samples was obtained when only those patients considered "curable" were tabulated, or those patients studied before, during and after operation. The survival rate in the entire group of 767 patients was not different with regard to positive or negative blood samples, being 13 and 12 per cent respectively. The survival rate of "curable" patients with positive blood samples was no different than for those with negative blood samples, being 32 per cent for each category.

Although there was no apparent difference in the five- to ten-year survival rates of all 767 cancer patients, regardless of whether the blood samples were positive or negative, a definite trend was apparent in the *decreased survival of patients with a shower of circulating cancer cells during* or *after operation*. Only two of 23 patients (8%) with showers of cancer cells demonstrated *during operation* were alive and well five- to ten-years postoperatively, compared to a 16 per cent survival (26 of 182) of patients with negative blood samples at all times before, during, and after operation. Also, vascular metastases developed in 39 per cent of those patients with showers of circulating cancer cells during operation as compared to only 18 per cent in those patients with all negative blood samples.

As to the patients with ovarian carcinoma, 10 per cent of the 21 with negative blood samples survived five to ten years while the single patient with positive blood samples obtained during pelvic examination and operation died 11 months postoperatively with locally recurrent ovarian carcinoma, but with no clinical evidence of blood-borne metastases in the lungs or liver.

Discussion

J. Graham said that undoubtedly malignant cells can be found occasionally in the blood draining the area of the tumour or in the peripheral blood. He had collected blood from the uterine vein in a series of about one hundred patients with carcinoma of the uterine corpus, Stage I, Group I, and only one patient had malignant cells in the blood.

In this case, the preoperative evaluation was erroneous, because the patient had tumour in the parametrial area, as well as in the uterus. She died within a year of recurrent disease.

It was disappointing, he said, that there was no close correlation with prognosis, and little difference in the resting blood samples and those taken during operation. In his opinion, he said, the significance of finding cancer cells in the absence of demonstrable metastasis was that free cancer cells do not always produce metastasis and other factors influence their development.

DAVIDSOHN said that long before there was interest in the cells in the circulating blood, pathologists who tried to isolate cancer cells in tissue sections had the same difficulties as cytologists have at present in trying to identify the cells in the blood.

The problem of bone marrow embolism has been reported, DAVIDSOHN said, but there is another situation which has not yet been fully explained — bone marrow embolism not caused by trauma or neoplastic invasion. A fat embolism is the most common, possibly because many patients, particularly older persons, have considerable fat in the marrow or have acute hyperplasia such as occurs when a pernicious anemia patient is given liver therapy. Since the bone marrow is surrounded by a rigid capsule which does not permit expansion under pressure, intravasation of the fat or sometimes even bone marrow embolus occurs.

R. GRAHAM said that the investigation described by J. GRAHAM was made because of the suggestion that manipulation of the tumour during dilatation and curettage might force tumour cells into the blood stream. These patients had a dilatation and curettage within three weeks of the time that the blood was drawn from the uterine vein. She thought that the problem of identifying the cancer cells was one of technique, specifically the concentration technique.

DAVIDSOHN said that one cell which can be identified well in the peripheral blood is the megakaryocyte. These can be seen in the peripheral blood in myelofibrosis with sufficient frequency to arouse the suspicion of myelofibrosis when megakaryocytes are found in the peripheral blood.

LENZ said that Roberts' work emphasized the importance of how the tumour was removed. He had been impressed by reports that showers of tumour cells were found if the tumour was roughly manipulated. In the Radiumhemmet experience, he said, patients who had ovarian cancer with fixed adhesions or any condition which required rough manipulation for removal died within 20 months.

SCULLY inquired of the Grahams if any conclusion was reached about the danger of dilatation and curettage. He had often seen thrombosed blood vessels in pathological specimens after dilatation and curettage, he said, and he wondered how many tumour cells were introduced into the blood stream in this way and how many tumour cells were pushed through the Fallopian tube to implant possibly on the peritoneum.

R. GRAHAM said that the patients were all Stage I, Group 1 corpus carcinoma, which meant that the disease was confined to the uterus. Since only one case had malignant cells, the conclusion was that the dilatation and curettage was not as dangerous as had been thought.

GENTIL asked ROBERTS how he would interpret the mechanism of metastases formation since (1) patients who had "a shower of cancer cells" during operation had a higher incidence of vascular metastases and a lower survival rate, (2) the peripheral blood usually contained a much smaller incidence of cancer cells as compared to that in the regional circulation, (3) the number of circulating cancer cells going into the hepatic and pulmonary circulation is much larger than the number of those coming out of these two organs. How could these phenomena be interpreted, he asked, and was there any correlation between these and the development of metastases. He also asked what Roberts' opinion was about the effect of chemotherapy at the time of operation — the action of drugs in preventing circulating cancer cells from forming clumps which eventually might form a metastasis.

ROBERTS said that he agreed that concentration was the key to the problem, and added that now a method had been developed by which 95 per cent of the cells can be recovered. In 715 patients, he said, seven per cent of the samples were "positive" and 93 per cent were "negative." Thirty per cent (212) of these patients developed blood-borne metastases. This discrepancy results possibly from a difference in time when the blood samples were done, or an inadequate sample, because 10 cc. is an insignificant percentage of a blood volume of 5,000 cc.

As to pathogenesis, he referred his audience to Sumner Woods' *in vivo* studies of the ear chamber and the mesentery chamber of rabbits; these studies showed that in the arterial or capillary vein, an important but not invariable finding is the firm adherence of the tumour cells to the capillary endothelium with the surrounding intravascular thrombus formation. Woods' experiments showed that within two hours the tumour cell could be in the extravascular position by passing through actual defects created by white cells that

would migrate or emigrate through the walls. He anticipated, he said, that probably a time period of from several days to weeks was required for intravascular proliferation and a break through the wall would occur.

These observations have significance in chemotherapy, Roberts said. KINSEY reported that no tumour cells were present in the extravascular position in what appeared to be an abortive attempt at metastasis formation and that was certainly true in the intravascular position, particularly when there was no firm adherence to the endothelial wall. He thought that probably what did happen was that these tumour cells formed a firm adherence to each wall of the blood vessel and then migrated, perhaps in as little as two hours. Therefore, timing was important in adjuvant chemotherapy, and drugs given in the recovery room would be given too late to prevent metastases formation.

The idea is appealing, he said, that a drug could be given at a time when the cells which might cause metastases could be attacked cytologically in the intravascular position. Once the cells are in the extravascular position, there is less chance of prevention. Eventually, it will be evident that certain things can be done with surgery or with irradiation, with or without chemotherapy, in various combinations, so that by these various combinations, the survival rate will be increased.

The cytologic criteria are now solid, ROBERTS said, and when a competent cytologist made a diagnosis of Class IV in any type of fluid, tumour was present.

He wished to emphasize, ROBERTS said, that although the study of tumour cells in the circulating blood provided interesting research, it should not affect the clinical management of the patient. The circulating cancer cell cooperative study members had cautioned physicians that curative therapy should not be withheld or treatment changed because of the presence or absence of cancer cells in the blood. He had not withheld curative therapy because tumour cells were present. The two applications which had been made in his own institution were to avoid manipulation with soap and water during preparation for surgery and to attempt to tie off the veins early.

Acknowledgements

Supported by a Grant from USPHS, 9594.

References

ENGELL, H. C., Cancer cells in the blood; a five to nine year follow-up study. *Ann. Surg.* **149**, 451 (1959).

GOLDBLATT, S., and NADEL, E. M., Cancer cells in the circulating blood: A critical review. *Acta cytol. (Philad.)* **9**, 6 (1965).

LONG, L., ROBERTS, S., McGRATH, R., and McGREW, E., Simplified technique for separation of cancer cells from blood. *J. Amer. med. Ass.* **170**, 1785 (1959).

McGRATH, R., VALITIS, J., McCREW, E. and S., Separation of cancer cells from blood by differential filtration. In preparation.

ROMSDAHL, M. M., CHU, E. W., HUME, R., and SOUTH, R., Method for cytological detection of tumor cells in vitro. *J. Amer. med. Ass.* **26**, 19 (1961).

ROBERTS, S., Vascular dissemination of cancer, in COLE, W., McDONALD, G., ROBERTS, S., and SOUTHWICK, H., *Dissemination of cancer, prevention and therapy,* p. 61. New York: Appleton-Century-Crafts, Inc. 1961.

— WATNE, A., McGRATH, R., McGREW, E., and COLE, W. H., Technique and results of isolation of cancer cells from circulating blood. *Arch. Surg.,* **76**, 334 (1958).

WATNE, A. L., SANBERG, A. A., and MOORE, G. E., Prognostic implications of tumor cells in the blood. *Cancer Res.* **3**, 160 (1960).

WOOD, S., Pathogenesis of metastases formation observed *in vivo* in the rabbit ear chamber. *Arch. Path.* **66**, 550 (1958).

YOUNG, J. S., and GRIFFITH, H. D., The dynamics of parenchymatous embolism in relation to the dissemination of malignant tumors. *J. Path. Bact.* **62**, 293 (1950).

Clinical Staging in Ovarian Carcinoma

H. L. KOTTMEIER, M. D.

Professor of Gynecology, Radiumhemmet, Stockholm, Sweden

Introduction

Evaluation of treatment methods is possible only by comparing therapeutic results. Consequently, it is of vital importance that international agreement is reached on nomenclature and on a uniform staging of all cases of ovarian cancer. The purpose of clinical staging is to facilitate the accurate, concise description of the apparent extent of the neoplasm.

Clinical staging implies an estimate of the anatomic extent of growth on careful clinical examination prior to the application of therapy. The clinical staging should not consider findings made after treatment or after microscopic examination of operative specimens. Often, however, it is impossible to form an opinion as to the nature of an ovarian mass by clinical examination. Laparoscopy, needle biopsy and cul-de-sac aspiration (GRAHAM *et al.*, 1964; RUBIN and FROST, 1963) may assist in the determination of the nature of the growth but are, in our experience, unreliable. Therefore, the clinical staging should be based on clinical examination and on findings at laparotomy. However, surgical exploration may not be performed in all cases. This occurred in 7.5 per cent of the Radiumhemmet series and in 6 per cent of the cases reported by MUNNELL and TAYLOR (1949). Although such cases cannot be accurately staged, it is important to report them.

Several methods of clinical staging have been developed. HEYMAN (1930), HELSEL (1946), MONTGOMERY (1948) and others based the staging on operability criteria while DAVIS *et al.* (1956), MUNNELL and TAYLOR (1949), RANDALL (1955), PEARSE and BEHRMAN (1954) and others determined the stage in regard to the anatomic extent. Munnell and Taylor's proposal has been used by many authors. Their criteria for staging were
— Stage I, one ovary only involved; Stage II, both ovaries involved; Stage III, extension to pelvic peritoneum and/or pelvic viscera; Stage IV, extension to abdominal peritoneum and/or viscera. A different staging has been proposed by the Mayo Clinic (TURNER, 1957). To Stage I are allotted only cases with intracystic excrescenses; cases with extracystic excrescenses are defined as Stage II irrespective of whether they involve one or both ovaries, tubes or uterus. According to the Radiumhemmet experience, staging based on the presence of extracystic excrescences can be carried out only if many sections are taken from the ovary.

The International Federation of Gynecology and Obstetrics adopted, in 1964 (KOTTMEIER, 1966), a clinical staging as follows:

Stage I: Growth limited to the ovaries.

Stage Ia: Growth limited to one ovary, no ascites.

Stage Ib: Growth limited to both ovaries, no ascites.

Stage Ic: Growth limited to one or both ovaries, ascites present with malignant cells in the fluid.

Stage II: Growth involving one or both ovaries with pelvic extension.

Stage IIa: Extension and/or metastases to the uterus and/or tubes only.

Stage IIb: Extension to other pelvic tissues.

Stage III: Growth involving one or both ovaries with widespread intraperitoneal metastases to the abdomen.

Stage IV: Growth involving one or both ovaries with distant metastases outside the peritoneal cavity.

Special category: Unexplored cases which are thought to be ovarian carcinoma.

Material and Methods

To determine the prognostic significance of the anatomic extent of the carcinoma, all cases of ovarian carcinoma treated at the Radiumhemmet in the years 1958 through 1962 have been reviewed. Ninehundred and thirty-one patients have been followed up for 3 or more years and 720 patients for at least 5 years.

A series of ovarian carcinomas has a limited value in assessing results if cases of low potential malignancy, sometimes referred to as possibly malignant neoplasms, are not reported separately. These tumours, as well as obvious carcinomas, give rise to ascites and metastases. Histologically the epithelium and the epithelial cells of the low potential malignant neoplasms resemble those of real carcinomas, but evidence of infiltrative destructive growth in the more or less abundant stroma of the possibly malignant tumour cannot be found. The prognosis is different in these two types of epithelial neoplasms. Unfortunately,

many clinicians do not realize this fact; consequently there is great variation in the end results presented from different institutions. Although this observation is not really a matter for the present discussion, it is important and cannot be kept separate from the discussion of clinical classification. In the Radiumhemmet series of 720 cases followed for five years and 931 cases of ovarian carcinoma followed for three years, 599 and 775 cases respectively are real carcinomas. Further discussion will be restricted to these cases.

Results and Discussion

Ovarian Carcinoma with Microscopic Verification. To elucidate the prognostic significance of anatomic spread, cases are divided with regard to the findings on surgical exploration and to the presence of ascites, in accordance with the definitions proposed by the Federation. A growth fixed by firm adhesions to surrounding tissues has been considered as incompletely removed, provided microscopic examination of the tumour demonstrated extracapsular extension of the cancer. The histologic type of the growth has not been considered in the following discussion:

Growth Limited to One Ovary. (No ascites. Stage Ia. 90 cases treated 5 years and 105 treated 3 years previously.) The survival rates amount to 65.6 and 73.3 per cent respectively. Extracystic excrescences have been described in a few of these cases. There is nothing to prove that the presence of extracystic excrescences has affected the outcome.

Growth Limited to Both Ovaries. (No ascites. Stage Ib. 11 cases treated 5 and 19 treated 3 years previously.) The survival rates are 36.4 and 52.6 per cent respectively.

Growth Limited to One or Both Ovaries. (Ascites present. Stage Ic. 26 cases treated 5 and 34 patients 3 years previously.) The survival rates are 50 and 64.7 per cent respectively. With regard to the unilaterality or bilaterality of the tumour, the 5-year survival rate for unilateral growth is 52.1 per cent and for bilateral tumours 42.8 per cent. The corresponding 3-year survival rates are 66.7 and 60 per cent.

implants to pelvic tissues. A growth was considered incompletely removed if it was fixed to surrounding tissues by firm adhesions and microscopic examination showed extracapsular extension. Possibly cases with varying degree of malignancy have been allotted to this stage even though attention is drawn only to the anatomic extent of the growth. There-

Table I. *5-year and 3-year survival rates in cases of ovarian carcinoma with extension to other pelvic tissues than the uterus and/or tubes only*
Stage II b

Type of lesion	Cases treated			
	5 years ago		3 years ago	
	No. of cases	Survival rate	No. of cases	Survival rate
Primary tumour fixed (unilat.)	81	53.1	102	67.6
No metastases (bilat.)	30	16.7	39	35.9
Primary tumour movable (unilat.)	15	53.3	21	61.9
Metatstases present (bilat.)	20	35.0	26	46.2
Primary tumour fixed (unilat.)	18	33.3	30	30.0
Metastases present (bilat.)	17	11.8	30	26.7
Total	181	39.2	248	50.4

Growth Limited to One or Both Ovaries. Extension to the Uterus and/or Tubes Only. (Stage II a. 34 cases treated 5 years and 34 patients treated 3 years previously.) The survival rates are 61.8 and 85.3 per cent respectively. Bilateral tumours were seen in 5 cases. Two patients survived 5 years; 5 survived for 3 years. Ascites was found in only three instances. Two of these three patients survived more than 5 years.

Growth Involving One or Both Ovaries with Extension to Other Pelvic Tissues. (Stage II b, 181 cases treated 5 years and 248 patients treated 3 years previously.) The survival rates amount to 39.2 and 50.4 per cent respectively. This series includes patients with completely and incompletely removed primary tumours, as well as cases with or without metastatic

fore, the cases have been divided with regard to the fixation of the tumour and the presence of metastases (Table I).

Table I demonstrates that a growth involving both ovaries has a poorer prognosis than a unilateral one. This fact is in accordance with the corresponding results obtained in cases of carcinoma limited to the ovaries (Stage I). Furthermore, the survival rate is the same whether the growth is fixed to surrounding structures without visible metastases or is movable and metastases are present.

The records state that ascites was found in 44 and 67 respectively of the 181 and 248 cases. The 5-year survival rate in these cases amounts to 36.4 per cent, the 3-year survival rate to 44.8 per cent. Ascites evidently does not have a deleterious effect on the prognosis.

Metastasis to the uterus was diagnosed in 27 (14.9 per cent) and 44 (17.9 per cent) respectively of the cases followed up for 5 and 3 years. The survival rate in these cases was 44.4 and 54.5 per cent respectively.

Growth Involving One or Both Ovaries with Widespread Intraperitoneal Metastases to the Abdomen. Stage III. (169 cases treated 5 years, 218 cases 3 years ago.) The

Special Category: Unexplored Cases which are Thought to be Ovarian Carcinoma. (44 cases traced at least 5 years and 58 cases traced 3 or more years.) Excluded were 4 patients with an ovarian mass clinically considered to be malignant but who are symptom free 5 years after treatment.

All cases of true ovarian carcinoma treated at the Radiumhemmet in the

Table II. *5-year and 3-year survival rates in cases of ovarian carcinoma with widespread intraperitoneal metastases*

Type of lesion	Cases treated			
	5 years ago		3 years ago	
	No. of cases	Survival rate	No. of cases	Survival rate
Primary tumour (unilat.)	13	2	14	3
Movable (bilat.)	44	1	54	6
Primary tumour (unilat.)	26	2	30	4
Fixed (bilat.)	86	1	120	3
Total	169 *	6 = 3.6%	218 *	16 = 7.3%

* Metastases to the uterus diagnosed in 12 and 15 respectively of the 169 and 218 cases of Stage III. Three of the 12 patients with intrauterine metastases survived 5 years.

survival rates are 3.6 and 7.3 per cent respectively. The difference in the survival rate is striking between cases in which the carcinoma had extended beyond the ovaries, but is still limited to the pelvis and those with cancer extending into the upper abdomen. The cases allotted to Stage III have been studied with regard to the status of the primary growth (Table II). It does not seem to make any difference whether the growth is movable or fixed. Again, bilateral tumours show poorer prognosis.

Growth Involving One or Both Ovaries with Metastases Outside the Peritoneal Cavity. Stage IV. (44 cases treated 5 years and 59 cases treated 3 years previously.) Four patients have survived 3 years. Metastases to the uterus were diagnosed in 3 cases.

years 1958 through 1962 are shown in Table III.

The study of a series of true ovarian carcinomas has demonstrated a good correlation between the increasing anatomic extent of the disease, as it is reflected in the clinical staging, and the survival rate. Carcinomatous involvment of both ovaries signifies a rather poor outcome, at least if the survival rate is compared with that in cases of unilateral growth. The presence of ascites does not affect the survival rate. The present investigation supports the original proposal by the Cancer Committee of the Federation that the presence of ascites should not influence the staging. A further interesting observation is that extension of the carcinoma to the uterus does not seem to affect the prognosis in the Radium-hemmet series.

I have pointed out that the clinical staging adopted by the Federation of Gynecology and Obstetrics considers the anatomical extent of the disease but does not always keep cases with metastases separate.

The International Union against Cancer has adopted a technique of descrip-

TP3. Tumour extending into the uterus or Fallopian tubes.
TP4. Tumour extending to other surrounding anatomical structures.
Note. No regard is paid to the presence of ascites.
N.   Regional Lymph Nodes
NX. As it is impossible to assess the pelvic lymph nodes, NX will be used permitting eventual addition

Table III. *Ovarian carcinoma treated in the years 1958 through 1962. A presentation of the cases with regard to anatomical extent of the growth*

Stage	Cases treated 5 years ago			Cases treated 3 years ago		
	No. of cases	5-year survivals		No. of cases	3-year survivals	
		No. of cases	Per cent		No. of cases	Per cent
Ia	90	59	65.6	105	77	73.3
Ib	11	4	36.4	19	10	52.6
Ic	26	13	50.0	34	22	64.7
IIa	34	21	61.8	34	29	85.3
IIb	181	71	39.2	248	125	50.4
III	169	6	3.6	218	16	7.3
IV	44			59	4	6.8
Special category	44			58		
Total	599	174	29.1	775	283	36.5

tion and clinical classification that involves three symbols:

T = extent of primary tumour;
N = condition of regional lymph nodes;
M = distant metastases.

The T classification, which is based as a rule on simple clinical examination, is inappropriate. Accordingly TP, which takes into account the findings at operation, should be used. The Committee on Clinical Stage and Classification of the International Union has proposed a classification of the ovarian cancer as follows:

TP-Extent of Primary Tumour

TP1. Tumour involving one ovary which remains mobile.
TP2. Tumour involving both ovaries, both of which remain mobile.

of histological information thus: NX— or NX+.
M.   Distant Metastases
M0. No distant metastases.
M1. Implantation or metastases are present.
   M1a. In the true pelvis only.
   M1b. Within the peritoneal cavity including the omentum, small intestine, mesentery, liver or other viscera.
   M1c. Outside the peritoneal cavity.

This classification makes it possible to designate precisely by number the extent of the disease. An attempt was made to classify the 775 cases of ovarian carcinoma in accordance with the T.N.M. system.

Table IV demonstrates that it is evidently the extent of metastases which determines the prognosis.

At the beginning, I stated that the purpose of this paper was to discuss the significance of the clinical staging of true ovarian carcinoma disregarding the histopathologic type of the tumour. SAN-

information for an estimate of prognosis and planning of therapy. The conclusions, however, that can be drawn from this table may be misleading since the cases have not been divided in regard to the histopathologic type of the growth. Such an investigation will be seen in Tables V and VI.

Table IV. *Ovarian carcinoma treated in the years 1958 through 1962 classified in accordance with the T.N.M. system*

Classification	Cases followed up for			
	5 years		3 years	
	No. of cases	Survival rate	No. of cases	Survival rate
TP 1 NX M 0	109	63.3	129	72.1
TP 2 NX M 0	18	38.9	29	55.2
TP 3 NX M 0	34	61.8	35	82.9
TP 4 NX M 0	111	43.2	141	58.9
TP 1 NX M 1 a	12	50.0	16	56.3
TP 2 NX M 1 a	19	36.8	25	44.0
TP 3 NX M 1 a	4	50.0	5	80.0
TP 4 NX M 1 a	35	22.8	60	28.3
TP 1 NX M 1 b	13	15.4	14	21.3
TP 2 NX M 1 b	40	—	49	10.2
TP 3 NX M 1 b	4	25.0	5	20.0
TP 4 NX M 1 b	112	8.7	150	4.7
TP 1 NX M 1 c	1	—	2	50.0
TP 2 NX M 1 c	9	—	9	—
TP 4 NX M 1 c	34	—	48	6.0
Total	555		717	

TESSON has, among others, emphasized the importance of classifying ovarian carcinoma in regard to the histologic type of the lesion and he has called special attention to carcinomas that are similar to the adenocarcinoma of the endometrium. This tumour has been termed endometrioid carcinoma in the histopathological grouping of epithelial ovarian tumours proposed by the International Federation of Gynecology and Obstetrics. In Table III, the cases of true ovarian carcinoma were staged clinically in regard to the anatomical extent of the growth. This table affords valuable

Table V demonstrates clearly that the over-all survival rate is much better in cases of mucinous and endometrioid carcinomas than in cases of serous tumours. There are several reasons for this fact. Although I do not intend to discuss them in detail, I will refer to the faster growth and greater tendency to metastasize of the serous carcinomas in comparison with the mucinous and endometrioid tumours (Tables V and VI).

Of the serous carcinomas, only 19.9 per cent were allotted to Stage I and II a; 26.8 per cent to Stage II b; 41.3 per cent to Stage III, and 12 per cent to Stage IV.

The corresponding figures in mucinous cases were 58.8 per cent in Stage I and IIa; 23.5 per cent in Stage IIb; and 17.6 per cent in Stage III. Of the endometrioid carcinomas, on the other hand, formation. Forty of 194 patients with serous carcinoma (20.6 per cent) that had spread to pelvic or intraperitoneal tissues are living after 5 years, while the corresponding figure for endometrioid tu-

Table V. *Ovarian carcinoma. Five-year follow-up. The cases are divided regarding the histo-pathological type of lesion and anatomical extent of disease*

| Stage | Histo-pathological type | | | | | | | |
| | Serous | | Mucinous | | Endometrioid | | Unclassified | |
	No. of cases	Survival rate	No. of cases	Survival rate	No. of cases	Survival rate	No. of cases	Survival rate
Ia	33	45.5	21	85.7	24	79.2	12	58.3
Ib	5	one case	2	one case	2	two cases	2	two cases
Ic	11	36.4	6	66.7	7	71.4	2	—
IIa	6	50.0	1	—	25	72.0	2	one case
IIb	74	21.6	12	58.3	81	55.6	14	21.4
III	114	1.8	9	—	24	16.7	22	—
IV	33	—	—	—	5	—	6	—
Total	276	14.8	51	62.7	168	55.4	60	21.7

Table VI. *Ovarian carcinoma. Five-year follow-up. Number of cases in various histo-pathological groups*

| Stage | Histo-pathological type | | | | | | | |
| | Serous | | Mucinous | | Endometrioid | | Unclassified | |
	No. of cases	Per cent	No. of cases	Per cent	No. of cases	Per cent	No. of cases	Per cent
Ia+Ib+ Ic+IIa	55	19.9	30	58.8	58	34.5	18	30.0
IIb	74	26.8	12	23.5	81	48.2	14	23.3
III	114	41.3	9	17.6	24	14.3	22	36.7
IV	33	12.0			5	3.0	6	10.0
Total	276	100.0	51	100.0	168	100.0	60	100.0

34.5 per cent were allotted to Stage I and IIa; 48.2 per cent to Stage IIb; 14.3 per cent to Stage III, and 3 per cent to Stage IV. These facts are significant prognostically and for the planning of therapy. Important also is the observation that patients with serous carcinomas have often had symptoms for only a short period of time. The analysis of the cases also permits other important in-

mours is 67 of 130 patients (51.3 per cent).

The conclusion to be drawn from the presentation of the Radiumhemmet series of true ovarian carcinoma, as far as clinical staging and classification are concerned, is that statistical analysis of the results of treatment of ovarian carcinoma demands a histo-pathological classification and a clinical staging regarding the anatomical extent of the growth. Staging of all cases must be done by the same method. The criteria proposed by the International Union against Cancer should be adopted. The staging recommended by the Internatio-

staging of malignant tumours, these proliferating ovarian neoplasms should be allotted to Stage 0 or be designed as TIS if the T.N.M. system is applied. The cases are presented in Table VII. The T.N.M. system has been suitable for

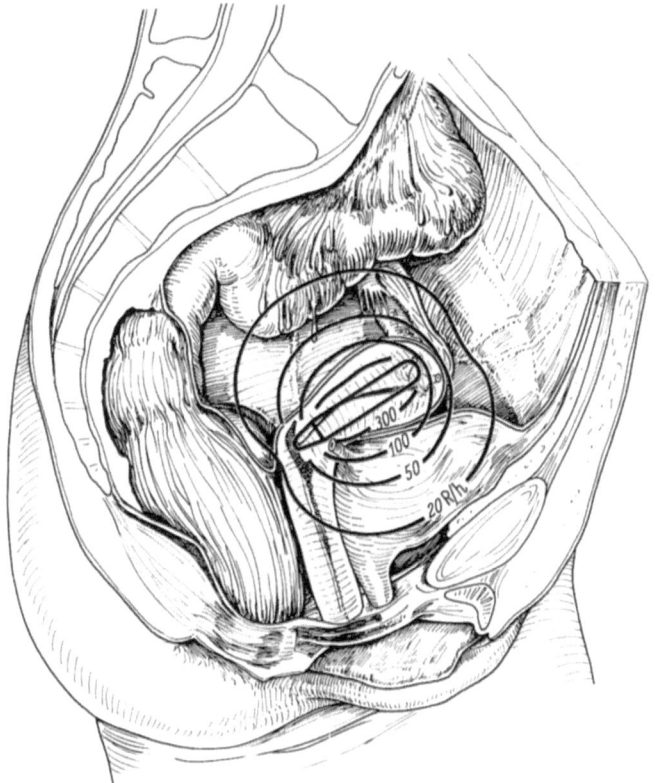

Fig. 1. Isodose curves of radium introduced into the uterine cavity

nal Federation of Gynecology and Obstetrics should be applied universally.

Ovarian Carcinoma of Low Potential malignancy. Earlier I drew attention to these tumours which may also be designated as "proliferating cystadenomas without stromal invasion". I pointed out the importance of separating these cases from the true invasive carcinomas though they may give rise to ascites and metastases. In accordance with the general rules accepted for classification and

these cases since metastases were found in the pelvis (M 1 a), the abdomen (M 1 b) and outside the abdominal cavity (M 1 c).

The review of 121 cases of low potential malignancy treated 5 years and 156 treated 3 years ago has shown that these tumours should be considered and treated as malignant neoplasms. However, the prognosis of these tumours is quite different from that in real carcinomas. Consequently, it is essential to separate these two types of carcinoma in statistics.

Summary

Although the term "clinical staging" implies an estimate of the anatomic extent of the neoplasm by careful clinical examination before the application of therapy, clinical staging for ovarian tumours should be based on both clinical examination and findings at laparotomy. The extent of ovarian disease cannot always be determined accurately by clinical examination alone. It is most important that a universally accepted method of staging be adopted so that therapeutic results can be compared. To examine the usefulness of the various classifications proposed, all Radiumhemmet ovarian cancer patients treated in the years 1958 through 1962 were staged according to anatomical extent as proposed by the International Federation of Obstetrics and Gynecology in 1964 and according to the T.N.M. system adopted by the Internatinal Union against Cancer. These patients were also staged according to the histopathologic type of the neoplasm and the extent of the disease. This latter method provides the most accurate information in regard to prognosis and treatment.

Table VII. *Ovarian carcinoma of low potential malignancy, treated in the years 1958 through 1962*

Classification	Cases followed-up for			
	5 years		3 years	
	No. of cases	Survival rate	No. of cases	Survival rate
TIS NX M 0	72	93.6	89	92.1
TIS NX M 1 a	27	88.9	38	92.1
TIS NX M 1 b	19	68.4	25	76.0
TIS NX M 1 c	3	66.7	4	75.0
Total	121	87.6	156	89.9

Discussion

RUTLEDGE listed three requirements for an international system of staging for carcinoma of the ovary: (1) simplicity, (2) close correlation between each stage and the progressive gravity of the prognosis and (3) applicability to the therapeutic problem. The classification presented by KOTTMEIER showed that the prognosis is poorer with disease outside the pelvis, with bilateral disease, local metastasis, and combinations of an adherent primary mass and local metastases, and also that there was correlation between the histologic type and prognosis.

KOTTMEIER had clarified several puzzling points in the system of staging proposed, RUTLEDGE said. For example, the primary mass is described as adherent if there is microscopic invasion of the tumour capsule. He had also demonstrated that papillary excrescences on the primary lesion were not important prognostically and that ascites is not always important. However, RUTLEDGE asked, would it be more informative if, instead of discounting ascites, it was required that the fluid be designated as malignant or benign? There were several other points to be clarified : (1) the importance of spillage and (2) whether small bowel or omentum adherent to the primary lesion in the pelvis represented pelvic or upper abdominal disease. He also inquired as to the significance of inguinal lymph node spread and mentioned that occasionally the only evidence of extra-abdominal spread would be disease in an inguinal node.

DAVIDSOHN asked whether it was true that chorioepithelioma or pseudomucinous carcinoma of the ovary regresses spontaneously more often than other types of tumours. He had also heard said that occasionally, when ascites is present, removal of the ovary is followed by regression of the ascites.

KOTTMEIER, in closing, remarked that many difficulties existed in the staging of ovarian carcinoma, but an agreement on histopathology, and to some extent on clinical staging, would represent a great advance. In reply to RUTLEDGE's question, he said that fixation of the small bowel and the omentum to the tumour in the pelvis represented tumour adherent to surrounding organs, not primary disease above the pelvis. When the omentum is fixed to the tumour, the classification should be Stage IIb, if there is no grossly detectable metastasis in the upper abdomen.

Others had also questioned the action of the Federation in not attaching prognostic significance to ascites, and eventually the Federation adopted the classification of Ic for ascites with malignant cells.

The natural history of the disease was important he agreed. The difference between the endometrioid and serous tumours he believed was the result of the natural history of the disease. However, many problems remain unsolved. He could not say definitely whether postoperative radiation had something to offer for those patients with the low potential malignant tumours. Most patients in his own series had been treated by radiation and, in general, good results had been obtained. In some instances marked radiation damage could be demonstrated. As to DAVIDSOHN's question, undoubtedly if the primary tumour was removed the metastasis sometimes disappeared. Also, if the primary lesion was removed, the ascites sometimes disappeared. He himself preferred to remove the omentum if there was a large mass present but only if a cancer-free margin of tissue could be obtained.

References

ALLAN, M. S., and HERTIG, A. T., Carcinoma of ovary. *Amer. Obstet. Gynec.* **58**, 640–653 (1949).

BUKA, N. J., and MACFARLANE, K. T., Malignant tumors of the ovary. *Amer. J. Obstet. Gynec.* **90**, 383—387 (1964).

COUNSELLER, V. S., Ovarian neoplasms. *Amer. J. Surg.* **49**, 284—289 (1940).

DAVIS, B. A., LATOUR, J. P. A., and PHILPOTT, N. W., Primary carcinoma of ovary. *Surg. Gynec. Obstet.* **102**, 565—573 (1956).

GEIST, S. H., *Ovarian tumors.* New York: Paul H. Hoeber 1942.

GRAHAM, J. B., GRAHAM, R. M., and SCHUELLER, E. F., Preclinical detection of ovarian cancer. *Cancer (Philad.)* **17**, 1414—1432 (1964).

HELSEL, F. V., Review of 100 cases of ovarian cancer. *Amer. J. Obstet. Gynec.* **52**, 435—439 (1946).

HERTIG, A. T., and GORE, H., *Tumors of the female sex organs,* sect. IX, fasc. 33, part. 3. Armed Forces Institute of Pathology, Washington, D. C. 1961.

HEYMAN, J., Die Strahlentherapie als vollständiger oder teilweiser Ersatz der Operation bei der Behandlung von Karzinomen des Uterus, der Vagina und der Ovarien. *Strahlentherapie* **37**, 254—265 (1930).

KENT, W., and MCKAY, D. G., Cancer of ovary: Analysis of 349 cases. *Amer. J. Obstet. Gynec.* **80**, 430—438 (1960).

KERR, H. D., and ELKINS, H. B., Carcinoma of the ovary. *Amer. J. Roentgenol.* **66**, 184—189 (1951).

KOTTMEIER, H. L., The classification and treatment of ovarian tumours. *Acta obstet. gynec. scand.* **31**, 313—363 (1952).

— The classification and clinical staging of carcinoma of the uterus and vagina. *J. int. Fed. Gynaec. Obstet.* **1**, 83—93 (1963).

— *Problems relating to classification and stage-grouping of malignant tumours in the female pelvis. Krebs-Dokumentation und Statistik maligner Tumoren* (G. WAGNER). Stuttgart: F. K. Schattauer 1966.

LONG, M. E., and TAYLOR jr., H. C., Endometrioid carcinoma of the ovary. *Amer. J. Obstet. Gynec.* **90**, 936—950 (1964).

MILLER, J., *Die Krankheiten des Eierstockes.* In: Handbuch der speziellen pathologischen Anatomie und Histologie von O. LUBARSCH u. F. HENKE, Bd. VII. Berlin: Springer 1937.

MONTGOMERY, J. B., Malignant tumors of the ovary. *Amer. J. Obstet. Gynec.* **55**, 201—217 (1948).

MUNNELL, E. W., JACOX, H. W., and TAYLOR jr., H. C., Treatment and prognosis in cancer of ovary: With review of new series of 143 cases treated in years 1944—51. *Amer. J. Obstet. Gynec.* **74**, 1187—1200 (1957).

—, and TAYLOR jr., H. C., Ovarian carcinoma: A review of 200 primary and 51 secondary cases. *Amer. J. Obstet. Gynec.* **58**, 943—959 (1949).

ORDEN, D. E. VAN, MCALLISTER, W. B., ZERNE, S. R. M., and McLEAN MORRIS, J., Ovarian carcinoma. The problems of staging and grading. *Amer. J. Obstet. Gynec.* **94**, 195—202 (1966).

PEARSE, W. H., and BEHRMAN, S. J., Carcinoma of the ovary. *Obstet. and Gynec.* **3**, 32—45 (1954).

PRIBRAM, E. E., Zur Pathologie und Therapie maligner Ovarialtumoren. *Z. Geburtsh. Gynäk.* **88**, 134—151 (1924).

PUROLA, E., Serous papillary ovarian tumours. A study of 233 cases with special reference to the histological type of tumour. *Acta obstet. gynec. scand.* **42**, Suppl. 3 (1963).

RANDALL, J. H., Treatment of ovarian carcinoma. Evaluation of results at State University of Iowa Hospitals. *Obstet. and Gynec.* **5**, 445—451 (1955).

RUBIN, D. K., and FROST, J. K., The cytologic detection of ovarian cancer. *Acta cytol. (Philad.)* **7**, 191—195 (1963).

SANTESSON, L., Personal communication.

SCHÄFER, P., Über Dauerheilung bei Ovarialkarzinomen. *Z. Geburtsh. Gynäk.* **85**, 613—624 (1922/23).

TAYLOR jr., H. C., The diagnosis and treatment of ovarian carcinoma. *Clin. Obstet. Gynec.* **1**, 1078 (1958).

— Studies in the clinical and biological evolution of adenocarcinoma of the ovary. *J. Obstet. Gynaec. Brit. Emp.* **66**, 827 (1959).

—, and LONG, M. E., Problems of cellular and tissue differentiation in papillary adenocarcinoma of the ovary. *Amer. J. Obstet. Gynec.* **70**, 753—765 (1955).

TURNER jr., J. C., REMINE, W. H., and DOCKERTY, M. B., A clinicopathologic study of 172 patients with primary carcinoma of the ovary. *Surg. Gynec. Obstet.* **109**, 198—206 (1959).

VARA, P., and PANKAMAA, P., A clinical-statistical investigation of ovarian tumours operated at the Helsinki University Clinic. *Acta obstet. gynec. scand.* **26**, Suppl. 4 (1946).

WALTER, R. I., BACHMAN, A. L., and HARRIS, W., The treatment of carcinoma of the ovary. *Amer. J. Roentgenol.* **5**, 403—411 (1941).

Surgical Management - Conservative Surgery

Indications According to the Type of the Tumour

H. L. KOTTMEIER, M. D.

Professor of Gynecology, Radiumhemmet, Stockholm, Sweden

Introduction

Surgery is the keystone in the treatment of ovarian carcinoma. In his brilliant way PARSONS (1962) has discussed the surgical approach. BRUNSCHWIG has described the value of superradical operations in another paper in this book. The question remains: is simple oophorectomy ever proper therapy?

Ovariau Tumours related to the Germinal Epithelium

Preservation of one Ovary. The primary problem when dealing with a unilateral encapsulated tumour in the young patient is to establish whether the growth is malignant. Frozen sections during the operation may help in the determination, but is, in our experience, an unreliable method. A simple unilateral oophorectomy is adequate therapy if the patient is young. There should be no hesitancy in performing a second operation for a patient conservatively treated in the belief that the ovarian tumour was benign if the tumour later proves to be malignant.

However, there might be cases of ovarian cancer in which preservation of the normal ovary could be considered justified. In this respect, the observation of MUNNELL and TAYLOR (1949) in 46 patients with a unilateral ovarian neoplasm is of interest. The uninvolved ovary was preserved in 23 cases, while a bilateral salpingo-oophorectomy had been performed for the other 23 patients. The 5-year survival rate for the two groups was essentially the same.

The tendency of malignant ovarian tumours to be bilateral has to be taken into consideration in the discussion as to whether it is justified to leave *in situ* an apparently uninvolved ovary. MILLER (1937) reported that of 1,791 cases of ovarian cancer, both ovaries were involved in 50.5 per cent. HEIMANN gives a figure of 21.9, KERMAUNER, of 36.2 and FRANKL (1920), of 36.8 per cent. Ovarian carcinoma is, however, a group of diseases, which is why an analysis of the cases with regard to the histo-genetic type is essential. Many authors have pointed out that both ovaries are affected more frequently in serous tumours than in mucinous tumours. PUROLA (1963) reported bilateralism in 42 of 77 cases of serous cystadenocarcinomas.

Material and Discussion

In the years 1958 through 1962, 718 cases of true ovarian carcinoma and 156 cases of proliferating tumours with no stromal invasion, so called carcinomas of low potential malignancy, have been treated at the Radiumhemmet. The cases in question have been tabulated regardig the to histo-genetic type and frequency of unilateral or bilateral tumours (Table I). In this respect it should be mentioned that all cases of carcinoma in which the growth is massive and wide-spread — at least throughout the pelvis — are classified as bilateral even was confined to the ovaries, the uterus and/or the tubes (Table II). This same fact holds valid for these cases, i.e. bilateralism occurring in 36 per cent of serous carcinomas, but only in 10 to 12 per cent of mucinous and endometrioid car-

Table I. *Frequence of unilateral and bilateral tumours in regard to the histogenetic type of the carcinoma*

	Total No. of cases	Unilateral No. of cases	Bilateral No. of cases	Per cent
True ovarian carcinoma				
Serous tumours: Ic	359	124	235	65.3
Mucinous tumours: IIc	59	48	11	18.7
Endometrioid tumours: IIIc	215	150	65	30.2
Unclassified tumours: IV	85	39	46	54.1
Total	718	361	357	49.7
Carcinomas of low potential malignancy				
Serous tumours: Ib	106	42	64	60.4
Mucinous tumours: IIb	48	37	11	22.9
Endometrioid tumours: IIIb	2	1	1	
Total	156	80	76	48.7

Table II. *Frequency of unilateral and bilateral tumours in regard to the histogenetic type of the carcinoma. Cases of carcinoma confined to the ovaries, the uterus and/or the tubes*

	Total No. of cases	Unilateral No. of cases	Bilateral No. of cases	Per cent
Serous	71	52	19	36.5
Mucinous	32	29	3	10.3
Endometrioid	71	62	9	12.7
Unclassified	19	15	4	26.7
Total	193	158	35	18.1

though, occasionally, the description in the records does not always furnish proof of this. Involvement of both ovaries was seen in more than 60 per cent of serous carcinomas, in about 20 per cent of mucinous and in 30 per cent of endometrioid neoplasms. Thus, the great tendency in ovarian carcinoma to be bilateral is why the preservation of one ovary is only exceptionally appropriate. Bilateral frequency was less common if account was taken only of cases in which the tumour

cinomas. As a consequence, re-operation with removal of the other ovary should be carried out — irrespective of the age of the patient — in all cases of unilateral serous ovarian carcinoma in which an apparently uninvolved ovary was not removed. This is important as in serous carcinomas an ovary of normal appearance may harbor a microscopic focus of cancer. Eight such cases were diagnosed at Radiumhemmet in 1940 to 1948.

Microscopic foci of cancer in an apparently normal ovary, however, have not been observed in any cases of mucinous or endometrioid tumours. The tendency of these neoplasms to be bilateral is evidently less common than that of serous tumours. This is why it may be adequate to leave the normal ovary if the patient is young and wants to have children. This demands, however, that

ovaries. The Radiumhemmet has, for several years, advocated leaving the uterus in order to apply radium into the uterine cavity following the removal of the anexa. In this manner it is possible to apply a rather heavy dose of radiation to the area of the pelvis, where metastases or recurrences from ovarian carcinoma are most frequently seen. MAYER (1926), HEINRICHS (1899) and ABT (1946)

Table III. *Extension of ovarian carcinoma to the endometrium. Survival rate*

Ovarian carcinoma	No. of cases	Living after 5 years	
		No. of cases	Per cent
All cases	555	174	31.4
Cases with carcinomatous infiltration of the endometrium	76	31	40.8
Cases of endometrioid type	168	93	55.3
Cases of endometrioid type with cancer in the endometrium	61	27	44.3
Cases of carcinoma limited to one or both ovaries	127	76	59.8
Cases of carcinoma limited to one or both ovaries with extension to the uterus	33	22	66.7
Cases of endometrioid carcinoma limited to one or both ovaries	33	26	78.8
Cases of endometrioid carcinoma limited to one or both ovaries with extension to the uterus	25	18	72.0

the patient be kept under observation for many years. This conservatism in treatment is applicable also to unilateral neoplasms of low potential malignancy, as in the experience of HERTIG of the Radiumhemmet and others, such a growth will rarely develop into a true carcinoma. In recent years several cases of unilateral carcinoma of low potential malignancy, with metastases to the peritoneum, have been treated successfully by unilateral oophorectomy and supervoltage radiation therapy. No radiation therapy was given to the ovary left *in situ*. Three such patients have given birth to healthy children.

Preservation of the Uterus. Clinicians stress usually that the principal treatment of cancer of the ovary is total hysterectomy with removal of both tubes and

have demonstrated that metastases occur foremost in the posterior and anterior cul-de-sac. The contribution of the uterine source of radiation to these areas cannot be neglected. It is true that metastases to the uterus occur in ovarian carcinoma, especially in cases of endometrioid tumours. LYNCH and DOCKERTY (1945) report a 6 per cent involvement of the endometrium in patients with cancer of the ovary. The material of the Radiumhemmet in respect of carcinomatous involvement of the endometrium is presented in Table III. Extension to the uterus was diagnosed in 76 of 555 cases of true ovarian carcinoma (13.7 per cent). Thirty-one of these patients survived for 5 years, i.e. 40.8 per cent. The cancer was of endometrioid type in 61 of 76 cases. Twenty-seven of

these 61 cases survived for 5 years, i.e.
44.3 per cent. Carcinomatous involvement
of the endometrium was diagnosed in
33 cases in which the primary growth
was otherwise limited to one or both
ovaries (33.8 per cent). Twenty-two of
these 33 patients survived for 5 years,
i.e. 66.7 per cent. The cancer was of the
endometrioid type in 25 of 33 cases.
Eighteen of these 25 patients survived
for 5 years, i.e. 72.0 per cent.

Thus, the interesting observation is
made that, provided radium is applied in-
tracavitarily and the dosage given is adequate, the survival rate is not influenced
by the extension of the cancer to the endometrium. A 5-year survival rate of 61.3
per cent was attained in 119 cases of
carcinoma restricted to one or both
ovaries in which the uterus was left *in
situ*. In 6 of 46 patients who died from
the cancer, the first sign of recurrence
was in the pelvis.

A panhysterectomy had been performed in 8 similar cases. Three of these
8 patients survived for 5 years. The
initial recurrence appeared in the pelvis
in 4 cases. These results were achieved
at the Radiumhemmet in the years when
an external treatment was given only by
conventional x-ray therapy. I admit that
supervoltage radiation has improved our
facilities for application of cancericidal
doses to the entire pelvis. Yet I consider
the application of radium into the uterine
cavity of value in cases of ovarian carcinoma restricted to pelvic tissues.

Dysgerminoma is the most common
germ cell tumour. The material of
the Radiumhemmet is composed of 60 patients treated in the years 1921 through
1959. Dysgerminoma is a tumour that
is seen especially in women less than
40 years of age. Sixteen patients were
less than 20 years old; 30 patients were
between the ages of 20 and 29 years.
Involvement of both ovaries was seen in

7 of 60 cases. This tumour is obviously
malignant and has a strong tendency to
metastasize and to recur. Opinions differ
as to the best treatment for dysgerminoma. Bilateral salpingo-oophorectomy
and hysterectomy are considered as adequate therapy by some authors, while
others prefer to restrict the operation to
unilateral oophorectomy if only one
ovary is involved by the growth. PEDO-
WITZ *et al.* (1955) have collected a series
of 102 cases treated exclusively by surgery. The 5-year cure rate is 27.1 per cent.

At the Radiumhemmet we have chosen a combined treatment of surgery and
irradiation with small doses in all cases
of dysgerminoma. The operation is restricted to a unilateral oophorectomy in
cases of a unilateral growth. Radiation
is directed towards the area of retroperitoneal lymph nodes. Forty-four of the
60 patients, i.e. 73.3 per cent, treated are
living 5 years after initial therapy. Four
of 12 cases with extensive metastases
above the pelvis were cured. In 19 patients no irradiation was directed towards
the normal ovary. Eleven of these 19 patients have given birth to healthy children.

Functioning Tumours. Granulosa cell
tumour is the most common functioning
neoplasm. Most granulosa cell tumours
are potentially malignant. SANTESSON,
among others, has stressed the importance of separating the undifferentiated
sarcomatous granulosa cell tumour from
the folliculoid and the cylindroid types,
as the former is undoubtedly more
malignant than the others. The rate of
growth is apt to be slow. Many times
recurrences do not occur until 10 to
20 years after initial therapy. Recurrences
have developed in 18.5 per cent of folliculoid and cylindroid tumours and in
70 per cent of sarcomatoid lesions treated
10 to 20 years earlier. Bilateral tumours
are rare. A conservative operation with

removal of the involved ovary is the treatment of choice in patients less than 40 years of age with functioning ovarian tumours.

Summary

The use of conservative surgery in the treatment of malignant ovarian tu-mours in young women is discussed. The author considers conservative sur-gical intervention indicated in cases of mucinous and endometrioid carcinoma, as well as in cases of tumours of low potential malignancy, dysgerminomas and granulosa cell tumours.

Discussion

RUTLEDGE commented that KOTT-MEIER's new statistics showing that con-servative management was permissible for some patients with unilateral ovarian disease of certain histologic types were reassuring. Former statistics were based largely on patients with advanced dis-ease, and it was important that new statistics on early cases showed that the disease is not always bilateral, parti-cularly in the mucinous tumours. How-ever, he added, the frequency of bilateral disease is still an important factor in the management of the serous and unclassi-fied adenocarcinomatous groups.

Intracavitary radium in the retained uterus is not often used at the University of Texas M. D. Anderson Hospital and Tumour Institute, he said. This method meant that radiation could be given to the cul-de-sac area and metastasis to this site may be controlled by intracavitary radium.

The special tumours, the dysgermi-nomas and the granulosa cell tumours, do have certain characteristics that make conservative management possible. Se-venty-five per cent of the dysgermino-mas, for example, are estimated to be unilateral. Recurrence develops within the first year in about 75 per cent of the patients treated. The microscopic pattern is also helpful in planning treatment. Teratomatous and choriomatous elements are more serious. Age also is a factor in the choice of therapy.

The granulosa cell tumours are also frequently unilateral and metastasis to the uterus is unusual. These lesions evolve slowly so that repeated opera-tions to remove recurrent disease are frequently successful. Gross tumours had been removed at least twice from some patients in his series.

His own experience, however, with 20 patients who had dysgerminomas and 28 with granulosa cell tumours was less satisfactory than that at the Radium-hemmet. Only one of the six patients with dysgerminomas who had Stage Ia disease was considered suitable for uni-lateral oophorectomy without irradia-tion. Two others had unilateral oophor-ectomy with radiation to one side; the remaining patients had total hysterec-tomy and bilateral salpingo-oophorec-tomy. The stage of disease was advanced in many instances and the survival rate was not good.

Twelve of the 28 patients with gra-nulosa cell tumours had Stage Ia dis-ease. Treatment was with surgery only. Two died of tumour after nine, and one after 13 months; three died of other causes. Six are well; two are ten-year sur-vivors and four are five-year survivors. Of the 15 patients who had more advanced disease and received postoperative irradiation, nine have died of the disease. Three were five-year survivors. Five are well after 54, 48, 79, and 84 months respectively. The remaining patient in this series is well but treatment was relatively recent.

J. GRAHAM said that, at his institution also, experience with the granulosa cell tumours was less satisfactory than at the Radiumhemmet. Most of the patients had advanced disease which progressed rapidly and behaved in a different fashion. He had some reservations, he said, about the use of unilateral oophorectomy for patients with mucinous and endometrioid carcinoma because of the frequency with which abnormalities could be found in the second ovary when it appeared normal. In the last few years, cul-de-sac aspirations had been used to follow patients who had been treated elsewhere and then referred. If malignant cells were present in the peritoneal fluid, the second ovary was removed.

SCULLY remarked that although frozen section diagnosis was unreliable to some extent, this method has been much improved recently, especially with the advent of the cryostat. He inquired of KOTTMEIER as to whether, when the opposite ovary was examined during the surgical procedure, a biopsy specimen was obtained, if the ovary was actually split or whether examination consisted only of palpation and observation. He also inquired as to what percentage of the serous carcinomas were bilateral, because a patient occasionally would take a minor risk so that she could have children.

He thought that KOTTMEIER's series was not really comparable to that of PEDOWITZ because the latter series consisted of a collection of isolated case reports from the literature. The Radiumhemmet series seemed more com-

parable with one from the Mayo Clinic in which the results of unilateral oophorectomy and radical operation were compared for patients who had unilateral encapsulated dysgerminomas grossly confined to one ovary. These investigators found, SCULLY said, that in the cases treated with conservative surgical intervention, without postoperative radiation, they had a 40 per cent recurrence, but in most instances re-operation was possible. As a result, the five-year survival rate was reduced to only about five per cent for those patients who did not receive postoperative irradiation. In his opinion, SCULLY said, patients with these tumours should be treated conservatively when the disease was unilateral, because he had seen no evidence that radical operation added anything to the salvage rate.

KOTTMEIER replied that in the series he presented, frozen section diagnosis was not used, because formerly it was considered unreliable by the Swedish pathologists. Recently, however, this attitude had changed and the modern method for frozen section diagnosis was in use.

In most of the patients with unilateral serous tumours, he said, the other ovary was considered normal on gross examination. Although a biopsy specimen was obtained in some instances, usually the ovary was not cut. As to PEDOWITZ' series, he realized it was not comparable; it was used because of its size and because the treatment was surgical only. The dysgerminomas, he said, should be removed without rupture; if the neoplasm is a cyst, an effort should be made to remove the tumour without emptying the cyst. Under these circumstances, he was not completely convinced that irradiation should be given. At the Radiumhemmet, irradiation was given in small doses, but he agreed that the therapeutic plan described by Scully of performing unilateral oophorectomy, giving no irradiation but keeping the patient under observation, might be useful. If there was recurrence, then irradiation might be used.

Kottmeier then asked two questions in regard to surgical treatment in general. Was it always possible for the pathologist to tell the surgeon if the tumour had penetrated the capsule? Swedish pathologists find this difficult. To Gentil, he directed the question of what should be done when the carcinoma was really fixed to the sigmoid colon, small bowel, urinary bladder, or pelvic wall. Some surgeons try to resect the tumour from the sigmoid colon and the intestine, but inevitably cancer recurs and the patient does not respond to other treatment. In such circumstances, then, would the best plan be to explore only, treat the patient with either irradiation or chemotherapy, and then perform a second laparotomy, or should the bladder be resected, for instance, if the tumour had invaded it?

Gentil replied that if a malignant ovarian lesion was infiltrating by direct extension as, for example, a mass was adherent to the sigmoid loop or to the dome of the bladder, without evidence of dissemination, every possible effort should be made to remove *en bloc* the entire lesion without attempting to separate the mass from the bladder or the sigmoid colon. If seeding is present, then only the primary lesion should be removed.

Another important question, Gentil said, is how, if gross tumour is present in only one ovary, the identification of histologic type can be made, since most pathologists will not give a definite report on the frozen section. What, he also asked, is the proper management if one ovary is removed and the final pathologic reports shows the lesion to be serous carcinoma?

Kottmeier said that many times the type of lesion, serous, endometrioid, or mucinous, could be identified by frozen section. At the Radiumhemmet, the plan was to remove the tumour; and if one ovary was left and microscopical examination revealed a serous carcinoma, irradiation was given. With supervoltage therapy, it is easy to give 4,000 to 5,000 rads to the pelvis. Intracavitary radium is used at times, especially if metastasis is present in the true pelvis. If the disease was identified histologically as serous carcinoma, resurgery is performed after completion of the radiation. A hysterectomy is then carried out. If, however, the tumour proved to be mucinous, which is frequently unilateral, slow growing and does not respond to irradiation, no irradiation would be given. When the surgical specimen showed endometrioid carcinoma, future therapy was discussed with the patient. No irradiation was used if the patient was young and wanted children. If she did not want children, then treatment would be the same as for serous carcinoma, i.e. irradiation and re-exploration. This plan has been followed also for patients with mesonephric carcinoma.

References

Abt, K., Beitrag zur Klinik und Therapie der Ovarialcarcinome. *Gynaecologia (Basel)* 122, 75—109 (1946).

Brody, S., Clinical aspects of dysgerminoma of the ovary. *Acta radiol. (Stockh.)* 56, 209—230 (1961).

Corscaden, J. A., *Gynecologic cancer* (ed. 3). The Co. Baltimore: William & Wilkins 1962.

Frankl, O., Beiträge zur Pathologie und Klinik des Ovarialkarzinoms. *Arch. Gynäk.* 113, 29 (1920).

Funck-Brentano, P., Le traitement du cancer de l'ovaire. *Gynaecologia (Basel)* **149**, 383 (1960).

Heinrichs, M., Karzinome. Die Krankheiten der Eierstöcke und Nebeneierstöcke. In: Martin, A., *Handbuch der Krankheiten der weiblichen Adnexorgane*, Bd. 2. Leipzig: A. Georgi 1899.

Hertig, A. T., and Gore, H., *Tumours of the female sex organs*, sect. IX, fasc. 33, part. 3. Armed Forces Institute of Pathology, Washington, D. C. 1961.

Kottmeier, H.-L., The classification and treatment of ovarian tumours. *Acta obstet. gynec. scand.* **31**, 313—363 (1952).

— Radiotherapy in the treatment of ovarian carcinoma. *Clin. Obstet. Gynec.* **4**, 865—874 (1961).

Long, M. E., and Taylor jr., H. C., Endometrioid carcinoma of the ovary. *Amer. J. Obstet. Gynec.* **90**, 936—950 (1964).

Lynch, R. C., and Dockerty, M. B., Spread of uterine and ovarian carcinoma with special reference to role of Fallopian tube. *Surg. Gynec. Obstet.* **80**, 60—65 (1945).

Mayer, A., Klinik der Ovarialtumoren. In: Halban und Seitz, *Biologie und Pathologie des Weibes*, Bd. 5/2, S. 799. Berlin u. Wien: Urban & Schwarzenberg 1926.

Mengert, W. F., Carcinoma of the ovary. *Sth med. J. (Bgham, Ala.)* **47**, 118 (1954).

Miller, J., Die Krankheiten des Eierstockes. In: *Handbuch der speziellen pathologischen Anatomie und Histologie* (Lubarsch O. u. F. Henke, Bd. VII. Berlin: Springer 1937.

Morris, J. Mc. L., and Scully, R. E., *Endocrine pathology of the ovary*. St. Louis: C. V. Mosby Co. 1958.

Mueller, C. W., Topkins, P., and Lapp, W. A., Dysgerminoma of the ovary. An analysis of 427 cases. *Amer. J. Obstet. Gynec.* **60**, 153—159 (1950).

Munnell, E. W., and Taylor jr., H. C., Ovarian carcinoma: A review of 200 primary and 51 secondary cases. *Amer. J. Obstet. Gynec.* **58**, 943 (1949).

Orden, D. E. van, McAllister, W. B., Zerne, S. R. M., and Morris, J. McLean, Ovarian carcinoma. The problems of staging and grading. *Amer. J. Obstet. Gynec.* **94**, 195—202 (1966).

Parsons, L., and Sommers, S. C., *Gynecology*. Philadelphia: W. B. Saunders Co. 1962.

Pedowitz, P., Felmus, L. B., and Grayzel, D. M., Dysgerminoma of the ovary. Prognosis and treatment. *Amer. J. Obstet. Gynec.* **70**, 1284 (1955).

Purola, E., Serous papillary ovarian tumours. A study of 233 cases with special reference to the histological type of tumour. *Acta obstet. gynec. scand.* **43**, Suppl. 3 (1963).

Randall, C. L., Ovarian carcinoma; risk of preserving the ovary. *Obstet. and Gynec.* **3**, 491—497 (1954).

Santesson, L., Clinical and pathological survey of ovarian tumours treated at Radiumhemmet. I. Dysgerminomas. *Acta radiol. (Stockh.)* **28**, 644—668 (1947).

Taylor jr., H. C., and Munnell, F. W., Treatment of tumours of the ovary. In: *Treatment of cancer and allied diseases* by G. T. Pack and I. M. Ariel, vol. 6, p. 254. New York: Harper & Brothers 1962.

Varangot, J., *Les tumeurs de la granulosa. Folliculomes de l'ovaire*. Paris: L. Arnette 1937.

Woodruff, J. D., Bie, L. S., and Sherman, R. J., Mucinous tumors of the ovary. *Obstet. and Gynec.* **16**, 699 (1960).

—, and Novak, E. R., Papillary serous tumours of the ovary. *Amer. J. Obstet. Gynec.* **67**, 1112—1126 (1954).

Intestinal Surgery for Advanced Cancer of the Ovary

ALEXANDER BRUNSCHWIG, M. D.

Memorial-James Ewing Hospitals, New York, N.Y., U.S.A.

DON G. C. CLARK, M. D.

Memorial Hospital for Cancer and Allied Diseases, New York, N.Y., U.S.A.

Introduction

The patient with cancer of the ovary requiring extensive operation is one who has had recurrent or persistent disease or is seen for the first time in an advanced stage.

The surgical problem is that of affording palliation with the hope that due to host resistance she may be afforded longer survival in comfort, or indeed "cure" lasting many years.

The patient presents herself clinically desiring relief from mechanical disturbances which are the result of 1. enlarged abdomen due to ascites and/or large tumour masses pressing upward against the diaphragm and interfering with respiration, and 2. varying degrees of intestinal obstruction.

Laparotomy is indicated for extensive evacuation of ascites. Recurrent ascites may develop, in which case paracentesis is carried out as indicated.

At the time of laparotomy, a large omental mass is often present (unless it has been previously removed). The mass should be resected as completely as possible by total omentectomy, because it contributes to ascites. In addition, time and effort should be spent in removing scattered masses of metastatic cancer over peritoneal surfaces.

Intestinal obstructions may be due to several causes. Heavy infiltrations of the small bowel mesentery and of the walls of the intestines themselves produce a vascular stasis which impairs motility and results in ileus (carcinomatosis ileus). There may be actual constriction of the lumen of the bowel at one or more points, producing mechanical obstruction or kinking due to metastasic deposits, (Fig. 1). Mechanical interference with gastrointestinal motility may be due to varying proportions of these factors. Our policy has been, at the time of laparotomy, to be prepared to resect or by-pass, by intestinal anastomoses, the levels of obstruction, if such resections are feasible and it is obvious that sufficient relatively uninvolved bowel remains to permit satisfactory continued survival in relative comfort for a while. When or when not to resect bowel and how much to resect are matters of judgment and experience. Written directions for such surgery cannot be given. Unless the surgeon is experienced, willing and able to perform these operations, he would do well not to perform laparotomy at all but to refer the case to one who could do the operations. Too often, surgeons will carry out exploratory laparotomy only to find what is obvious on clinical examination, i.e. advanced ovarian cancer. They then do nothing but close the abdomen, feeling righteous that they at least "explored" when, in the first place, they would not carry out the intestinal surgical procedure that might be done.

of cancer of the ovary seen on the Gynecological Service of Memorial-James Ewing Hospital, New York City (Table I). The large majority of these had advanced and recurrent disease after treatment elsewhere. In 94 cases, segments of large intestines were resected.

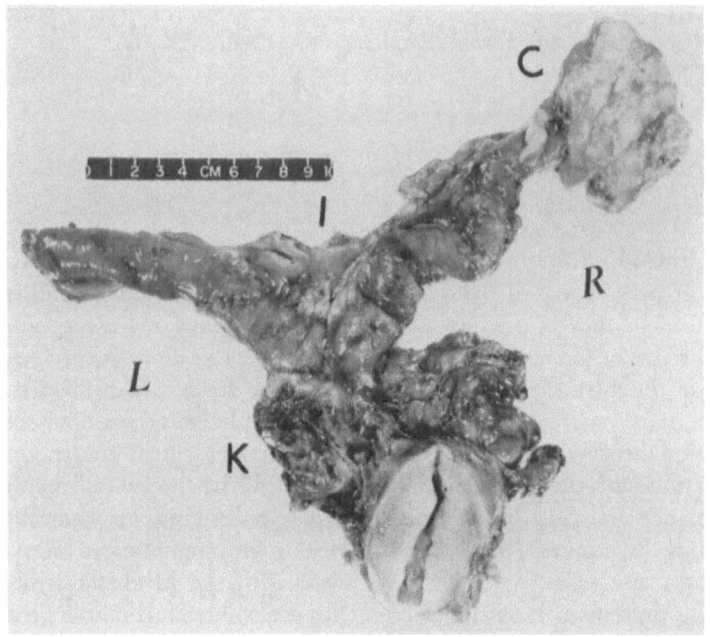

Fig. 1. Example of resection of terminal, ileum (*I*), and cecum (*C*) with panhysterectomy for cancer (*K*) of left ovary involving ileum producing acute angulation (impending obstruction). Specimen viewed from posterior; *L* left side, *R* right side

The question then arises: can anything be gained by operations on the intestine in the presence of carcinomatosis from the ovaries? Except for our own experience, I know of no reports based upon appreciable series of cases in the literature. One hears gynecologists and surgeons speak of "taking out all they can", obviously leaving cancer behind, and achieving palliation. But in how many cases and palliation for how long? Accurate documentation of the latter is not available.

During the period September 1947 to January 1, 1960, there were 614 cases

Included in this group were right colectomies with the terminal ileum also excised. Eight patients were living and well after five years (8.5%). In these cases, laparotomy showed the cancer to be confined to a region; excision necessitated colonic resection but there was no widespread disease. Such fortuitous circumstances are discovered only at laparotomy. There were, in addition, 42 instances of small bowel resection as the main form of intestinal resection. There were no five-year survivors. The average length of survival in the latter group was 8 months, with 22 months being the longest survival period. I believe that in at least one-half some degree of effective palliative response, albeit brief in certain cases, was achieved. Thus, the outlook for palliation is better when large bowel resection seems indicated and is done than when small bowel resection seems indicated and is done. It would appear preferable to side-track an involved segment of small bowel to relieve obstruction than to resect it. However, for palliation, I would not hesitate

Case 1. Vaj, 61 years. In October 1947, she underwent panhysterectomy for solid anaplastic cancer of the left ovary; at the same time, elliptical excision of metastasis, 3 cm in diameter, in the anterior vaginal wall just proximal to urethra was removed. In November 1947, a large solitary nodal metastasis in left superficial inguinal region was excised. Five years later, she had a resection of transverse colon for a mass about half the size of a fist, in the transverse

Table I. *Cancer of the ovary*

	No.	5-year survival	%
All cases s̄ intestinal resection	467	101	21.6
Large intestinal resection	94	8	8.5
Small intestinal resection	42	0	0
Total	603	109	18.1

to resect small bowel, even though I recognize the bad prognosis. One does not hesitate to perform colostomy as palliation for non-resectable colonic cancer. Experience has amply justified this procedure. Indeed, in our series, colostomy has been performed 25 times for ovarian cancer. In 21 instances small intestinal by-pass was done. In seven instances segments of urinary bladder were excised (Table II).

Surprise Findings at Laparotomy for Apparently Hopeless Recurrent Ovarian Cancer

If the surgeon pursues an agressive attitude in regard to treating ovarian cancer, aggressiveness always tempered by sound surgical judgment, certain apparently hopeless situations will be encountered at laparotomy that turn out to be curable. The following are four examples among others from my own experience:

Table II. *Visceral surgery for ovarian cancer*

Small intestine resection	42
Large intestine resection	94
Colostomy	25
Intestinal bypass	21
Resection segment of bladder	7
Pelvic exenteration	15
Total operations	204

Total cases 614; 204/614 = 33.2% incidence of complementary visceral surgery.

mesocolon causing, obstruction of colon. She was alive and without evidence of cancer in 1966, at 80 years of age, 19 years after initial operation.

Case 2. Sark, 50 years. Right ovarian cancer was excised in 1949 elsewhere. Postoperative roentgen therapy was given and repeated in 1951 because of a recurrent left pelvic mass which did not regress after this treatment. In March 1952, with the clinical diagnosis of probable abdominal carcinomatosis, laparotomy was again performed and the palpable mass was found to be carcinoma of the left ovary adherent to sigmoid. A panhysterectomy, with excision of adherent loop of sigmoid, was done together with omentectomy; the omentum did

Case 4. Saund, 57 years. This obese patient had a large mass in the left pelvis. At laparotomy carcinoma of the left ovary, 18 cm diameter, infiltrating an

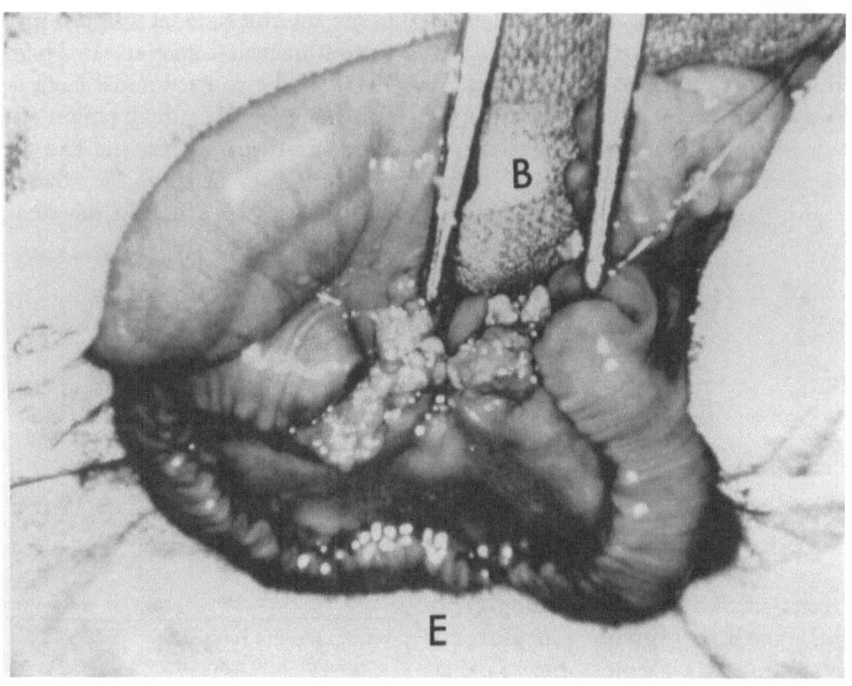

Fig. 2A. Enteroenterectomy. Photograph at operation showing (*E*), segment of jejunum isolated from continuity with its blood supply preserved and mucosa everted. B, final step with re-establishment of continuity by enteroenterostomy

not contain metastases. The patient remains well 14 years following the last operation.

Case 3. D., 55 years. In 1948, she had supracervical panhysterectomy for a malignant ovarian cyst with subsequent roentgen therapy. In 1951 there was a large pelvic mass, for which laparotomy was done with excision of the mass the cervical stump and resection en masse of an infiltrated adherent loop of pelvic colon. In June 1957 and February 1958, repairs of minimal incisional herniae were carried out and no recurrences were noted in the pelvic or abdomen. The patient remains well in 1966, fifteen years later.

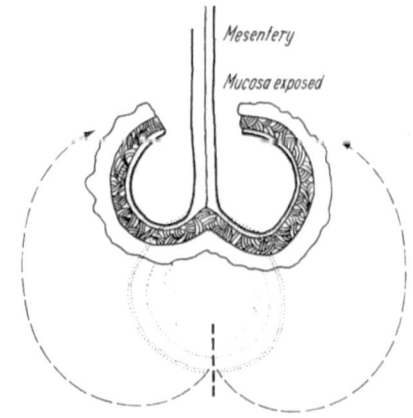

Fig. 2B. Diagramm showing method of eversion of small bowel mucosa. Catgut sutures only should be used and no sutures should include mucosa itself — only serosa and muscularis

attached loop of sigmoid and adjacent left ureter was found. Radical hysterectomy and en masse resection of the invaded colon (8 inches) were done; the histologic diagnosis was malignant granulosa cell tumour. End-to-end colocolostomy with diverting transverse colostomy was performed. The colostomy was later closed. The patient is well 7 years after treatment.

Pelvic Exenteration

In view of the tendency of ovarian cancer to spread widely over the peritoneal surfaces of the pelvis, omentum and upper abdomen, it would appear that the question of pelvic exenteration would not arise, if and when pelvic colon and bladder were invaded, so as to require this operation. The justifiable assumption is that by the time bladder and rectal invasion had occurred, upper abdominal spread would have developed and thus the operation would not encompass the disease. Yet in 22 cases, pelvic exenteration was carried out because at laparotomy all cancer appeared grossly to be confined to the pelvis. All but one were recurrences. There were 14 cases done prior to 1960, with one survivor for 71 months, who died of uremia. Among the 8 patients operated upon after 1960, one is living and well over 5 years.

Thus when pelvic exenteration for ovarian cancer spread to (but limited to) the pelvis is performed, the outlook for five-year survival is rather dim; yet, when 2 among 22 cases afford satisfactory results (9%), the situation is still not absolutely hopeless.

Ileo-Enterectopy

Finally there is the problem of recurring ascites in the presence of advancing ovarian cancer. As already stated, a thorough evacuation of the abdominal fluid at laparotomy, together with omentectomy and resection of metastatic masses, often result in delay of the re-accumulation of ascites as compared with the frequency of such accumulations prior to operation when only paracenteses are done as symptoms demand. A time comes, however, when paracentesis becomes frequently necessary and each one does not afford the relief desired.

In studies carried out on dogs by NEUMANN, a plastic surgeon, he demonstrated that if a segment of small bowel, whose natural function is fluid absorption from the lumen, is isolated and opened longitudinally, its mucosal surface everted, the continuity of the small bowel re-established and the whole dropped into the abdominal cavity with tight closure of the wound, ascites produced by artificial means will be absorbed. I have applied this principle in attempts to bring about resorption of ascites from ovarian cancer (Fig. 2). Six patients were operated upon but the initial cases were poor choices because of the large amount of tumour present; also the ascites was loculated. The feasibility of the operation was demonstrated in patients with ascites and ovarian cancer. It became evident that the ideal case was one in which there was no loculation of fluid. Among the 6 patients operated upon, there was one such ideal case, a patient with scattered small metastases over the entire peritoneal surfaces and one large collection of fluid in the left abdomen without loculation. The patient has survived over one year in excellent general condition and still has no accumulation of fluid. Obviously only a minority of patients would be suitable for this procedure, but it is well worth further trial.

Discussion

While advanced ovarian cancer cannot be "cured", an aggressive surgical attack, tempered by judgment, may afford appreciable palliation in some patients lasting from months to many years.

The variables in these cases are numerous and this precludes setting forth, in a clear-cut manner, a series of directions that may be followed by others. The principal prerequisite for surgical attack upon advanced ovarian cancer is that the surgeon possess the qualifications for carrying out any type of abdominal and pelvic surgery, and not be "psychologized" to limit himself to dealing with any one organ system. He must also be fully cognizant of gastrointestinal physiology and methods of alleviating organic situations which may impair normal gastrointestinal function.

The objectives of radical surgery in advanced ovarian cancer are to 1. reduce as much as possible the amount of cancer present, 2. evacuate all accumulated fluid, and 3. restore as well as possible gastrointestinal function.

Summary

In the palliative treatment of advanced ovarian cancer, resection of segments of small bowel and/or colon have a definite place. When to carry out these procedure is a matter of judgment based upon experience.

On the writer's service there were 94 instances of colonic resection and 42 instances of small bowel resection carried out among 603 patients followed between September 1947 and January 1, 1960, inclusive. Among the patients undergoing colonic resections, eight were living and well five years after operation. The five-year survivors were patients who were thought to have widespread ovarian cancer, but, at laparotomy, the disease was localized and excisable, providing segments of colon were also resected. No five-year survivors were observed among those who received small bowel resections, as in these cases cancer was widespread and the small bowel was resected to relieve intestinal obstruction. It would appear that side-tracking procedures would be preferable to small bowel resection, if relief from obstruction is envisaged for the small bowel.

Pelvic exenteration may be carried out for advanced locally spread ovarian cancer when there are no metastases outside the pelvis. Among 22 patients, 2 are five-year survivors.

Entero-enterectopy is described as a procedure, still experimental, to deal with large accumulations of abdominal fluid in selected cases.

Abdomino-pelvic visceral surgery involving both small and large bowel has a definite place in the management of cancer of the ovary, both as palliative treatment and in some cases as definitive treatment envisaging "cure".

Discussion

Gentil supported Brunschwig's recommendation of omentectomy and added that he always advised removal of the omentum, even in early disease, because even when the omentum was apparently normal, examination often showed clusters of cancer cells. He also stated that unless there was widespread seeding in the peritoneum, he made an effort to remove "*en bloc*" all tumour infiltrating by direct extension, including sometimes a segment of the bladder or of the large intestine. He commented on the value of complementary treatment with radiotherapy or chemotherapy, and added that he considered chemotherapy especially important in this disease. Often in advanced disease, he said, he began treatment with chemotherapy and performed laparotomy at a later date. He would hesitate to perform pelvic exenteration for ovarian cancer since this disease responds well to radiation and chemotherapy. As to the relief of small bowel obstruction, he had had better results with a by-pass operation than when he resected loops of ileum or jejunum.

GENTIL expressed interest in the operation, described by BRUNSCHWIG, for absorbing ascites and added that this might present an excellent means of controlling the accumulation of fluid which shortens the life of the patients with advanced cancer of the ovary. He ended his discussion with the recommendation that attention be given to the training of pelvic surgeons, i.e. surgeons who would be trained to deal with any problem which arose during an operation for any disease in the pelvis.

J. GRAHAM emphasized the importance of an aggressive surgical approach for patients with far-advanced ovarian cancer because, he said, often more can be done surgically than is realized. For example, patients sometimes have large masses which are really pseudocysts and which can be resected successfully. The

results which were achieved depended to some extent on the growth potential or characteristics of the tumour. For example, the lack of long-term survivors in patients who underwent small bowel resection reflected the growth pattern of the tumour. The presence of small bowel obstruction demonstrated that the tumour was disseminated and therefore could not be successfully removed.

R. GRAHAM asked if there was any evidence of the value of omentectomy. In animals, she said, the omentum contains large number of mast cells and histiocytes, the cells of host response. BRUNSCHWIG replied that although the omentum was a "strong defense" organ, cancer present in this organ would continue to grow. He cited as evidence of the value of omentectomy, a series of 145 patients who underwent omentectomy; only 52 (35.8 per cent) developed ascites and the average survival time was 43.2 months. In a series of 184 patients who did not undergo omentectomy, 75 (40.8 per cent) developed ascites and the average survival time was 43.2 months. Although the differences in the percentages of those who developed ascites and the average survival time are slight, they are significant because the first group of patients had obvious disease, but the second group, those who did not undergo omentectomy, had no evidence of disease in this organ at operation.

References

NEUMANN, C. G., BRAUNWALD, N. W., and HINTON, J. W., The absorption of ascitic fluid by a pedicled flap of intestinal mucosa exposed within the peritoneal cavity. *Plast. reconstr. Surg.* **17**, 189 (1956).

Seropapillary and Endometrioid Carcinoma of the Ovary: Survival Rate after Surgery and Radiotherapy

Maurice Lenz, M. D.

Professor Emeritus of Clinical Radiology, Columbia University, New York;
Consultant Radiotherapist, Presbyterian, Delafield and Montefiore Hospitals,
New York, N.Y. U.S.A.

Introduction

The effectiveness of surgery and radiotherapy of seropapillary and endometrioid cancers is limited strictly to the treated region, and cancer cells outside this area may continue to grow despite regression in the treated portion of the neoplasm. The cancer may often be entirely excised, if treatment is given while it is still confined to the ovaries. Growth may at times be restrained and survival prolonged by postoperative radiotherapy used after the cancer has extended beyond the ovaries and is still limited to the pelvis. This combined treatment has little influence on survival, once the cancer has extended into the upper abdomen, where cancerocidal radiation dosage is not well tolerated. Finally, the clinical course of the disease remains unaffected by treatment to the pelvis if the cancer has genrealized. Clinical progress at this stage depends more on the resistance of the host to the growth of the metastases than on the result of treatment to the pelvis.

It seems, therefore, that the anatomic extent of cancer at laparotomy before active treatment is started has more influence on the outcome of surgery and radiotherapy of seropapillary and endometrioid ovarian cancer than do the details of treatment.

Material

The relation between the pretreatment extent of these cancers and posttreatment survival, has been investigated by a number of authors: e.g. Munnell and Taylor (1957), Kent and McKay (1960) and many others. Nevertheless, it was thought that further clarification of this problem may result from a review in 1963 and 1964 of 562 patients with seropapillary and endometrioid ovarian cancer, who had been treated at the Radiumhemmet, Stockholm, from 1915 to 1959 inclusive. This analysis was undertaken at the suggestion of Professor Hans Ludwig Kottmeier, Director of Gynecology of the Radiumhemmet, in whose service these patients were treated.

Before I started my study, Professor Lars Santesson, Director of the Department of Pathology of the Radiumhemmet, microscopically classified 359 seropapillary and 276 endometrioid ovarian cancers. Of these 635 cases, 73 were excluded from the present investigation as we believed that they could not contribute to the clarification of the relation of survival to the exact anatomic extent of the pelvic disease. The cases excluded were those in which precise description of the pretreatment extent of the disease at laparotomy was lacking, or patients who, at the time of laparotomy, had distant metastases and in whom, therefore, the results of treatment to the pelvis had no bearing on survival. There remained 314 seropapillary and 248 endometrioid cases available for analysis of the survival rate.

Microscopic Classification

The histologic criteria for the diagnosis of serous or endometrioid adenocarcinoma of the ovary in this study have been those given in the "histologic classification of the common primary epithelial tumours of the ovary" by the Cancer Committee of the International Federation of Gynecology and Obstetrics, September, 1964. According to this definition only those neoplasms were classified as cancer, in which the epithelium showed obvious infiltrative and destructive growth. Tumours of low potential malignancy without such infiltrative and destructive growth were not accepted as cancer, even though they showed proliferating activity of the epithelial cells and nuclear abnormalities; they were placed in a separate group.

Endometrioid cancers showed epithelial structures similar to adenocarcinoma in the endometrium. This diagnosis was made by Prof. SANTESSON more often in the present series than is usually seen in other series of reported cases. The endometrioid cancers grow more slowly than the seropapillary variety (LONG and TAYLOR, 1964). It may be significant (LONG and TAYLOR, 1964) that the nucleolus in endometrioid cancer cells is smaller than in seropapillary types; most ribonucleic acid (RNA) in the cancer cells is concentrated in the cytoplasm and the nucleolus and considerable protein synthesis takes place here.

Anatomic Classification — Staging

As the effectiveness of surgery and radiotherapy of cancer is limited strictly to the treated cancer cells, this treatment becomes progressively less effective with increasing anatomic extent of the disease before therapy. Unfortunately, in the present series most patients, especially those with seropapillary cancer, did not arrive for treatment until the disease had become extensive. The reasons for this extensiveness were many: the possibility of ovarian cancer was not thought of clinically; there were no characteristically diagnostic symptoms or signs; pelvic and abdominal examinations were often inconclusive; expert laparoscopy, which at times may be helpful, was not generally available; there was a reluctance to submit patients to exploratory laparotomy. Yet, exploratory laparotomy not only permits biopsy, and delineation of the clinical limits of the cancer by direct vision and palpation of the growth, but also allows multiple biopsies beyond the clinical limits in the search for silent metastases. All staging was only of approximate accuracy and silent extensions may have escaped detection even with the abdomen open.

Various methods have been developed for staging ovarian cancers. The one used in the present discussion was suggested by the Cancer Committee of the International Federation of Gynecology and Obstetrics in 1964 and uses the following criteria:

Stage I. Growth limited to the ovaries.

Stage Ia. Growth limited to one ovary.

Stage Ib. Growth limited to both ovaries.

Stage II. Growth involving one or both ovaries with pelvic extension.

Stage IIa. Extension and/or metastasis to the uterus and/or tubes only.

Stage IIb. Extension to other pelvic tissues.

Stage III. Growth involving one or both ovaries with widespread intraperitoneal metastasis to the upper half of the abdomen (the omentum, the small intestine and its mesentery).

Stage IV. Growth involving one or both ovaries with distant metastasis outside the peritoneal cavity.

Special Category. Unexplored cases which are thought to be ovarian carcinoma (surgery, explorative or therapeutic, not having been performed).

Note. The presence of ascites should not influence the staging.

The accuracy of staging varied with the thoroughness with which the surgeon searched for silent extensions and metastases.

Search for silent extensions may be facilitated if, instead of attempting to investigate the entire body, this search is at first confined to the usual routes of extension. Knowledge of these routes may also assist in better planning of the fields to be irradiated. Tolerance of cancerocidal radiation dosage is insufficient for seropapillary and endometrioid cancer if applied to large volumes of the body. Restriction of the irradiated areas to the usual routes of extension increases the likelihood that the necessary dosage will be tolerated. These routes will now be reviewed.

Routes of Extension

SCHOTTLAENDER (1913) and KER-MAUNER (1932) chiefly on the basis of postmortem findings, believed that from its primary site in the peritoneal covering of the ovary, seropapillary cancer extended to the pelvis, upper abdomen, etc. equally, by transplantation to the peritoneum and through the lymph capillary system.

In a small series of exploratory laparotomies for ovarian cancer observed by me in various Stockholm hospitals during 1964, the surgeons, at my request,

kindly palpated the paraaortic lymph node region in each patient. The only cases in which these nodes were palpably enlarged were those in which, at laparotomy, there was already extensive pelvic involvement. In several instances of early limited pelvic disease, in which there were no palpably enlarged lymph nodes, microscopic examination of the paraaortic lymph nodes failed to disclose any metastases. The number of my observations was small, yet they suggest that transplantation to the peritoneum may precede invasion of the lymphatic system. It may be worth while, in the future, to check at the operating table how often paraaortic metastases can be found in early cases, to get a clearer understanding of the frequency of this involvement.

Spread by transplantation in seropapillary cases may start early in the disease. An intracystic ovarian cancer may grow through the thin wall of the cyst and present itself on its peritoneal covering as a papillary excrescence; this excrescence may be rubbed off on to the peritoneum as it glides past during breathing. The cancer cells may adhere to the peritoneum if this is roughened, e.g. by inflammation, and grow locally or drop into the pouch of DOUGLAS, because of gravity in the upright position of the patient, and develop there (WILLIS, 1934).

HERTIG and GORE (1961) believe that "the ease of endometrial transplantability is in proportion to its proliferation and lack of differentiation".

If ascites is present, the ascitic fluid itself may serve as a culture medium (TAYLOR, 1959); the cancer may thus be transported to various portions of the abdominal cavity.

At first, such superficial peritoneal transplants are not well vascularized and may, at times, be eradicated by superficially acting Beta rays or intraperitoneally placed radioactive gold (MÜLLER, 1959) or by chemotherapy. With advancing growth and improved vascularization, however, the cancer tends to become invasive and no longer disappears after such surface treatment.

Invasion through the peritoneal mesothelium into the subjacent lymph spaces is especially serious. These lymph spaces extend under the entire peritoneal surface and intercommunicate with each other, the pleura, and the mediastinum (YOFFEY and COURTICE, 1956). The spaces may thus act as conduits for the silent yet rapid spread of ovarian cancer not only over the entire abdomen, but also into the pleura and, more rarely, into the mediastinum. Supraclavicular lymph node metastasis may be the first clinical evidence of retroperitoneal involvement and should be looked for routinely if ovarian cancer is suspected. The sentinel group of the supraclavicular nodes are situated near the jugulo-subclavian venous angle; from the sentinel nodes connecting tubules enter directly into the jugulo-subclavian confluence on the right and into the thoracic duct on the left (HAAGENSEN, 1956). The thoracic and right lymphatic ducts also drain into the jugulo-subclavian confluence near this point. Cancer cells may therefore enter the venous system either via the direct efferents from the sentinel nodes, the right lymphatic or the thoracic ducts. ACKERMAN and DEL REGATO (1962) mentioned that metastases from ovarian cancers to the lungs and liver may follow mediastinal and supraclavicular involvement. At postmortem examination, however, WILLIS (1953) found that blood borne metastases in seropapillary cancer were uncommon. Clinically, we have often seen pleural involvement, but much more rarely pulmonary metastases in these growths.

The flow of lymph and probably the progress of cancer cells along the lymph spaces are enhanced by breathing; YOFFEY and COURTICE emphasize that these lymph spaces are alternately compressed and decompressed by changes in the intra-abdominal pressure due to the contraction and relaxation of the diaphragm. Breathing actually raises and lowers abdominal organs, e.g. the omentum, thus facilitating contact between an excrescence of an ovarian cancer and the surface of the omentum. This increases the likelihood that the omentum will be invaded. Removal of part or most of the invaded omentum is at times recommended as this may be followed by temporary suppression of ascites. Transsection across a microscopically invaded omentum, however, may open venous and lymphatic channels and, smear cancer cells over the peritoneum, thus disseminating the disease and shortening survival.

The danger of dissemination from incomplete cancer surgery also makes it questionable whether lymphadenectomy of the paraaortic lymph nodes really helps survival. In early cases, these metastases are probably absent, and in late cases they represent only part of a wider involvement, the greater portion of which is left unremoved.

The above review of the usual routes of extension may improve the accuracy of planning treatment fields and help to clarify the reason for some of the failures of surgery and radiotherapy in these cancers.

Treatment Methods

Shortly before admission to the Gynecological service of the Radiumhemmet, most patients had an exploratory laparotomy for microscopic corroboration of the diagnosis and anatomic staging of the extent of the cancer. At the same time, as much cancer was re-

moved as possible and a bilateral, or
more rarely a unilateral, oophorectomy
was done. There is no definite proof
that complete suppression of ovarian
function by bilateral oophorectomy prolongs survival of these patients, but this
operation was done as a routine part of
the cancer surgery. It may be worth
recording for future reference that, in
a few of these castrated patients, with
generalized metastases, survival was
extraordinarily long.

In contrast to the usual treatment of
ovarian cancer in other hospitals, the
uterus in the present series was left in
place and was later used to hold radium
applicators.

On admission to the gynecological
service of the Radiumhemmet, additional
investigations of the various body systems were done by clinical, x-ray and
laboratory methods so as to have a
complete picture of the patient's status
before beginning active treatment. When
this preliminary investigation had been
completed, a plan was set up for radiotherapy. This usually consisted of ex-
ternally applied orthovoltage x-ray therapy to the pelvis, less often to the upper
abdomen and, in practically all cases,
intrauterine radium therapy.

All intracavity and external radiotherapy was started within a few days
after admission to the Radiumhemmet
and finished within less than 3 months
from inception of this treatment. In a
small number of patients the pelvis and,
at times, the upper abdomen were irradiated *preoperatively* as well as postoperatively. In a few of these instances, radiotherapy was continued as the sole method
of therapy; cases treated preoperatively
and those treated solely by radiation,
however, were too few to permit reliable evaluation. Discussion of radiotherapy will therefore be limited mainly
to patients treated postoperatively.

External Radiotherapy
Radiation Fields

External radiotherapy in our cases
was applied chiefly to the pelvis. The
upper abdomen was irradiated only when
there was strong suspicion or proof that
it was involved. Radiation tolerance of
the upper abdomen is not sufficient to
support high radiation dosage. The reasons for this lesser tolerance are many:
1. the small intestine and stomach are
more radiosensitive than the colon and
rectum; 2. the kidney does not support
intensive irradiation. 3. absorption from
the peritoneal cavity takes place chiefly
high up in the abdomen through the
lymph spaces of the peritoneal covering
of the muscular portion of the diaphragm
(YOFFEY and COURTICE, 1956). Here, the
usual toxic substances resulting from
breakdown of irradiated cells, are likely
to be a absorbed more readily than they
are in the pelvis "Radiation sickness"
is therefore notoriously worse after irradiation of the upper abdomen, than when
only the pelvis is irradiated.

Various expedients have been tried
to increase the radiation tolerance of the
upper abdomen, yet the administration
of high cancerocidal dosage to this
region, remains one of the most difficult
problems in the treatment of these cancers by irradiation. Thus, the abdomen
has been divided into a number of narrow horizontal strips which overlap each
other, and one of these strips has been
irradiated daily until the entire abdomen
has thus been covered (DELCLOS et al.,
1966). Accurate calculations of the tumour doses at the point of overlap of
the fields has proved very difficult.
Attempts have been made to spare the
intestines by reducing the tumour dose
to below cancerocidal levels; but this
fails to destroy the cancer. The period
of irradiation has been prolonged without increasing the tumour dose. This

tends to spare the intestine, but may also reduce the efficacy of irradiating the cancer, unless personally supervised by an experienced radiotherapist familiar with this method. In the present series, two large opposing fields, with or without compression tubes, were employed at first. This delivered too much radiation to the bladder, small bowel, rectum, head and neck of the femur, and a considerable (integral) dose to the whole body. More recently, a 3-beam technic has been developed to suit the shape of the probable tumour volume; this reduced the unwanted radiation to the organs just listed, and diminished the integral dose. Only in cases with cancer in the upper abdomen are two opposing portals used at present.

Voltage of External X-Ray Therapy

Most x-ray therapy used for external irradiation in the present series was orthovoltage with 200—250 KV, and a half value layer, 1—2 mm Cu. In a few cases, during the earlier period, radium beam and, more recently, cobalt beam or supervoltage x-ray therapy have substituted the orthovoltage. In the early days, the radiation technic varied greatly but, during the last few years, it has become more standardized.

Intrauterine Radium Therapy

In planning intrauterine radium therapy, the length of the uterine canal was determined first by the use of the uterine sound. Dilatation and curettage was then done and, depending on the length of the canal, one to three standard Radium-hemmet radium tubes were inserted, the radiation reaching the posterior bladder wall and the anterior rectal wall measured directly by an intracavity ionization chamber. The radium was left in place for the required dosage and then removed. This treatment was repeated once or twice, at two- and three-week-intervals.

The intrauterine radium was most useful in cases in which cancer involved the uterine mucosa, e.g. in many cases of endometrioid cancer of the ovary. Because of the marked reduction in radiation intensity with increasing distance from the intrauterine radium, however, the contribution from this source has been of less importance in cancer foci outside of the uterus. Further reduction in the significance of the intrauterine radiating source for extrauterine cancer foci has resulted from the use of cobalt beam and supervoltage irradiation in place of orthovoltage x-ray therapy. Nevertheless, one may deliver by the intrauterine radium source, 3,000—3,500 gamma r, to the pouch of Douglas, while only 2,400 gamma r of this will reach the anterior rectal wall. On the gynecological service, they found intrauterine radium a useful addition to external irradiation of ovarian cancer.

Tumour Dose

The local cancerocidal effect of radiotherapy is influenced by the radiation dosage absorbed by the cancer, i.e. — the tumour dose. This cancerocidal effect is restricted to the irradiated tissue and may not influence survival, unless the entire cancer is included in the irradiated area. Calculation of tumour dosage, especially in large masses, is at best approximate and errors in estimating the distance between the source of irradiation and a cancer site probably occur quite often. Thus, clinically, it may not be appreciated that a particular cancer site has been displaced by fluid in the urinary bladder, in an ovarian cyst, or by air in the intestine, etc. Mistakes in estimating this distance, while calculating tumour dosage in a lateral direction from an intrauterine radium applicator, may amount to as much as 50% for each centimeter of error. Notwithstanding these possible inaccuracies, an attempt should at least be made to estimate tumour dosage so as to have a better appreciation of the effect of a specific tumour dose on the individual cancer.

While tumour doses in the pelvis are probably best measured *in situ*, a recent study of pelvic measurements of patients on the gynecological service at the Radiumhemmet showed that most patients have an anteroposterior pelvic diameter between 17 cm and 24 cm, or an average of 20 cm; this information helped in the consideration of the "average tumour dose" in the present series. In x-ray pelvimetry studies of 1,600 patients by SNOW (1952), the anteroposterior distance from the mid-sacrum to the posterior wall of the pubic symphysis averaged 11—12 cm, while the interspinous distance in these patients was 10—11 cm.

The central axis depth dose tables, published in *The British Journal of Radiology, Supplement* No. 10, 1961, were used by RANUDD in his study of the average tumour dose used. These calculations assumed an anteroposterior diameter of 20 cm, and were about — 25% for the radiation quality of 1.0 mm Cu and field sizes 15 × 15 cm and 20 × 20 cm. For higher radiation energies, the variation was less: about — 20% for H. V. L. of 2.0 mm Cu and about — 10% for Cobalt-radiation. The method of calculation of these dose distributions has been described by RANUDD (1966).

The charts on the gynecological service of the Radiumhemmet prior to 1964 gave only skin doses and did not state the anteroposterior or transverse diameters of the pelvis of each patient. Since 1964, all pelvic measurements have been routinely recorded on admission and tumour doses have been carefully estimated. RANUDD constructed the dose distribution for each patient with the help of the recorded skin doses and the average pelvic measurements given in the literature.

The significance of mistakes in calculating individual tumour doses in the present series is somewhat reduced by the large number of patients studied. The isodose curves from each radium applicator were known, as these applicators had been used for years and had, of course, remained practically unchanged, as they contained radium element. A survey of the common combinations of radium applicators used on the gynecological service and consideration of the physical accuracy of these combinations have been published by WALSTAM (1954) and RANUDD (1964).

The tumour dose in the present series was calculated at a point in the parauterine tissues, 2 cm lateral to the central axis of the intrauterine radium applicator and at a depth of 10 cm from the skin surface. The reason for choosing this particular region, was that "recurrences" after treatment appeared most frequently in this area. For calculation of the tumour dose, we combined the dosage contributed to this point from the intrauterine and external radiating sources and assumed an anteroposterior pelvic diameter of 20 cm.

Postoperative Tumour Dosage

The bearing which differences in tumour dosage of postoperative x-ray therapy may have on survival has been studied by a number of authors.

KENT and MCKAY (1960) quoted definite prolongation of survival in their follow-up of 5 to 20 years, after midpelvic doses of 1400—2600 r, orthovoltage x-ray therapy, in 12—20 daily exposures.

HOLME (1962) reported an increase from 4.8% to 17% five-year survivors when he compared 206 extensive cases treated only surgically with 141 similar patients who, in addition, had post-operative radiotherapy. The mid-pelvic dosage in 4 to 5 weeks in these cases was 3,000—3,500 r when limited to the pelvis, and 2,500—3,000 r when the upper abdomen was included.

LATOUR and DAVIS (1957), on the other hand, doubt the value of post-operative x-ray therapy. They base their opinion, however, on only 56 irradiated, as compared to 146 non-irradiated patients. Their average tumour dose was 3,000 r, through two opposing pelvic fields of 10 × 25 cm.

MUNNELL, JACOX and TAYLOR (1957) compared their five-year survival after surgery and postoperative orthovoltage x-ray therapy, treated between 1924 to 1943, with those of surgery and post-operative supervolt x-ray or cobalt beam given from 1944—1951. They concluded that there was "no significant improvement" in the results of the more recent series of cases. In their earlier orthovoltage series, the mid-pelvic dose was 3,500—4,000 r, if limited to the pelvis, and 2,000—3,500 r if the upper abdomen was included; in their later cases treated with 2,000 KV or cobalt beam, the mid-pelvic dose was raised to 4,500—5,000 r when limited to the pelvis, and to 3,500—4,000 r if the upper abdomen was included. The main technical difference between patients whose therapy was given with orthovoltage x-ray therapy and the others, treated with super-voltage x-ray or cobalt beam, was that with the two latter modalities a higher tumour dose was administered because of the lesser absorption of the radiation in the intervening tissues. The surgery in both series preceded radiotherapy and the principle of "removing as much cancer as possible", had been thoroughly followed. It is significant

that survival was not affected by the higher tumour dose in their second series.

In 1961, KOTTMEIER, reviewing his extensive experience with surgery and radiotherapy in ovarian cancer, advised against "forcibly removing growths fixed to surrounding tissues by firm adhesions or even by sharp dissection of those attached to the intestinal or pelvic walls"; all patients, operated on under these circumstances, died within 21 months after operation. He therefore counselled in such cases only exploratory laparotomy and radiotherapy. These observations on the poor results of incomplete surgery and postoperative radiotherapy raised the question as to whether survival could be improved in similar cases if radiotherapy were given before, instead of after, excisional surgery. If laparotomy had been performed, would pre-excisional radiotherapy increase survival?

Preoperative Radiotherapy

Sporadic attempts at such "preoperative" radiotherapy have been tried for years in small series of cases. Thus, PARKS (1945) at the Presbyterian Hospital, New York, delayed excision of three extensive seropapillary cancers, seen at exploratory laparotomy, until after radiotherapy had reduced the size of the growths, making them more operable. In the interval, between the first and second laparotomy, a few months later, there was marked reduction in the size of these neoplasms. LONG and SALA (1963) reported eight year survival in 8 extensive ovarian cancers, which after laparotomy had each received 4,000 rads tumour dose and then had excisional surgery. This type of preoperative radiotherapy should now be tried in a large series of cases to investigate the possibility of increasing survival in advanced ovarian cancer cases.

Results in Present Series

The results of surgery and postoperative radiotherapy in Stages I—III of the present series, staged according to the method suggested by the Cancer Committee of the International Federation of Gynecology and Obstetrics, are presented in Table I.

The figures in Table I emphasize the influence of the stage at the time of the first exploratory laparotomy on the proportion of patients living and well after treatment. The cases were usually in a more advanced stage in rapidly growing seropapillary cancers than in the slower advancing endometrioid growths. Death within a year after laparotomy in Stage I occurred in 7% of seropapillary and 6% of endometrioid cancers. In Stage III, however, deaths within a year after laparotomy were seen in 65% of patients with seropapillary cancer and in 46% with the endometrioid variety. The percentage of patients living and well five years after treatment in Stage I was 45% for the seropapillary and 76% for the endometrioid cases. In Stage III, on the other hand, this survival in the seropapillary variety was only 3%, but was 15% in the endometrioid type. If one now examines the relative frequency of the various stages with which patients with these two microscopic varieties were admitted to laparotomy, the difference in growth rate and its influence on prognosis becomes clearer. In Stage I, there were seen only 17% seropapillary as compared to 32% endometrioid cases. On the other hand, 59% of seropapillary and 30% of the endometrioid patients were not admitted until they were in Stage III.

The proportion of patients admitted in Stage III who were living and well five years after treatment was very small. It is the predominance of Stage III and the paucity of Stage I cases in the seropapillary variety which explain the difference in the overall survival figures of 14% for seropapillary and 50% for patients with endometrioid cancer. As in most other types of cancer, it is the extent of the disease before treatment, rather than the details of local therapy, which primarily decides the outcome of the treatment.

Operability and Survival

Operability of ovarian cancer depends primarily on the stage of the

Table I. *Survival and stage at first laparotomy*

Seropapillary: 314 patients Survived: 1 year — 142 patients — 45% 5 years — 45 patients — 14.3%							Endometrioid: 248 patients Survived: 1 year — 46 patients — 18% 5 years — 124 patients — 50%							
Frequency			Survived				Frequency			Survived				
Stage	No.	%	1 year 142 patients		5 years 45 patients		Stage	No.	%	46 patients 1 year		124 patients 5 years		
			No.pts.	%	No.pts.	%				No.pts.	%	No.pts.	%	
I	55	(17)	4	(7)	25	(45)	I	79	(32)	5	(6)	60	(76)	
II	75	(24)	18	(24)	14	(19)	II	95	(38)	7	(8)	53	(56)	
III	184	(59)	120	(65)	6	(3)	III	74	(30)	34	(4)	11	(15)	

I: Limited to the ovaries. II: Extension to the uterus and tubes or other pelvic structures. III: Extension above the pelvis, e.g., omentum, mesentery, small intestine.

disease and secondly on the skill of the surgeon. At times, it is difficult to decide whether operability should be judged on the stage or the surgeon's judgment.

The classification of I a in Table II, which denotes limitation of the cancer to one ovary, indirectly suggests that these cases are completely operable, and should survive 5 years — yet 56% of seropapillary I a patients died prior to

younger when admitted. Among the older age group, however, relatively more patients were admitted in Stage III, than among the younger patients. Thus, the stage on admission and not only the age, influenced the outcome of the treatment.

The influence of stage also interfered with an unbiased evaluation of the effect of other factors on survival. Such factors

Table II. *Stage and survival: I, a and b; II, a and b*

Stage	Seropapillary			Stage	Endometrioid		
	Total No.	5 years No.	% 5 years		Total No.	5 years No.	% 5 years
I	55	25	45.5	I	79	60	76
I a	36	16	44	I a	63	49	78
I b	19	9	47	I b	16	11	69
II	75	14	19	II	95	53	56
II a	—	—	—	II a	36	27	75
II b	75	14	19	II b	59	26	44

It will be recalled that I a is limited to one, and I b to both ovaries. II a signifies extensions which are confined to the uterus and tubes, while II b denotes extension to other pelvic structures. The difference in survival figures in II a and II b are significant in the endometrioid cases.

5 years. Was this an error in staging, in surgical judgement or failure of postoperative radiotherapy?

The value of postoperative irradiation is shown more clearly in Stage II, especially in Stage II b. In these cases there cannot be any doubt that cancer persisted in the pelvis postoperatively, yet 19% of the patients with seropapillary and 44% with endometrioid cancer were well at the end of 5 years after treatment. It seems fair to assume that these patients lived 5 years after incomplete surgery, because of postoperative radiotherapy.

Age and Survival after Treatment

Patients who on admission were 50 years or older lived 5 years after treatment less often than those who were

were: 1) the significance of excrescences on the peritoneal surface or rupture of carcinomatous cysts, 2) the value of castration and 3) the importance of endometrial involvement in endometrioid cancer. Valid conclusions could therefore not be made on the influence of these factors and they will therefore not be discussed any further.

Preoperative Radiation and Stage

The stage on admission also affected the outcome of treatment when preoperative irradiation was given so that conclusion as to the value of this therapy could not be made on the basis of the available material. Among the preoperatively irradiated cases, there were 43 seropapillary and 26 endometrioid types. Of the seropapillary, 30 were in

Table III. *Age and survival rate*

Seropapillary			Endometrioid		
Total	Over 50	Under 50	Total	Over 50	Under 50
314	206	108	248	136	112
5 years 14%	12%	19%	5 years 50%	43%	59%
Stage III 184 pts.	69.5%	30.5%	Stage III 74 pts.	58%	42%

Table IV. *Five-year survival and tumour dosage, Stage II*

No. survivors Seropapillary	Tumour dose	No. survivors Endometrioid
4/18 pts. 22%	0—3,500 rads	15/29 pts. 52%
4/28 pts. 14%	3,600—5,500 rads	23/39 pts. 59%
6/26 pts. 23%	5,600—7,500 rads	8/16 pts. 50%

Stage III, 10 in Stage II and none in Stage I. Only one of the forty three lived 5 years and she was admitted in Stage II. Among the endometrioid cases, 9 were in Stage III, 13 in Stage II and 4 in Stage I. Two of Stage III, 9 of Stage II and 4 of Stage I were free from clinical evidence of cancer at the end of five years. These figures are small, and not significantly better than survival rates among patients who did not have preoperative irradiation. It should be mentioned, however, that none of these patients received the now usually employed tumour dosage of 5,000 to 6,000 rads to the pelvis.

Radiation Fields and Tumour Doses

Because of the intolerance of the upper abdomen for intensive irradiation, this region was treated only when its involvement was strongly suspected or in Stage III.

Tumour doses given in Table IV were calculated only in Stage II, where there was likelihood that cancer persisted after the operation, yet was still limited to the pelvis. Stage I cases could not be used for this purpose, as it was uncertain

whether some growth remained post-operatively. Stage III cases presented so few 5-year survivors that the effect of various tumour doses on survival could not be deduced from this scarce material. It is therefore only Stage II in which convincing information was available; this is shown in Table I. The bearing on survival of higher tumour doses appears to have a relatively minor role in the experience of MUNNELL *et al.* (1957). In the present series, survival rate in Stage II arranged according to the tumour dosage, did not support the bearing of the differences of these doses on five year survival. These variations could be attributed chiefly to differences in microscopic type and stage on admission.

Acknowledgments

The present investigation was suggested by Professor HANS LUDWIG KOTTMEIER, whose help and encouragement were of inestimable value.

I am indebted to Professor LARS SANTESSON. He made all microscopic material available to me and, by friendly discussions, clarified the pathological aspect of this problem. He also assigned to me two junior pathologists, CLAES SILFERSWART and STEN FRIBERG; they assisted me with abstracting the patients' histories, written in Swedish. I greatly appreciate their help.

All calculations of tumour dosage were done by NILS ERIK RANUDD of the Department of Physics of the Radiumhemmet, to whom I am very grateful for his cooperation. He is now in charge of Clinical Physics in the Central Lasarett, Karlstad, Sweden.

I thank Mrs. FORSTNER and her staff in the Record Room, who kindly provided me with the records I used for this study.

I would also like to express my appreciation to the other members of the gynecological staff of the Radiumhemmet. Their spirit of cooperation and tolerance helped me to overcome initial difficulties with the language, etc.

Discussion

Radical surgical removal of the cancer, including bilateral salpingo-oophorectomy, is probably the most effective treatment of seropapillary and endometrioid cancers of the ovary, but only if at the time of the laparotomy the entire cancer is thus completely excised. This is most likely to occur in Stage I, in which the cancer is still limited to one or both ovaries. Postoperative irradiation of the pelvis, preferably with supervoltage x-ray or cobalt beam, to a tumour dose of 5,000—6,000 rads in 7—8 weeks, should be added, in case a mistake in staging has been made, and if, microscopically, the cancer has extended beyond the limits of excision.

In Stage II, when there is great likelihood of postoperative persistence of the cancer in the pelvis, radiotherapy should follow immediately after laparotomy and precede any attempt at excisional surgery. Incomplete surgical excision before radiotherapy may open lymph and blood channels, smear cancer over the peritoneum and disseminate the cancer; this type of surgery tends to make postoperative radiotherapy less and not more efficient.

Preoperative radiotherapy has displaced postoperative radiotherapy in other cancer sites, and should now be tried in a large series of Stage II of these ovarian cancers. The tumour dose should usually not be less than 5,000 rads in seven weeks to the pelvis if a prolonged result is desired. Radiotherapy, of course, must be preceded by laparotomy; this is needed not only for microscope classification of the cancer, and anatomic delineation of the clinical borders of the growth by direct visualization and palpation, but also to permit multiple biopsies in a search for silent eatensions and more accurate determinxtion of the limits of the neoplasm. Expert laparoscopy, when available, may be helpful in this problem.

Excisional surgery, especially in Stage II a cases, may be reconsidered about 2 to 3 months later, after radiotherapy has had a chance to reduce the activity and perhaps the size of the growth, thus making it more operable. Even in cases of no, or very little, reduction in the size of the growth during this period, excisional surgery may still be considered at the end of 2 or 3 months after treatment.

Sudden shrinkage of a cyst after radiotherapy most likely signifies that it has ruptured into the peritoneal cavity; reduction of the growth due to radiotherapy is usually more gradual. Increase in the volume of a cyst may either be due to greater fluid content within the cyst because of radiation reaction or may represent actual growth of the cancer.

In Stage III, in which five-year survival in the present series was only 3% in seropapillary and 15% in endometrioid cases, surgery is needed for biopsy, for ascertaining the anatomic stage of the cancer, occasionally to relieve intestinal obstruction by cancer, but does not prolong survival in the average case. Excision of the cancer in Stage III is always incomplete and the benefit of postoperative radiotherapy under these circumstances is less than if it is given alone or at least preoperatively. Ordinarily radiotherapy in Stage III produces only temporary growth restraint. It is questionable whether excisional surgery before radiotherapy in this Stage ever prolongs survival, or whether what appears to be prolongation is really a naturally slow course of the disease. Excision in Stage III cuts across lymph and blood channels and smears cancer cells across the peritoneum, disseminating the disease. Radiotherapy under such circumstances is likely to be less efficient than when the vascularization of the area has not been disturbed by surgery. The aim of radiotherapy in Stage III should be palliation. Tumour dosage should not be influenced by unrealistic hope of permanent arrest, but by consideration of the patient's comfort.

Stage IV cases were not included in the present investigation; their survival does not depend on the therapeutic effect within the pelvis, which was the subject of this study, but on the relation between the resistance of the host and the aggressiveness of the distant metastases. The over-all survival rate in Stage IV is very poor in most large series of cases, irrespective of the form of local therapy. The occasional patient who survives a long time after treatment, in spite of being in this Stage, only serves to support this rule.

Summary

This is a retrospective study of the survival rate after surgery and radiotherapy of 314 patients with seropapillary and 248 with endometrioid cancer of the ovary. The patients were treated at the Gynecological Service of the Radiumhemmet, Stockholm, Sweden, between 1915 and 1959; they were reviewed in 1963 and 1964.

The purpose of the investigation was to study the relation between survival, anatomic extent before therapy and details of treatment. Cases in which a clear description of the pretreatment extent of the cancer was lacking, were excluded from the study.

Microscopically, all cases in this series showed obvious infiltrative destructive growth, those neoplasms considered as of low potential malignancy were not included. Endometrioid cancers manifested epithelial structures similar to adenocarcinoma of the endometrium. At times this similarity was incomplete.

The growth rate was faster and fewer patients with seropapillary cancer survived 5 years than those with endometrioid cancer. Thus, 14% of the former and 50% of the latter were living and well five years after the end of treatment.

The anatomic extent of the cancer at exploratory laparotomy was staged according to the method suggested by the Cancer Committee of the International Federation of Gynecologists and Obstetricians: — Stage Ia, as cancer limited to one and stage Ib as cancer limited to both ovaries; Stage IIa, extension to uterus and tubes only and Stage IIb, cancer also involving other pelvic structures; Stage III — widespread pelvic metastases and cancer extending above the pelvis, to the omentum, small intestine, mesentery; Stage IV — cancer with distant metastases, outside peritoneal cavity.

Patients in Stage IV were excluded from the study as their survival rate depended mainly on the resistance of the host to the aggressiveness of the distant metastases and not on the therapy for the disease in the pelvis.

If the proportion of patients judged free from clinical evidence of cancer five years after treatment is classified according to the stage on admission, with seropapillary neoplasms first and endometrioid second, there were respectively: — in Stage I — 45% and 76%; in Stage II — 19% and 56%, and in Stage III — 3% and 15%. Of the seropapillary cases, however, only 17% were admitted in Stage I, 24% in Stage II and 59% in Stage III disease. The corresponding figures in endometrioid cases were: 32% in Stage I, 38% in Stage II and 30% in Stage III.

The influence of stage on the survival rate so overshadowed the possible effect of other factors, e.g. age, that investigation of these factors was inconclusive.

As a result of this study we think that incomplete surgery tends to cut across lymph and blood channels and spread cancer; it does not prolong survival. We believe that the following indications apply to the treatment of the patients according to stage:

Stage I: Radical surgery remains the treatment of choice, to be followed by radiotherapy if microscopic examination reveals persistent disease.

Stage II a: If complete surgical removal at laparotomy appears to be possible, radical resection and postoperative radiotherapy may be considered; otherwise the treatment should be as in Stage II b.

Stage II b: Laparotomy, followed by radiotherapy to the pelvis, and second laparotomy 2—3 months later with or without resection of the remaining cancer, depending on its extent. The radiotherapy should preferably consist of supervoltage x-ray therapy or cobalt beam with a daily tumour dose of 150 to 175 rads a day, i.e. 700—800 rads a week, continued for 7 weeks.

Stage III: Laparotomy, followed by radiotherapy with palliative dosage, perhaps 4,000 rads tumour dose to the pelvis and 3,000 rads to the upper abdomen. Surgery for acute complications, such as intestinal obstruction due to pressure of the tumour, must of course be done if the need arises. Removal of cancerous masses, however, is not likely to have any effect on survival, but may be done for palliative purposes when indicated.

Discussion

SCULLY asked if the better results attributed to postoperative irradiation in patients with the so-called borderline tumours could actually be the result of the natural history of the disease. He also inquired if, when a patient has an endometrioid carcinoma of the ovary and a similar tumour in the uterus, the classification should be Stage II or, more accurately, Stage I ovary and Stage I uterus. The exception would be the serous tumours since these often spread from the ovary to the uterus. Therefore, the Stage II endometrioid and Stage II serous may not be strictly comparable. He also asked if any attempt to use hormone therapy for endometrioid tumours had been made.

JUNQUEIRA commented that one aspect often overlooked in planning treatment is the natural history of the disease. When chemotherapy is considered, he said, it is useful to classify the tumours into two groups: (1) those which grow and disseminate locally and permeate the lymphatic vessels but do not usually give rise to distant metastasis, and (2) those which metastasize early in the disease. In this last group chemotherapy should play an important role as an adjuvant to surgery with the purpose of reducing the circulating cancer cells and, consequently, the distant metastasis.

LENZ agreed with the importance that the natural history of the ovarian cancer should play in the prognosis and treatment.

References

ACKERMAN, L. V., and DEL REGATO, J., *Cancer,* ed. 2, p. 922—959. St. Louis: C. V. Mosby Co. 1962.

ARIEL, I. M., The treatment of ovarian cancer with radioactive isotopes. *Amer. J. Roentgenol.* **88**, 877—885 (1962).

DALLEY, V. M., Is preservation of the uterus worthwhile? *Amer. J. Roentgenol.* **88**, 867—876 (1962).

DELCLOS, L., and MURPHY, M., Evaluation of clinical effectiveness of cobalt 60 moving strip. *Amer. J. Roentgenol.* **96**, 75—80 (1966).

DOCKERTY, M. B., Pathologic features of certain ovarian carcinomas. *Amer. J. Roentgenol.* **88**, 841—845 (1962).

ELLIS, F., Malignant disease of the ovary and radiotherapy. *J. Fac. Radiol. (Lond.)* **7**, 1—10 (1955).

End results and mortality trends in cancer. National Institute of Cancer Monograph No 6. United States Department of Health, Education & Welfare, Washington, D. C. 1961.

HAAGENSEN, C. D., *Diseases of the breast.* Philadelphia: W. B. Saunders Co. 1956.

GRICOUROFF, G., Sur L'endométriose des ganglions pelviens. *Bull. Ass. franç. Cancer* **49**, 292—299 (1962).

HERTIG, A. T., and GORE, H., *Tumors of the female sex organs,* sect. IX, fasc. 33, part 3. Armed Forces Institute of Pathology, Washington, D. C. 1961.

HOLME, G. M., Prognostic factors in malignant ovarian disease. *Acta Un. int. Cancr.* **19**, 1135—1138 (1963).

KENT, S. W., and McKAY, D. G., Primary cancer of the ovary. *Amer. J. Obstet. Gynec.* **80**, 430—438 (1960).

KERMAUNER, F., and NURNBERGER, L., Die Erkrankungen der Eierstöcke und Nebeneierstöcke und Geschwülste der Eileiter. München, J. F. Bergmann, 1014 p., 1932.

KOTTMEIER, H. L., Radiotherapy in the treatment of ovarian carcinoma. *Clin. Obstet. Gynec.* **4**, 865—874 (1961).

LATOUR, J. P. A., and DAVIS, B. A., A critical assessment of the value of x-ray therapy in primary ovarian carcinoma. *Amer. J. Obstet. Gynec.* **74**, 968—976 (1957).

LONG, M. E., and TAYLOR jr., H. C., Endometrioid carcinoma of the ovary. *Amer. J. Obstet. Gynec.* **90**, 936—950 (1964).

MALLOY, J. J., DOCKERTY, M. B., WELCH, J. S., and HUNT, A. B., Papillary ovarian tumors.

Amer. J. Obstet. Gynec. **93**, 867—879, 880—885 (1965).

MULLER, J. H., *First five year results of routine intracavitary administration of colloidal radioactive gold for treatment of ovarian cancer.* Medical science, vol. XI, p. 265—272. New York: Pergammon Press 1959.

MUNNELL, E. V., JACOX, H. S., and TAYLOR jr., H. D., Treatment and prognosis in cancer of the ovary. *Amer. J. Obstet. Gynec.* **74**, 1187—1200 (1957).

PARKS, T. J., Carcinoma of the ovary treated preoperatively with deep x-ray. *Amer. J. Obstet. Gynec.* **49**, 676—685 (1945).

PUROLA, E., Serous papillary ovarian tumors. *Acta obstet. gynec. scand.* **42**, Suppl. No 3 (1963).

RUBIN, P. A., A critical analysis of current therapy of carcinoma of the ovary. *Amer. J. Roentgenol.* **88**, 833—840 (1962).

SAGERMAN, R. H., HANKS, G. E., and BAGSHAW, M. A., Supervoltage radiation therapy. *Calif. Med.* **102**, 118 (1965).

SCHOTTLAENDER, J., Über die metastatischen Geschwülste des Weibes. In: FRANKL-HOCHWART, *Erkrankungen des weiblichen Genitales in Beziehung für innere Medizin,* vol. 2 (L. V. FRANKL-HOCHWART, C. V. NOORDEN, u. A. V. STRUMPEL). Wien and Leipzig, A. Hölder, pp. 254—266, 1913.

SNOW, W., *Roentgenology in obstetrics and gynecology.* Springfield (Ill.): Ch. C. Thomas 1952.

STONE, L., WEINGOLD, A. G., SALL, S., and SONNENBLICK, G., Factors affecting survival of patients with ovarian carcinoma *Surg. Gynec. Obstet.* **116**, 351—360 (1963).

TAYLOR jr., H. C., Studies in the clinical and biological evolution of adenocarcinoma of the ovary. *J. Obstet. Gynaec. Brit. Emp.* **66**, 827—842 (1959).

—, and MUNNELL, E. W., Treatment of tumors of the ovary. In: G. T. PACK and I. M. ARIEL (eds.), *Treatment of cancer and allied disease,* ed. 2, p. 264. New York, Hoeber-Harper, Vol. 6, pp. 254—266, 1962.

WILLIS, R. A., *The spread of tumors in the human body.* London: J. & A. Churchill 1934.

— *Pathology of tumors.* London: Butterworth & Co. 1953.

YOFFEY, J. M., and COURTICE, F. C., *Lymphatic lymph and lymphoid tissue.* Cambridge: Harvard University Press 1956.

Megavoltage Irradiation in the Management of Malignant Ovarian Tumours*

Luis Delclos, M.D.

Associate Radiotherapist, Associate Professor of Radiology, Department of Radiotherapy, The University of Texas, M. D. Anderson Hospital and Tumour Institute, Houston, Texas, U.S.A.

Introduction

Most of the malignant tumours of the ovary spread diffusely throughout the abdominal cavity and along the lymphatics of the periaortic chain. An accurate preoperative diagnosis is rarely possible and the majority of cases are referred to the radiotherapist after, at least, an exploratory laparotomy. Seventy-five per cent of patients referred to this institution have had, before referral, surgical procedures ranging from complete removal of gross tumour to biopsy of generalized abdominal carcinomatosis. Additional surgery is performed after referral, depending on the individual patient under consideration.

Peritoneal washings are almost always positive even when the tumour was limited to one ovary and it had been completely removed; there is, therefore, potential contamination of the peritoneal cavity.

A study of different reports shows wide variation in five-year survival (5 to 65 per cent) which can be explained by including tumours that are of different histopathological entities (Munnel and Taylor, 1949; Taylor and Munnel, 1962). One can say that the larger

* This investigation was supported by U.S. Public Health Service Grants No. CA 06294 and CA 05654.

the masses and the more extensive the disease, the less effective is the radiation treatment, irrespective of the modality.

Classification of Ovarian Tumours from the Standpoint of Radiotherapy

Except for the dysgerminoma, malignant ovarian tumours are tumours of limited sensitivity to ionizing radiation, that is, tumours that will require relatively high doses to be sterilized. There is a group of tumours histologically similar to the dysgerminoma but whose response to irradiation is questionable. For this study tumours have been divided into two main groups:

A. Dysgerminoma and dysgerminoma-like tumours (mixed, sarcomatous, unclassified). These are tumours which one would expect to be sensitive to ionizing radiation.

B. Papillary serous cystadenocarcinoma and undifferentiated carcinomas. These are tumours which belong to the less sensitive group.

The latter account for most of the patients referred to radiotherapy. Pseudomucinous cystadenocarcinoma, mesonephromas, embryonic tumours (excluding dysgerminoma), teratomas, and metastatic carcinomas are not included in this study because they were referred for radiotherapy in small numbers and they should not be grouped together as they belong to different histopathological entities.

Treatment Techniques Employed

Through the years different treatment modalities have been used. At the University of Texas M. D. Anderson Hospital and Tumour Institute, except for the few cases where postoperative irradiation of the pelvis was the only irradiation given, for the most part and for reasons discussed in the introduction, the whole abdominal cavity was irradiated with additional treatment to the pelvis or to residual masses.

For the dysgerminoma group, additional treatment was given to the mediastinum and the supraclavicular fossa, when either of these areas was involved.

Pelvic Treatment

Up to 4,000 r only parallel opposed fields (Fig. 1a) were used (15 × 15 cm

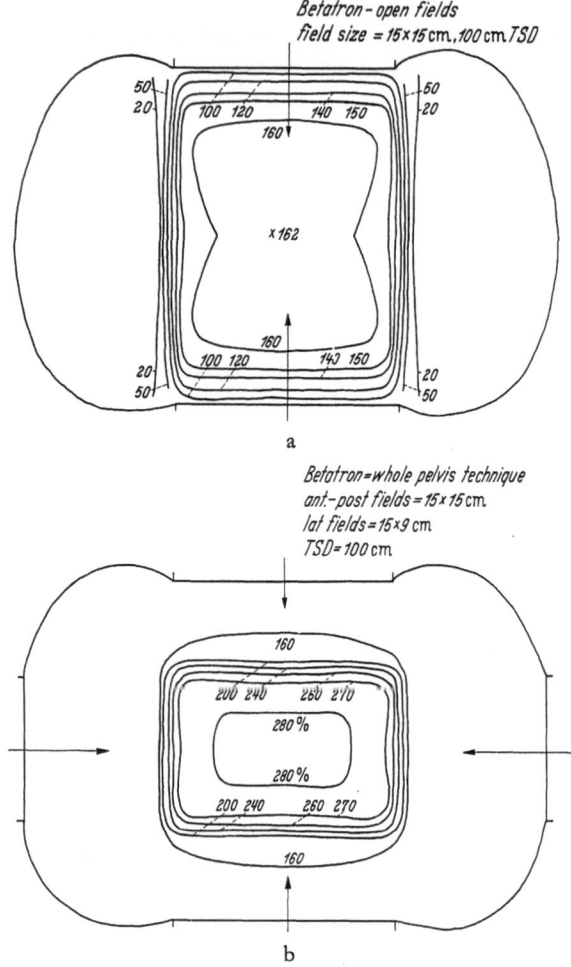

Fig. 1a and b. Isodose distribution for the pelvic treatment with a 22 Mev betatron. a Two parallel opposed fields. b Four fields. — Courtesy: FLETCHER, G. H., STOVALL, M., and SAMPIERE, V., Radiotherapy of cancers of the cervic uteri. In: *Carcinoma of the uterine cervix, endometrium and ovary.* Chicago: Year Book Medical Publ. Inc. 1962 by means of a 22 Mev betatron photon beam), but additional lateral fields were added (15 × 9 cm) with doses above 4,000 r (Fig. 1 b and 2 a). This dose was kept at 2,000 r (1,000 r tumour dose cause of its simplicity, it was easy to select any desired shape and to shield the kidneys. Homogeneity was excellent (Fig. 3 a) but because of the large volume irradiated *"in toto"* the dose was limited

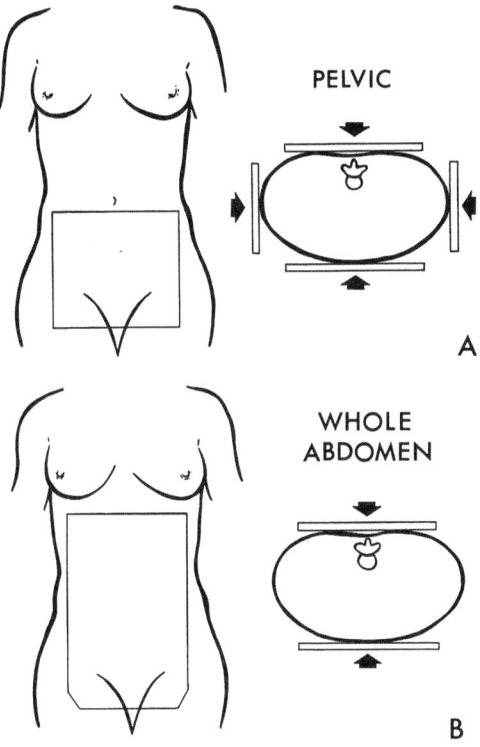

Fig. 2a and b. Volume covered with megavoltage irradiation. a Pelvic irradiation with four fields. b Parallel opposed fields to whole abdomen. — Courtesy: DELCLOS, L., and BURNS jr., B. C., Radiotherapy management of tumors of ovary. In: G. H. FLETCHER, *Textbook of radiotherapy.* Philadelphia: Lea & Febiger 1966

weekly) for additional treatment to the pelvis or to residual masses, but when the pelvic irradiation was the only modality of treatment, the dose was taken to 5,000 or 6,000 r (1,000 r tumour dose weekly).

Whole Abdominal Irradiation

Large Parallel Opposing Portals. These were used to cover the whole abdomen from the Douglas cul-de-sac to the diaphragm with a Co⁶⁰ unit (Fig. 2 b). Be-

to 3,000 r in six to seven weeks. Local and systemic reactions were very severe.

Four Oblique Fields. When it was desired to increase the central dose (*i.e.*, periaortic area), a four-angled field arrangement (Fig. 3 b) was used with a Co⁶⁰ unit. The set-up from day to day was simplified by the use of a "Manchester trunk bridge". Another advantage was that a set of isodose curves for different interfield distances and field sizes could be calculated, making unnecessary the repeated plotting of volume distribution (DELCLOS, 1966). Kidney shielding lacked absolute accuracy.

appropriate corrections of penumbra effect, depth dose, and by adjusting the dose to the resulting dose-time ratio.

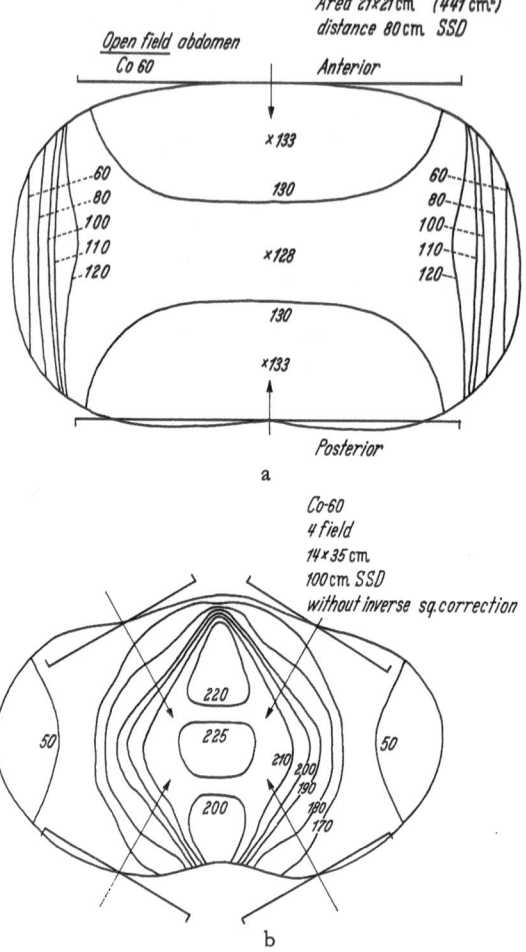

Fig. 3a and b. a Isodose distribution in the transverse diameter for parallel opposed fields, Co⁶⁰ gamma-ray therapy. b Isodose distribution for a four-field "trunk bridge" arrangement using Co⁶⁰ gamma-ray therapy. — Courtesy: DELCLOS, L., *et al.*, Whole abdominal irradiation by cobalt 60 moving strip technique. *Radiology* **81**, 632—641 (1963)

Co⁶⁰ Moving Strip. In an attempt to increase the dosetime relationship, the megavoltage moving strip technique was developed (based on a similar kilovoltage technique designed in Manchester for the treatment of generalized sensitive tumours). This technique is described in detail by DELCLOS *et al.*, 1963. It may be adapted to any megavoltage unit, by

The field is advanced daily from one end of the volume to the other, minimizing the risk of high or low dose effects at the junctional areas, which would occur if the whole volume were treated in separate segments (Fig. 4a—d).

With our units we were able to deliver to the abdominal cavity a dose of 2,500 to 3,000 r in two and one-half weeks (12 treatment days) and therefore the biological action should be greater than with open portals or three- or four-angled fields.

tolerance of the hemopoietic system, organs involved in the irradiated volume, and systemic reactions (DELCLOS and MURPHY, 1966).

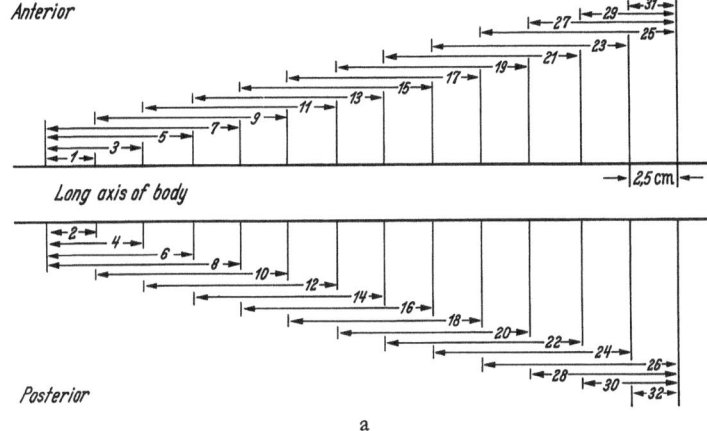

Fig. 4a—d. a Diagram showing the treatment sequence for the Co⁶⁰ moving strip. b Combined isodose distribution upon completion of treatment in the longitudinal axis of the body. c and d Photographs of patient showing skin marks during the treatment of the whole abdomen by the Co⁶⁰ moving strip. Lines are 2.5 cm apart. The kidney is shielded from the posterior beam by 2 HVL of lead placed on a "satellite platform" (this will reduce the total dose to the kidneys to about 50 per cent of the tumour dose). — a, c, d: Courtesy: DELCLOS, L., Segmental therapy. In: G. H. FLETCHER, *Textbook of radiotherapy*. Philadelphia: Lea & Febiger 1966. b: Courtesy: DELCLOS, L., *et al.*, Whole abdominal irradiation by cobalt 60 moving strip technique. *Radiology* 81, 632—641 (1963)

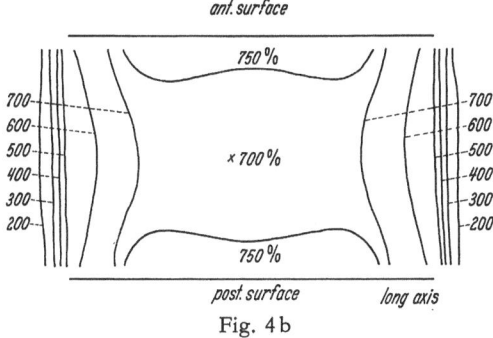

Fig. 4 b

Limiting Factors
with Whole Abdominal Irradiation

Irradiation of the whole abdominal cavity with megavoltage units is easier than with kilovoltage as the skin is no longer a limiting factor; the dose is more uniform but we still have to face the

The dose which we can deliver with any of the treatment modalities described in this paper is usually sufficient for the sensitive group of tumours (2,500 to 3,000 rads). In regard to the tumours of limited sensitivity, this dose is insufficient as far as cure is concerned; furthermore,

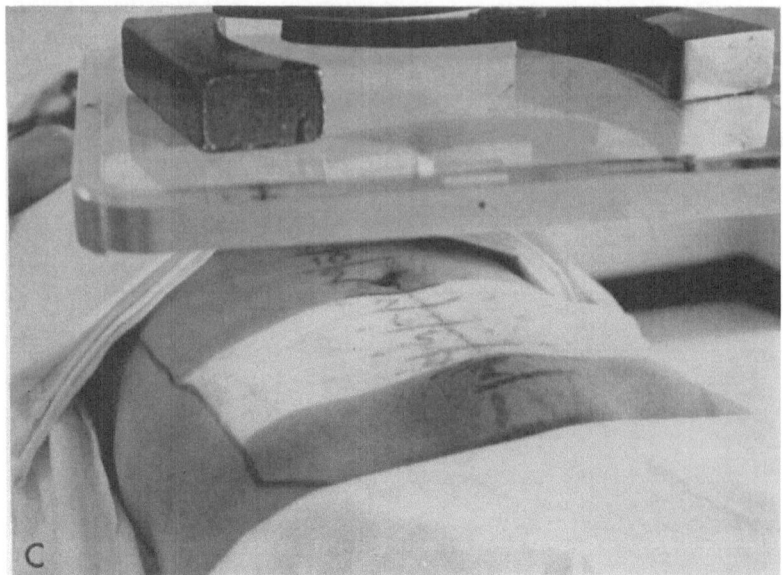

Fig. 4c

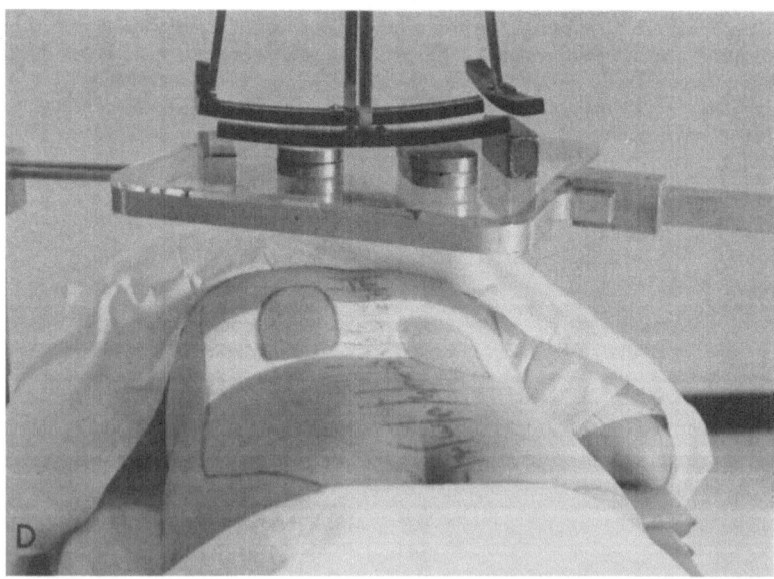

Fig. 4d

the kidneys have to be shielded in order to reduce the dose below a critical dose (about 2,500 rads) (KUNKLER *et al.*, 1952). Of course, these shields will also reduce the dose to potentially contaminated areas.

Intracavitary Radium

This type of therapy was only used as additional treatment when the uterine cavity was left in place at surgery or to treat residual disease in the vagina.

Ascites

No patients with massive ascites were treated postoperatively by means of external irradiation.

Analysis of Results
A. Dysgerminoma
and Dysgerminoma-Like Tumours

From 1952 to 1965, 19 patients with dysgerminoma and dysgerminoma-like tumours were treated with postoperative irradiation. The diagnosis was generally made late, when (1) the tumour had already attained a certain size, (2) the peritoneal cavity and/or the periaortic nodes were involved or (3) the tumour had metastasized to the left supraclavicular fossa.

In Table I it can be seen that 12 patients had dysgerminoma and 7 dysgerminoma-like tumours (difficult to classify, mixed, sarcomatous). It is important to separate these tumours because although the numbers are small, the well differentiated dysgerminoma has a better prognosis than the unclassified (of 12 patients, 8 are alive in the dysgerminoma group, 6 for more than five years, one for almost two years, and one for about six months); while in the dys-

Table I. *Dysgerminoma and dysgerminoma-like tumours treated by radiation therapy following different surgical procedures, 1952—1965, 19 cases*

	Incidence of postirradiation recurrence	Survival	
		2 years	5 years
Dysgerminoma: 12	2/12	6/12*	6/12*
Dysgerminoma-like (unclassified, mixed, et cetera): 7	5/7	0	0

* Two more patients are alive with no evidence of disease at 6 months and 20 months (less than 2 years).

Table II. *Carcinoma of ovary. Postoperative irradiation (all techniques), 88 patients (5 year minimum survival), 1953—1961*

	Number of patients	No evidence of disease	Expired
Papillary cystadenocarcinoma	67	19 (28.3%)	48
Undifferentiated carcinoma	21	0	21*
Total	88	19 (22%)	69 (78%)

* All expired before 2 years after completion of treatment.

Table III. *Carcinoma of ovary. Postoperative irradiation (all techniques) 88 patients (5 year minimum survial) 1953—1961*

	Total	5 year survival	
Tumour removed	4 ⎫		
Unknown extent	5 ⎬ 13	9/13	69%
Spillage	4 ⎭		
Residual tumour: pelvis	20	5/20	25%
abdomen	55	5/55	9.1%

germinoma-like group, all 7 patients expired within one and one-half years after treatment.

The sensitivity of these tumours to irradiation seems to be different also. In the dysgerminoma group, only 2 out of 12 patients recurred in the abdomen, while there were 5, out of 7, recurrences in the less differentiated group. Two of the patients in the dysgerminoma group had positive supraclavicular nodes and after comphrehensive treatment of these areas, are alive with no evidence of disease for more than five years.

B. Papillary Cystadenocarcinoma and Undifferentiated Carcinoma

Eighty-eight cases were treated from 1953 to 1961. In Table II it can be seen that all 21 patients with a pathological report of undifferentiated carcinoma died of their disease within two years after completion of their treatment. In the papillary cystadenocarcinoma group there are 19 patients out of 67 alive at five years (28.3%).

When we divide the patients according to the stage of their disease after surgery (Table III), we can see that the

Table IV. *Patients with widespread abdominal disease treated with*

Patient	Date of surgery and operative findings	Extent of surgery and residual tumour	Postoperative radiation technique
O. B. Age-68	April 1960: Involvement of both ovaries, omentum, peritoneal seedings.	Removal of tumour in ovaries and omentum. Residual: peritoneal seedings, pelvis + omentum. *Not palpable*	*Pelvis only.* 22 Mev photon beam 15 × 15 cm fields 4,000 r/28 days. *Intracavitary* radium 5,500 mg/hrs.
B. R. Age-41	October 1956: Involvement of both ovaries, omentum, outside sigmoid and urinary bladder dome. Peritoneal seedings	Removal of tumour masses. Residual: tumour throughout abdomen, induration in vault	*Abdomen* (kidneys not shielded): Co 60. Parallel opposed fields 35 × 30 cm, 3,000 r/63 days. *Additional to pelvis:* 22 Mev betatron, 15 × 15 cm fields, 2,000 r/12 days
M. C. Age-26	March 1954: Involvement of right ovary, left tube, omentum.	Removal of tumour masses. Single recurrent mass in pelvis (cul-de-sac)	*Pelvis only:* Co 60. Parallel opposed fields 14 × 14 cm, 3,500 r/43 days
F. C. Age-43	March 1960: Involvement of right ovary and omentum	Removal of tumour masses. *Not palpable*	*Abdomen* (kidney shielded): Co 60 moving strip 3,000 r/12 days. *Additional to pelvis:* 22 Mev betatron, photon beam, 15 × 15 cm fields 2,000 r
M.S. Age-44	June 1959: Involvement of both ovaries, omentum, cul-de-sac	Removal of larger masses. Residual: in pelvis and most likely omentum. *Not palpable*	*Abdomen* (kidneys shielded): Co 60 moving strip, 2,660 r/12 days

prognosis is directly related to the stage. Sixty-nine per cent of the patients survived five years when there was a chance of having removed all the tumour, 5 out of 20 when tumour was left in the pelvis, and 5 out of 55 when there was residual tumour in the abdomen above the pelvis.

Discussion

Analysis of treatment methods in carcinoma of the ovary will be possible when agreement is reached on the classification of the different histopathological groups and on the staging. It is beginning to be evident that the behavior of these tumours depends on the histological entity and degree of extension at the time of diagnosis.

Papillary cystadenocarcinoma accounts for the larger group of patients referred for postoperative irradiation. The dysgerminoma, less common, is seen less often but is the most radiosensitive. The prognosis is also better.

For the papillary cystadenocarcinoma group, prognosis seems to be better when a growth is limited to one or both

postoperative irradiation of different modalities; five years or more survival

Further treatment	Follow-up	Comments
None	August 1966: No evidence of disease	No major complaints since treatment
March 1964, developed metastasis to abdominal wall. April 1966, resected. Multiple seedings left in scar	April 1966: Alive with residual disease in abdominal scar. On chemicals now	Since treatment in 1956 several episodes of partial intestinal obstruction relieved by Levine and rectal tubes, on rest and diet only
Little regression. Surgery: tumour removed + hysterectomy	March 1966: No evidence of disease	Postoperative specimen showed marked radiation changes in tumour
None	June 1966 No evidence of disease	
None	August 1966: no evidence of disease	

ovaries and is removed, even when rupture and spillage of a cystic mass has occurred.

We may influence the natural behavior of some of these tumours by obtaining growth restraint in the more advanced cases. This, of course, is difficult to prove as it is well established that peritoneal seedlings have regressed after removal of the main tumour mass. We have 5 patients (out of 55 with abdominal carcinomatosis) treated with postoperative irradiation who have been comfortable for more than five years. They are analyzed in Table IV.

Summary

Malignant tumours of the ovary are found, in many instances, at time of surgery fixed to surrounding structures or already spread to the omentum. Even when a tumour has been completely removed, peritoneal washings are almost always positive.

The radiotherapy techniques that have been employed at the M. D. Anderson Hospital and Tumour Institute are discussed briefly.

Except for dysgerminoma, it is felt that because of the poor results obtained with present treatment modalities, it is warranted to try new methods, especially when tumour has spread beyond the pelvis. The importance of combining surgical, chemotherapeutic, and irradiation techniques in various sequences is stressed.

Résumé

A l'exploration chirurgicale, les tumeurs malignes de l'ovaire se trouvent souvent adhérentes aux voisinage, ou encore, avec une extension épiploique. Les lavages péritonéals sont presque-toujours positifs, malgré la résection totale de la tumeur.

Les techniques radiothérapeutiques pratiquées à l'hôpital M. D. Anderson sont brièvement présentées.

A l'exception des dysgerminomes, il est bien justifié, à cause des mauvais résultats obtenus selon les présentes modalités thérapeutiques, d'essayer des méthodes nouvelles; particulièrement, quand il s'agit d'une extension extra-pelvienne de la tumeur. On s'appuie sur l'importance de combiner des techniques chirurgicales, chemiothérapeutiques et radiothérapeutiques en une séquence variable.

Discussion

Fletcher said that when megavoltage became available at the University of Texas M. D. Anderson Hospital and Tumour Institute, attempts were made to use it in various ways for ovarian carcinoma. He pointed out that treatment for this kind of cancer is not as straightforward as it is for cervical cancer, in which the pathways of spread are well defined. The "strip" technique was begun in 1958 after a visit to Paterson in Manchester. A tumour dose of 2,500 rads could be given by this method in 12 days. Since any volume of tissue was treated 12 times in 12 treatments, the dose to any one part was 2,500 rads, which was significantly more than the 3,000 rads given by opposing portals in six to seven weeks. One advantage of the strip technique is the better tolerance.

Some patients had benefited by arrest of the disease for long periods of time. Fletcher added that, although cure was the ideal goal for any kind of active therapy for cancer, the fact that cure was not possible should not discourage all attempts at treatment.

FLETCHER suggested that a cooperative study should be established by several institutions so that, by combined experience, some of the unresolved questions about treatment for ovarian cancer could be answered.

LENZ said that he did not think the strip technique was superior to giving irradiation at a slower rate and using larger fields which covered the entire abdomen. He had also been told by physicists, he said, that the overlapping fields in the strip technique were difficult to measure.

MULLER added that he agreed with LENZ that a slower rate was better.

FLETCHER said that there was no discrepancy in the dose and that there was nothing wrong with the physics of the treatment. The strip technique was not regarded as a "miracle cure" by any means but it was a technique to be considered. As to its value, this was hard to establish, he said, but some patients are alive several years after treatment and there have been no late complications.

LUISI said that DELCLOS' classification (radiosensitive and limited radiosensitive tumours) was of interest because it was possible that some of the dysgerminoma-like tumours were endodermal sinus tumours, and nothing had been known of the effect of radiation on these tumours. The fact that some were responsive is important.

References

DELCLOS, L., Segmental therapy. In: G. H. FLETCHER (ed.), Textbook of radiotherapy. Philadelphia: Lea & Febiger 1966.

— BRAUN, E. J., HERRERA jr., J. R., SAMPIERE, V. A., and VAN ROOSENBEEK, E., Whole abdominal irradiation by Cobalt 60 moving strip technique. Radiology 81, 632—641 (1963).

—, and BURNS jr., B. C., Radiotherapy management of tumors of ovary. In: G. H. FLETCHER, Textbook of radiotherapy. Philadelphia: Lea & Febiger 1966.

—, and MURPHY, M., Evaluation of tolerance during treatment, late tolerance, and better evaluation of clinical effectiveness of the Cobalt 60 moving strip technique. Amer. J. Roentgenol. 96, 75—80 (1966).

FLETCHER, G. H., STOVALL, M., and SAMPIERE, V., Radiotherapy of cancers of the cervix uteri. In: Carcinoma of the uterine cervix, endometrium and ovary. Chicago: Year Book Medical Publ. Inc. 1962.

KUNKLER, P. B., FARR, R. F., and LUXTON, R. W., The limit of renal tolerance to x-rays. An investigation into renal damage occurring following the treatment of tumors of the testis by abdominal baths. Brit. J. Radiol. 25, 190—201 (1952).

MUNNELL, E. W., and TAYLOR jr., H. C., Ovarian carcinoma. A review of 200 primary cases and 51 secondary cases. Amer. J. Obstet. Gynec. 58, 943—959 (1949).

TAYLOR jr., H. C., and MUNNELL, E. W., In: G. T .PACK and I. M. ARIEL (eds.), Treatment of cancer and allied diseases, 2nd ed., vol. VI. New York: Paul B. Hoeber, Inc. 1962.

Intraperitoneal Colloidal Radiogold [198]Au Therapy in Ovarian Cancer

Its Unique RES-Bound Paraselective Effects
Emerging Need for a Differentiated Stage III Definition

Prof. J. H. MULLER, M.D.

Chief of the Departments of Radiology and Pathology
Universitäts-Frauenklinik, Zurich (Switzerland)

Internal Radiocolloid Therapy
Its Philosophy

The author began intraperitoneal radiocolloid administration in 1945 and intraperitoneal (also intrapleural) colloidal radiogold therapy in 1949. These developments have been reported in a sequence of earlier publications. We refer to the more recent presentations and to the bibliography indicated therein (J.H. MULLER, 1962 and 1965).

Radiocolloid therapy takes specific advantage of the different *vital* functions of the reticuloendothelial system (RES).

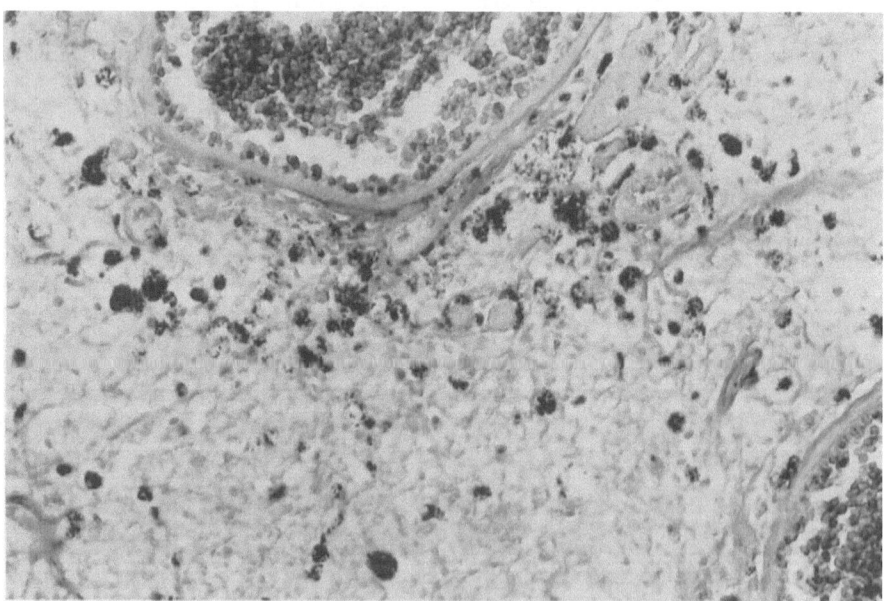

Fig. 1. Microscopic section of peritoneal biopsy performed at the "second-look" operation of a patient who had ovarian carcinoma and who had been treated by means of surgery, conventional radiation therapy and intraperitoneal administration of colloidal radiogold. Note numerous histio-cytic macrophages stuffed with large particles of flocculated colloidal radiogold at the site of a destroyed small metastasis. Only a few mesenchymal cellular elements have survived in the residual scar tissue of this heavily irradiated area, in which the ß-exposure was more than 200,000 R

These functions assist in the *paraselective* concentration of the radioactive particles as they become engulfed[1] by the *histiocytic macrophages around and within invasive cancer* (Fig. 1) and by the reticuloendothelial macrophages in the lymphatic channels and nodes, in the sense of a *radiotherapeutic lymphography* (Figs. 2 and 4).

of not only common radiochemical radicals, but also of immunologically active γ-globulin-bound antimitotic factors (MAURICE *et al.*, 1964).

After decay of the radioisotope, enhanced regenerative and reactive acti-

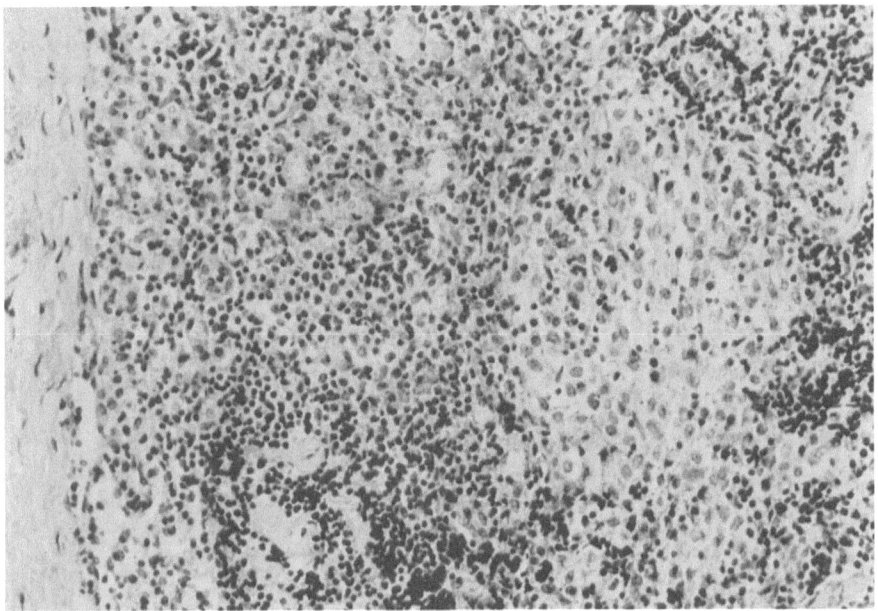

Fig. 2. Section of heavily irradiated axillary lymph node removed from a patient with breast cancer 14 months after preoperative therapeutic interstitial infiltration according to the author's original procedure (the patient had at first unexpectedly refused ablative surgery scheduled 14 days after this *interstitial colloidal radiogold* infiltration). *Abdominal and mediastinal lymph nodes would show the same aspects after intraperitoneal administration of the colloidal radiogold.* Part of the lymph node contains regenerating lymphatic tissue. Note the *increased proliferation of reticular cells.* Towards the left almost acellular scar tissue with residual macrocytic inclusions of flocculated collodial gold

Therapeutic procedures using radiocolloids may, in addition, tend to increase the intrinsic RES defense mechanisms against malignancy. The impact of radiocolloid radiation on the RES is indeed very likely to result in the release

vity of the RES is quite probable. This regenerative capacity is considerable. Even after massive radioactive deposits in lymph nodes, amounting in some areas to irradiation doses of the 100,000 R order of magnitude, lymphatic tissue will form anew, sometimes with increased reticular proliferation (Fig. 2).

These vital interactions with the RES play an important part in all paraselective localization procedures of radioactive particles by means of intravascular, interstitial and intracavitary administrations of radiocolloids. Intraperitoneal

---

[1] From electron microscope studies of phagocytosis by the RES of the liver, it is established that colloidal particles are deposited rapidly and concentrated in apparently specialized organelles of the RES cells (HALPERN, 1964).

or intrapleural administration of radio-colloids will then also contribute to the destruction of tumour cells floating and even multiplying in more or less abundant ascitic or pleural fluid (Fig. 3). It appears further, both from our clinical findings and from recent experimental work (PERKINS et al., 1966), that the engulfing and degradative capacities of

opinion, not quite reliable and well enough defined for routine clinical use. Some other radiocolloids are yet of but experimental interest.

The optimal particle size of colloids for intraperitoneal and intrapleural use is still slightly controversial. A certain variation of particle size is in our opinion likely to be an advantage when using

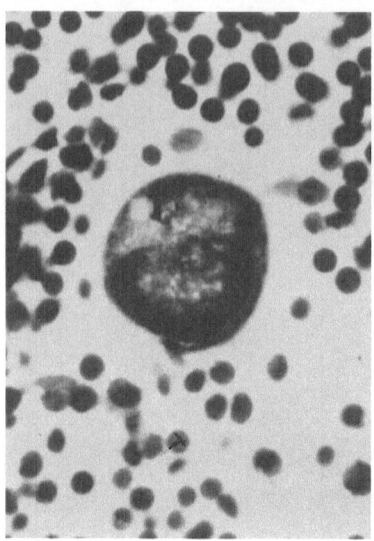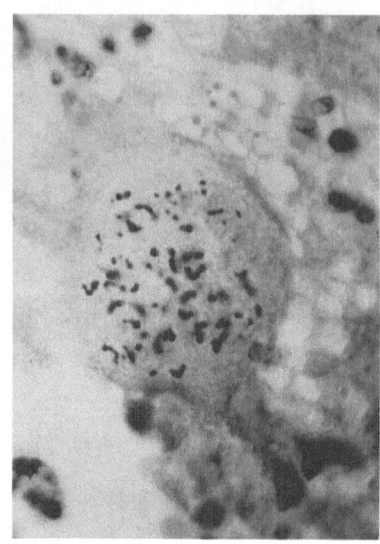

Fig. 3. Effects of intraperitoneal radiogold treatment on ascitic ovarian cancer cells, in a case of generalized abdominal carcinomatosis. *Left:* large, highly atypical cancer cell before treatment, surrounded by erythrocytes. *Right:* residue of such a cancer cell, about 5 weeks after two intraperitoneal administrations of colloidal radiogold (total amount 250 mCi). Observe the complete break-down of the chromatin structure. Only a few erythrocytes are left

peritoneal phagocytes are very radio-resistant (even to supra-lethal levels). This is also the case for other cells comprising the RES. Hence added conventional radiotherapy will not interfere with optimal paraselective effect of even repeated intraperitoneal radiocolloid administration.

Materials

The most frequently used radio-colloids are radioactive gold (^{198}Au) and to a lesser extent radioactive chromium phosphate (anhydrous Cr^{32}PO$_4$). Radioactive Yttrium (^{90}Y) is, in the author's

the intracavitary route, as well as for interstitial procedures. For intravascular (intravenous, direct intralymphatic and intraarterial) administration methods, on the contrary, colloids and suspensions with distinctly selected optimal particle sizes of different magnitudes have already emerged, *i.e.* —.005 μ for intravenous administration, for example in chronic leukemia, —.03 to —.05 μ for direct radiolymphography, 30 to 50 μ for intraarterial administration (MULLER and ROSSIER, 1951).

In our 20 years' clinical intraperitoneal administration work, we first pioneered the method by using colloids obtained from ground insoluble sulfide precipitates of cyclotron-produced radioactive zinc ([63]Zn *plus* some [65]Zn), and then, from 1949 on, we have invariably used the *classically* prepared red gold colloid. Most of the activity of this [198]Au colloid is carried by particles between —.009 μ and —.015 μ (the particles ranging in size from —.003 μ to .—035 μ). Consequently, vital histiocytic interactions are assured, with the resulting desired concentrations of radioactive particles within the large serosal surfaces and the lymphatic system. [198]Au is now a much used radioisotope with a half-life of 2.69 days, the energy levels of the emitted radiations being 0.96 Mev for the β-radiation and 0.411 Mev for the γ-radiation.

Methods and Therapeutic Management

The intraperitoneal (and intrapleural) administration of radioactive colloids became rapidly known after we had started it and became quite extensively used throughout the world for palliative treatment of malignant effusions. Useful, sometimes excellent, palliation can be obtained by this means in about one half of these generally hopelessly incurable cases. These palliative results were confirmed in a great number of papers and later also suggested the use of palliative intracavitary chemotherapy.

As soon as colloidal radiogold became available to us in 1949, I became specifically interested in the *curative* possibilities offered by this new approach. Hence I performed first intraperitoneal administrations of colloidal [198]Au in association with *artificial hydroperitoneum*, which were then used *routinely* in ovarian cancer patients from the fall of 1949 on. In 1950 this extensive indication of intraperitoneal radiocolloid became accepted and firmly established by Prof.

Held, as he took over the clinical direction of the Zurich Frauenklinik in 1950.

This principle of a combined surgical and radiotherapeutic cure of ovarian cancer, including routine intraperitoneal colloidal [198]Au (with the exception of the few cases that are primarily inadequate for radiocolloid administration) has since remained unaltered in this institution, in the sense of an optimal therapeutic tactic for obtaining the *maximal possible curative results* in the fight against this dreadful disease.

The indication for this extensive use of intraperitoneal radiogold appeared justified from the beginning of my intracavitary radiocolloid work, both from its specific rationale, as discussed above, and from the clinical experience I had of the well-known fact that even "radically operable and operated" ovarian cancer patients would strikingly often develop within the following months and years fatal generalised abdominal carcinomatosis. This clinical proof of obvious early desquamation and lymphatic spillage of tumour cells, even in the early stages of ovarian cancer, has also been confirmed by cytology of peritoneal washings (ELKINS and KEETTEL, 1956), as well as by the investigations on cul-de-sac aspiration cytology presented at this Conference (GRAHAM, 1966).

Tissue radiation dosimetry in intraperitoneal [198]Au colloid therapy is a quite difficult matter. Investigations by means of radiocolloids in tracer doses are of no value at all for such studies, which can be made with precision only on tissue specimens taken from patients (at "second look" operations or at autopsy), after intraperitoneal radiocolloid administration at full clinical dosage. For these studies we have used in particular microautographic methods and neutron activation analysis. We were thus able to establish that the previously discussed desirable concentrations of the colloidal radioactive gold at the level of the serous surface and in the lymphatic vessels, as well as in the retroperitoneal, mesentery and mediastinal lymph nodes are indisputably present (Fig. 4), all within the multikilorad dosage range for the β-radiation. Substantial added

mastery of this special therapeutic approach is now mandatory. Aspects of both the involved radiation safety problems and of technical and tactical factors that are of clinical importance must thus be briefly discussed.

The "nuclear" aspects do not involve great difficulties, since incidental contaminations with colloidal radiogold,

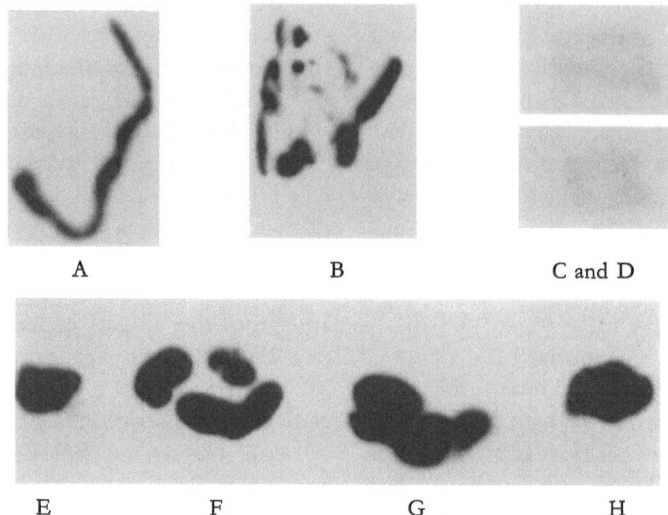

Fig. 4 A—H. Microautograms of tissues collected at autopsy from a patient, with severe ascitic abdominal carcinomatosis who died of heart failure seven days after palliative intraperitoneal administration of 150 mCi colloidal radiogold: A Serosa of small bowel (ileum); B Omentum (the deposits within the lymphatic vessels and the serosa are clearly visible; C Liver; D Spleen; Note the only low radioactivity levels in these two organs, averaging 200 R. E, F, G, H retroperitoneal and mediastinal lymph nodes, with heavy radioactive deposits therein

dosage from penetrating γ-radiation, amounting to about 500 R in the periphery and increasing rapidly to about 1000 R toward the central parts of the "abdominal sphere" — for one intraperitoneal dose of 125 to 150 mCi of colloidal ^{198}Au —, will further homogenize the irradiation effect throughout the abdomen.

Technique of Intraperitoneal Radiocolloid Administration

Intraperitoneal radiocolloid administration has now definitely outgrown the so-called experimental stage. Hence

that is by a nonmetabolizing material, are detectable and easy to control. The usual lead-protected devices are of course necessary when making the dose (100 to 150 mCi ^{198}Au) ready for intraperitoneal (or intrapleural) administration. For adequate personnel protection, lead panels of different types and sizes (Figs. 5 and 6) — with appropriate lead thicknesses — will suffice for proper protection during the radioactive phase of the administration procedure and in ward service. The latter will be greatly simplified by giving exact instructions to the ward personnel *and to the patient*, who will be from the beginning taught to spend a certain length of time out of bed, *i.e.* from about a total of one hour during the first day after administration up to several hours one week later; even

As to the problems involved in clinical management and administration technique, I discussed them at the last International Symposium on Radioactive Isotopes, January 1966 in Gastein,

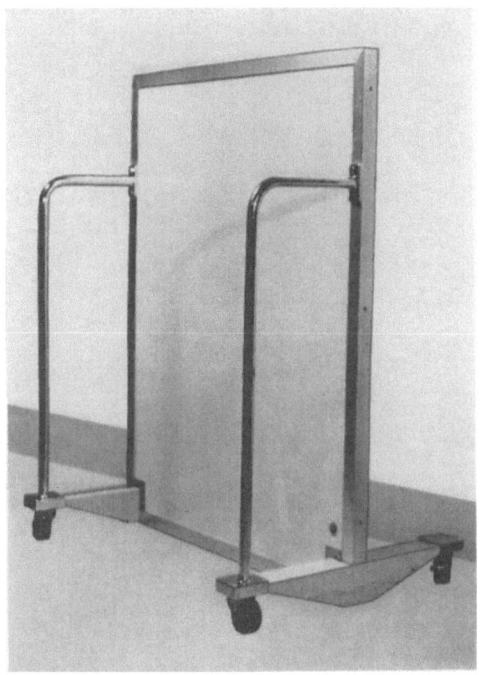

Fig. 5. Larger protection panel with 1 cm lead thickness (reduced to 0,5 cm towards the bottom). The whole radioactive phase of intraperitoneal radiogold administration is performed from behind this protecting device, which insures minimal exposure to operator and assisting personnel. Note smooth, easily decontaminable surface, in case spilling should exceptionally occur

right after administration, the patient will be allowed to rise if she needs to urinate; the patient will thus be perfectly capable, in most instances, of caring for herself within her own "hot area", the radius of which is 2 meters at the beginning of the radioactive decay of the incorporated therapeutic dose, and 1 meter a week later. Both ward personnel and the radioactive patients must be well instructed about these distance factors, important when the patient is allowed, from the third day on, to walk to the lavatories, etc. Almost all patients are quite willing to cooperate.

Austria (J. H. MULLER, 1966). I will recall here that there are possible pitfalls in routine postoperative intraperitoneal colloidal radiogold administration. These are, however, nearly always avoidable. It is thus quite clear that severe complications, such as necrosis of intestines followed by acute peritonitis, as well as necrosis of the abdominal wall, etc. are due to incorrect technique. Intraperitoneal radiocolloid administration is indeed by no means just a mere "injection", but rather an "intraabdominal intervention" that requires adequate skill and precision.

The principal clinical aspects involved are as follows: after adequate premedication (with the drug of preference plus —.25 to —.5 mg of atropine) and with the patient on a fasting stomach and emptied colon, local anesthesia is given (10 to 15 ml of a 1 per cent lido-

abdomen by forced pressure during the insertion of the trocar. Such ventral counterpressure insures against puncturing an intestinal loop, which will be displaced by the entering trocar, and it also makes it possible to penetrate the abdominal wall, layer by layer, with far

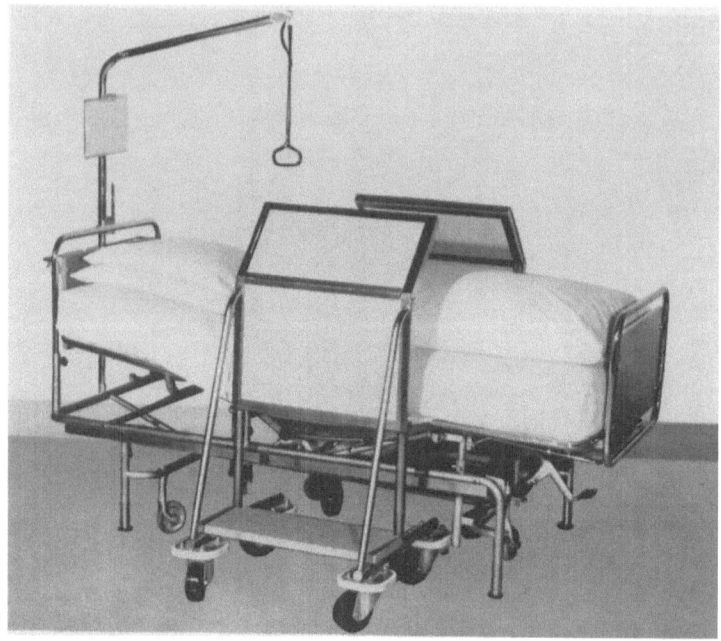

Fig. 6. Special construction for radioprotection "at the epicenter". The "radioactive belly" can thus be shielded from both sides. Lead thickness of 2 cm on the side, of 1 cm in the top parts. This device is also used for at least partial shielding in radium patients

caine plus epinephrine solution). The site of puncture is chosen after careful abdominal palpation has located a suitable *adhesion-free region* (which must be without *any* tenderness or deep infiltration), usually on the left, sometimes on the right side near the rectus abdominis muscle and 1 inch beneath the navel. Other sizes of puncture will be chosen in rare cases. As the paracentesis trocar (our special trocar [Fig. 7] has an outside diameter of 2.8 mm—thicker instruments are not recommendable) enters the abdominal wall, it is very *important* that the patient be asked to distend the

greater control and safety than when the patient's abdomen "lies slack".

As soon as the abdominal cavity is entered, a slight "give" is felt. A piece of polyethylene catheter is then introduced through the trocar about 15 cm deeper into the abdominal cavity and the trocar is gently withdrawn. Ventral counterpressure is then no longer necessary. A flask of physiologic saline solution is connected to the tubing in the manner of an intravenous perfusion. If the saline solution flows continuously by gravity into the abdomen (if there is a slow-down of flow the tubing must be slightly moved inwards or outwards), one can be certain that the polyethylene catheter is properly placed within the abdominal cavity. After administration of about 200 ml of saline solution, the colloidal radiogold, diluted with saline solution, is injected and saline is again given for final dispersion of the radio-colloid within the abdominal cavity, gold activity. In order to enhance even distribution, however, the patient is told to turn slowly in bed for about 8 hours. The fluid is thereby well dispersed within the whole abdominal cavity by the combined effects of capillary and hydrostatic pressure. In addition, the patient's bed should be inclined towards the feet (at an angle of about 15 degrees) for 3 days

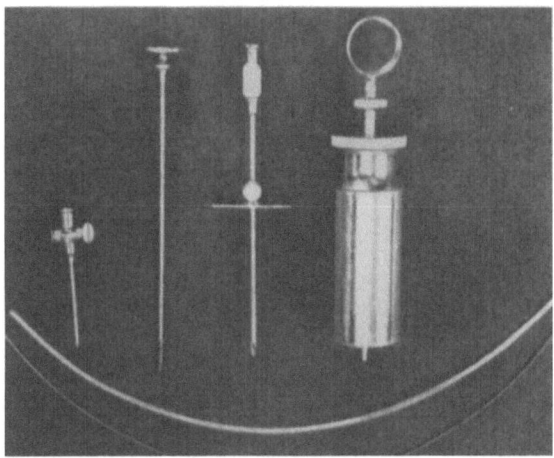

Fig. 7. Instruments used in intraperitoneal administration of colloidal radiogold. Note the thin trocar with adjustable supporting stem. Below: Thin polyethylene catheter with adapter and elastic "piano-cord" guide. To the right, lead-protected syringe used for injection of the diluted radiogold colloid

up to a total amount of about 400 ml fluid. In some sensitive and thinner patients, 5 to 8 ml of 1 per cent lido-caine (without epinephrine) will be added to the intraperitoneal saline.

As soon as the intraperitoneal administration is completed, the polyethy-lene tubing is removed, the puncture site massaged with a sterile cotton bud held by a long tongue and covered with a small adhesive bandage. The skin had of course been disinfected at the beginning of the procedure. A rapid monitoring of the radioactive abdomen is then performed with a smaller shielded Geiger counter held by means of a handling tongue or stick, which will in most instances demonstrate excellent primary distribution of the administered colloidal to allow for enhanced flocculation of the radioactive particles in the lower abdominal and pelvic areas.

This method of "sandwiching" the radioactive phase between substantial portions of plain physiological saline is a safe procedure, hazardous neither to the patient nor the operator, if carefully performed within a free peritoneal cavity. We have found that administration of the radiocolloid dose by means of a lead-protected syringe allowing colloid dilution up to at least 20 ml is the most suitable procedure, since it gives exact control and maximal reduction of the time required, which is the most important factor. Of course, such manual procedure must be performed swiftly from behind a lead protected wall, and with great precision. We have thus practically abandoned the use of remote control apparatus (which I had first constructed and employed from 1946 on).

Care must be taken not to allow significant amounts of air to enter the abdominal cavity together with the radiogold-saline mixture. Such artificial pneumohydroperitoneum would impair the even diffusion of the radioactive colloidal gold.

Important Special Clinical Factors

Cases with marked loculations of the abdominal cavity due to extensive adhesions are *not* suitable for such routine radiocolloid therapy. Such adverse conditions will be, in most instances, already known from direct observation at laparotomy. Hence it is mandatory to be *exactly* informed by a *detailed surgical report*. It will be also possible in some questionable borderline cases to ascertain the presence of loculation, improper for the administration of the therapeutic radiocolloid dose, when the first portion of plain physiological saline does not flow freely into the abdomen. Variation of drip speed when the patient is asked to inspire deeply will as a rule prove a free peritoneal cavity. In some instances we have also added a few millicuries of the ^{198}Au colloid to the saline for rapid hand scanning of the distribution pattern by means of a simple monitoring instrument. This is more reliable than scintiscans with tracer doses only.

Worth a special mention is the clinical observation that peritoneal irritation, sometimes tending to paralyze intestinal function, is not an infrequent complication with poorly nourished patients, as is secondary late fibrotic shrinkage of the omentum and mesentery. If there is no urgency, such as ascitic carcinomatosis, I have told thin pa-

tients to go home after the postsurgery hospitalization period — including in most cases also conventional radiotherapy — in order to recover well and fatten themselves up (but without using anabolic hormones, which might modify the functional capabilities of the RES). Four to six weeks later, such patients are then usually ready to undergo intraperitoneal radiogold administration without danger of such complications, which can be rather severe, since they may result in adhesive obliteration of the peritoneal cavity.

We have, since the beginning of routine administration of colloidal radiogold, organized the therapeutic management of the potentially curable ovarian cancer patients as follows:

In these potentially curable ovarian cancer patients *i.e.* Stages I, II and *early* III (see below), the postoperative recovery period will last for not less than 3 weeks. We will then usually first administer a part of our standard conventional radiation therapy before intraperitoneal radiogold application. Patients with exudative ascitic carcinomatosis, however, will of course receive first the intraperitoneal radiogold.

Conventional radiotherapy (J. H. MULLER, 1948; J. H. MULLER *et al.*, 1965) consists of fractionated 250 to 400 kev roentgen therapy over a period averaging 7 weeks with a total depth dose of up to 3000 R within the pelvic cavity and the adjoining lower abdomen. Exceptionally about 1000 R (rarely more) will be administered within the upper part of the abdomen in some advanced ovarian cancer cases. The irradiation period will then be substantially prolonged, no such penetrating radiation being given to immediately adjacent subphrenic structures. In addition, these patients receive, as a rule, a vaginal radium application (1800 mg/hr or less in 24 hours). Since the majority had either supravaginal or total hysterectomy, only few combined uterovaginal radium treatments were given (with from about one half to three quarters of the exposure used in cancer of the cervix).

When using intraperitoneal colloidal radiogold as a routine procedure in postoperative radiological treatment of ovarian cancer, one must be aware that this represents a major radiotherapeutic procedure. To avoid undue stress on the patient, single doses of more than 150 mCi in larger patients or 100 to 125 mCi in smaller women are never administered. Severe reactions are quite exceptional after *one* such administration, but repetition of the radiocolloid treatment may provoke them, especially when this is done at a shorter interval. In fact it is preferable to limit repeated treatments to selected patients because the danger of early complications due to intolerance and of late mesenteric fibrous contraction is enhanced when more than one administration is performed, most particularly in slender patients, as already said above. Stout women, on the other hand, will as a rule easily withstand two or even three radiogold treatments. Retreatment in patients from Stage I$_b$ on to Stage III (adopted staging of the *International Federation of Gynaecology & Obstetrics* — F.I.G.O. —) may thus be performed at an interval of 7 to 10 weeks and may be definitely gratifying. For advanced Stage III and Stage IV ovarian cancer patients, inasmuch as they appear to be incurable, both the dosage and the number of radiogold administrations are apt to vary greatly, since the purpose is to obtain prolongation of life with as little patient discomfort as possible. We have in more recent years also attempted chemotherapy in some of these advanced cases.

Clinical Results

The reason why I have endeavoured in the preceding sections of this paper to present at least a summarized synoptic view of the specific aspects involved in routine intraperitoneal [198]Au colloid administration in the framework of combined surgical and radiotherapeutic treatment of ovarian cancer is the now available evidence of its *curative* virtue. However such curative contributions appear to be limited to the rather earlier stages of this malignant condition, although these include cases with metastases throughout the whole peritoneal cavity, inasmuch as diffuse gross node generalization has not yet occurred. Let us point out, in this respect, that the surgical removal of a limited number of larger nodes from the visceral or parietal peritoneum, as well as resection of at least parts of the omentum containing such large deposits, may further enhance the curative range of the intraperitoneal radiogold, as we have experienced it in a few cases.

We are thus, in continuation of earlier reports given by invitation at the Tenth International Congress of Radiology at Montreal and at the University of Paris Gynecological Clinic (J. H. MULLER, 1963), in a position to present herewith the 5-year results obtained in our series of 230 unselected patients with true common ovarian carcinoma, all treated from the fall of 1949 on in the described manner. These results are summarized in Table III. In contradistinction to earlier presentations of results, we have now completely eliminated from the presented figures all epithelial ovarian tumours with proliferating activity of only low potential malignancy, *i.e.* of the $_b$-group of the now adopted F.I.G.O. histological classification. We had in fact contributed a first histopathological definition of these proliferating epithelial tumours, based on "histological grading" (J. H. Muller, 1945), that had been used at the Zurich Frauenklinik from 1945 on, until the F.I.G.O. classification became available and accepted (Kottmeier, 1965). There is a good correlation between the two classifications, as shown in Table I.

Table I. *Correlation of the author's previous histological grading with the F.I.G.O. histological classification of common primary epithelial tumours of the ovary*

Author's Grade A = F.I.G.O.-Groups I, II, III$_b$
Author's Grade B = F.I.G.O.-Groups I, II, III$_c$
Author's Grade C = F.I.G.O.-Group IV

The adjustment of the clinical staging we had introduced and used during the period of the reported results (late fall 1949 until end of 1961) to the accepted new F.I.G.O. staging, in use since 1965, can be made with enough accuracy to warrant exact evaluation of the figures, as shown in Table II. Such adjustment, however, made it necessary to introduce and use a *tentative subdivision of stage III* into stage III$_a$ and stage III$_b$. Such a differentiation of the "early" and "late" stages III does not in fact interfere with the basic viewpoint of the F.I.G.O. Cancer Committee and is indispensable for the scientific clinical understanding of the therapeutic results presented in this paper; such a subdivision would moreover appear of general value in the clinical management of common ovarian cancer.

The rationale of this tentative amendement of the F.I.G.O. Stage III definition is thus as follows:

From our 17 years of systematic clinical use of intraperitoneal radiocolloid administration in ovarian cancer therapy, we have learned that the limit of curability in this disease by all present available therapeutic means, *i.e.* surgery, all usual forms of radiotherapy, intraperitoneal radiogold and chemotherapy, is reached practically when *gross* widespread intraperitoneal metastasization has occurred. The suggested maximal size of diffusely scattered intraperitoneal secondaries of 1 inch (2.5 cm) in diameter for "Stage III$_a$" has proved useful in practice, this differentiated subdivision of Stage III being established *after completion of surgery*. Indeed, no 5-year cures were obtained in our series of true invasive common ovarian cancer when diffuse intraperitoneal deposits had clearly trespassed this suggested limit for "Stage III$_a$". Moreover almost all the "Stage III$_a$" cases of this series in which — essentially thanks to the intraperitoneal colloidal radiogold — 5-year cures were obtained, had shown at surgery only *smaller* widespread intraabdominal metastatic nodules, some of which were ascertained only by biopsies. Several years ago, Held introduced at this Institution the routine performance of biopsies from the omentum and the parietal peritoneum in all ovarian cancer operations. Though such biopsies will cover only very small areas of the huge peritoneal surface, incidental positive histological findings are very indicative for exact classification and further conduct of treatment. A few of these cases, that we have attributed to "Stage III$_a$" (since it represents a post-surgical definition of stage), are included in this presentation of results.

This more exact differentiation of the Stage III cases is not difficult to perform and will thus permit a correct selection of the potentially *curable* cases, for which a complete, energetic and systematic post-operative radiation treatment with a curative aim is *strictly indicated*, including one (or more) intraperitoneal colloidal [198]Au-applications.

Table II. *Comparison of the author's hitherto used common ovarian cancer staging with the newly adopted F.I.G.O. definitions of stages of primary ovarian carcinoma*

The author's previous definitions of stages	F.I.G.O.'s definitions of stages	The author's suggested amendment
	Stage I: Growth limited to the ovaries	
Stage I: Unilateral ovarian tumours without adhesions and/or metastases	Stage I$_a$: Growth limited to *one* ovary; no ascites	
	Stage I$_b$: Growth limited to both ovaries; no ascites	
	Stage I$_c$: Growth limited to both ovaries; *ascites* present, with malignant cells in fluid	
Stage II: Adherent unilateral tumours, *bilateral ovarian tumours*, cystic tumours ruptured before operation, tumours with metastasis limited to the pelvic area	Stage II: Growth involving one or both ovaries, with pelvic extension	
	Stage II$_a$: Extension and/or metastasis to the uterus and/or tubes only	
	Stage II$_b$: Extension to other pelvic tissues	
Stage III: Cases as in Stages I and II, but with additional metastases within the whole peritineal cavity, if the latter deposits do not exceed 2.5 cm (1 inch) in diameter	Stage III: Growth involving one or both ovaries with wide-spread intraperitoneal metastasis to the abdomen (the omentum, the small intestine and its mesentery)	III$_a$: Such cases, but with metastases *not greater than 1 inch in diameter* III$_b$: All other Stage III cases
Stage IV: All other cases of ovarian cancer	Stage IV: Growth involving one or both ovaries with distant metastasis outside the peritoneal cavity	

Table III. *Therapeutic results in true ovarian cancer—colloidal—*[198]*Au series (from fall of 1949 to end of 1961. Cases operated outside and referred for postoperative therapy are included)*

Author's staging	I	II	I+II	III	IV	Totals
F.I.G.O.'s staging	I_a	$I_{b,s}$, $II_{a,b}$	$I_{a,b,s}$, $II_{a,b}$	*III_a	*III_b IV	
Total number of treated cases						
B = F.I.G.O. histological groups I II III.	37	47	84} 99	56} 70	30	170} 230
C = F.I.G.O. histological group IV	1	14	15}	14}	31	60}
Alive without symptoms after 5 years						
B = F.I.G.O. histological groups I II III.	33	28	61} 63 = **64**%	22} 31%	0	83} 85 **49**% } **37**%
C = F.I.G.O. histological group IV	1	1	2}	0	0	2} **3**%
Deceased from carcinoma before 5 years						
B = F.I.G.O. histological groups I II III.	1	14	15} 26 = 26%	34	30	79} 135 59%
C = F.I.G.O. histological group IV	0	11	11}	14	31	56}
Deceased from intercurrent disease						
B = F.I.G.O. histological groups I II III.	3	—	8} 10 = 10%	0	0	8} 10 4%
C = F.I.G.O. histological group IV	0	—	2}	0	0	2}

Potentially *curable* ovarian cancer cases. Obtained 5-year cure rate = **50**%

* Amendment of definition suggested by the author.

The clinical management of all the other cases of common ovarian cancer, since they appear to be as a rule incurable, will follow rather variable trends, as already mentioned.

The therapeutic results thus obtained are summarized in Table III.

Discussion of Results

In Table III, 230 cases of true common ovarian cancer, exactly defined as explained above, are now presented.

It appears from this Table that *routine intraperitoneal administration of colloidal radiogold can and even must be considered an advance in the treatment of ovarian cancer.*

This advance is striking for the cases in Stages I and II (F.I.G.O. definition), since in 99 cases of these stages added together, of which many had only incomplete surgery, a 5-year cure rate of *64%* was obtained. Let us mention, for comparison, that this figure of 64% is about the same as had been obtained at the Zurich Frauenklinik, in the years preceding the routine use of colloidal radiogold, with the same surgery and the same conventional radiotherapy, *i.e.* 60%, in a group of cases in Stage I_a (the author's previous Stage I) only! In the present series, only one patient from 38 Stage I_a cases died from cancer. This single case is even questionable, since surgery had been performed elsewhere and the patient died at home from "liver tumour", which was not identified at autopsy.

Also most encouraging are the results obtained with the additional routine intraperitoneal [198]Au-therapy in the author's previous classification Stage III cases (suggested "Stage III_a"), of which 31% remained free of symptoms of disease after 5 years. This appears to be appreciable progress, since such cases, with proved dissemination throughout the whole peritoneal cavity, were but

exceptionally controlled before routine intraperitoneal radiogold administration.

The Stage III cases with 5 year survival were thus all alloted to "Stage III_a", but 3 cases were on the borderline of Stage "III_b". Repeated intraperitoneal radiogold treatments were performed in 60% of these 5 year survivors (average total dose 250 mCi [198]Au) and single administrations in 40% (average 130 mCi). Striking and, in spite of the relatively small number of these survivors, significant is the fact that more than 80% had had serous carcinomas of histological group I_c, the remaining cases having had mucinous carcinomas of histologic group II_c. Further, with the exception of one 70 years old patient of this group II_c, all survivors were relatively young patients, more than one third between age 20 and 40, none over age 60. This analysis indicates clearly that the paraselective intraperitoneal colloidal radiogold therapy operates under optimal specific and thus potentially curative conditions mainly in serous carcinomas with early abdominal disseminations, where the poorly vascularised metastatic nodules have a rather superficial neoplastic activity, whence the reactive interactions with the local peritoneal tissue histiocytes are enhanced. Moreover, unimpared general vitality of the patient's organism, as available in younger age, is likely to be a favorable additional factor for final curative success.

We have thus obtained a cure rate of 50% in the 169 cases of *potentially curable* true common ovarian cancer (*i.e.* F.I.G.O.'s Stages I, II plus suggested "Stage III_a").

The overall 5-year results (last figures to the right of Table 3) indicate that *37%* of the 230 patients of this series, including all the *a priori* incurable cases of Stage IV of the author's previous classification (F.I.G.O.'s Stage IV *plus* suggested "Stage III$_b$") remained alive without evidence of cancer after 5 years. This figure is about *the double* of other published overall cure rates in comparable unselected common ovarian cancer patients. This figure further compares favorably with published cure rate figures for patients, in which only "radical operations" were performed.

The prognostic significance of the histological grade of differentiation of the common ovarian epithelial cancers is further very striking, since only 3% of the poorly differentiated Grade C = F.I.G.O. group IV cases survived, whereas 49% of the more differentiated carcinomas (Grade B = F.I.G.O. groups I, II, III$_c$) were alive after 5 years without evidence of disease!

These routine intraperitoneal ^{198}Au administrations were performed with only low possibly related mortality, since only one patient (*i.e.* 0.45%) died without evidence of disease from septic peritonitis due to secondary colon perforation after ileus operation with Noble's technique — 1$^{1}/_{2}$ years after treatment for Stage II ovarian cancer. In the other cases of intercurrent death cardio-vascular disease is prevalent; several women, however, died from a second unrelated malignant tumour.

Routine intraperitoneal ^{198}Au administration is thus — taking into account its curative virtue — a quite reasonably safe procedure, if correctly employed. This is the reason why we discussed in a previous section of this paper the adequate therapeutic management and the technique of intraperitoneal radiogold administration.

A further point in clinical management that is worth a short discussion is the following:

In a number of patients who die from their ovarian cancer, terminal ileus will of course occur; these deaths are then incidentally attributed to the radiogold. But ileus or subocclusion may also occur in ovarian cancer patients who have *not* been treated with the gold. This is by no means exceptional.

In cases of intestinal subocclusion, the indication for surgical revision may be a difficult one. It is, as a rule, preferable to use first conservative procedures that will be successful in a large number of cases. However, prolonged conservatism in such syndromes may be harmful. As an example we will mention one of the Stage III ("Stage III$_a$") patients of this series, who had innumerable smaller metastatic nodes, mainly located around the right colon, and who developed subocclusion 2 years after full treatment with two intraperitoneal radiogold administrations. This girl, still in her twenties, returned to her home town, where the local surgeon operated upon her almost *sub finem*. He found a mechanical ileus caused by a single adhesive string, but no evidence of tumour. The patient recovered perfectly well and has now remained free of symptoms of the disease for 8 years.

Whilst the pallative efficacy of intraperitoneal colloidal radiogold in ascitic carcinomatosis has been confirmed throughout the world by a very great number of authors, only a few have hitherto, in spite of its obviously sound rationale, been adepts of the more extensive routine use of this paraselective radiocolloid therapy. A clear confirmation of our own original contribution in this respect and of the results thus obtained is the recently published statement of R. KEPP and H. CLEMENS (1965), who reported that the 5-year cure rate in 130 cases of ovarian cancer had been improved considerably by their *routine* use of intraperitoneal radiogold since 1958. Similarly confirmative survival figures for patients in the earlier stages of ovarian cancer had been also reported (1961) by LATOURETTE and have been published (1966) in a larger paper by W. C. KEETTEL, M. R. FOX, D. S. LONGNECKER and H. B. LATOURETTE, of the University of Iowa Medical School. These authors obtained a 5-year survival of 86% in their Stage I and II a ovarian cancer cases, which is much higher than a 52.3% survival from the same hospital in the same groups of patients *prior* to the use of radiogold.

In conclusion, the herewith presented evidence of the life-saving contribution of routine intraperitoneal administration of colloidal radiogold in ovarian cancer therapy may thus be considered as established.

Summary

The routine use of intraperitoneal colloidal [198]Au administration is an important addition to surgery and conventional forms of radiotherapy in the treatment of true common ovarian cancer. This approach presents unique specific qualities, since *paraselective* radiocolloid therapy takes advantage of its vital interactions with the reticuloendothelial system (RES). This provides means for combating efficiently *in situ* the often hidden foci of disseminating cancer. It is likely that radiocolloid therapy might also enhance other RES defense mechanisms against cancerous invasion.

Discussion of the factors involved in optimal clinical and technical management of intraperitoneal radiocolloid therapy and presentation of the 5-year results of its routine use in an unselected group of 230 patients, the hitherto largest available series of cases were given. These results indicate progress. This additional therapeutic means increases significantly the salvage rate of ovarian cancer patients with resectable primary lesions, even when surgery was not

radical and when metastases had already occurred in the pelvic area and/or started throughout the whole peritoneal cavity. Emphasis is laid upon exact definitions of histological groups and tumour staging. The author defines and uses, in this presentation of results, a suggested subdivision of F.I.G.O.'s. Stage III in III_a and III_b, since it appears mandatory to differentiate after surgery the potentially curable cases — radiocolloid therapy being strictly indicated in these cases, of which 50% remained cured after 5 years — from the as a rule *a priori* incurable advanced stages of ovarian cancer.

Résumé

L'administration intrapéritonéale «de routine» de l'or colloïdal radioactif [198]Au réalise, en adjonction à la chirurgie la plus radicale possible et à la radiothérapie d'espèce conventionnelle, un perfectionnement important de la cure radicale des cancers ovariens communs. Cette thérapie *parasélective* par radiocolloïde présente des qualités spécifiques remarquables, parce qu'elle tire singulièrement avantage de ses interactions vitales avec le Système Réticulo-Endothélial (SRE), ce qui permet une irradiation renforcée *in situ* au niveau des foyers de dissémination cancéreuse. Il est en outre très probable que cette thérapie par radiocolloïde déclenche en plus un renforcement d'autres mécanismes de défense du SRE contre l'agression néoplasique.

Discussion des facteurs cliniques et techniques dont la connaissance et le respect assurent un résultat optimum de l'administration thérapeutique intrapéritonéale de routine du radiocolloïde et présentation des résultats thérapeutiques ainsi obtenus chez 230 malades non sélectionnées (la plus grande série de cas réunis jusqu'à présent), atteintes d'un vrai cancer invasif de type commun, après

5 ans. Ces résultats apportent la preuve d'un progrès certain. En effet, cette thérapie combinée radicale augmente d'une manière significative le taux des guérisons à 5 ans des malades chez lesquelles l'ablation chirurgicale de la ou des tumeurs ovariennes était encore possible, même si cette chirurgie était de radicalité douteuse et même s'il se présentait déjà des métastases pelviennes, voire même si cette dissémination métastatique avait déjà commencé de se répandre dans la cavité péritonéale entière.

L'auteur insiste sur l'importance d'une définition exacte des groupes histopathologiques et des stades d'extension des cancers ovariens; il propose en outre une subdivision du Stade III, ainsi qu'il a été défini et accepté par la F.I.G.O., en un «Stade III$_a$» et en un «Stade III$_b$», subdivision qu'il utilise pour la présentation de ses résultats. Il apparaît en effet indispensable de différencier, après l'acte chirurgical, les malades potentiellement encore curables — l'administration du radiocolloïde étant strictement indiquée dans ces cas dont 50% sont resté guéris après 5 ans —, des malades aux stades avancés de leur cancer ovarien, qui restent, hélas, dans la régle *a priori* incurables.

The author is pleased to mention the support given by the "Fonds National Suisse de la Recherche Scientifique" in supplying the valuable cooperation of Dr. F. Levi, physicist.

Discussion

Burns reviewed data on the use of radioactive gold at the Universiy of Texas M.D. Anderson Hospital and Tumour Institute. Of the 919 patients with ovarian cancer examined at this institution since 1947, 101 were treated with radioactive gold. These patients have been divided into stages, according to the recommendations of the International Federation of Gynecology and Obstetrics.

The survival rate in 28 patients in Stages IA and IB was about 50 per cent. There were no survivors in Stage IC patients with ascites or in Stage IIA; in Stage IIIA, there was a 15 per cent five-year survival rate, and in Stage IIB, there was a 33 per cent five-year survival rate. There were no survivors in later stages of the disease. The over-all five-year survival rate in 101 patients was 23.7 per cent (24 patients).

Radioactive gold has not been used in the past five years in this institution because of the high incidence of complications which occurred. Instead, a combination of treatment with surgery, chemotherapy, and irradiation in sequence according to the individual situation of the patient has been used.

It was probable, said Burns, that the results achieved by radioactive gold or external irradiation therapy were similar in Stages IA and IB of the disease. At the present time, external irradiation would probably not be used for Stage IC disease with ascites at M.D. Anderson Hospital; instead a combination of chemotherapy and irradiation would be preferred. In the late stages, II, IIB, and III, he and his colleagues preferred to use chemotherapy in an effort to diminish the size of the mass so that irradiation could be more effective. In most instances, those patients with gross pelvic disease received irradiation with cobalt-60, using the whole abdomen strip technique. When large tumour masses in the pelvis or generalized abdominal disease was present, sarcolysin was used to reduce the volume of tumour. Patients with generalized carcinomatosis received sarcolysin only.

J. GRAHAM commented that from the viewpoint of irradiation, radioactive gold gave a nice distribution of irradiation to the peritoneal surfaces. But, in his experience, any further surgical intervention was extremely difficult. He inquired if possibly this was the result of the dose and if a more modest dose would be useful without creating problems for the surgeon.

KOTTMEIER remarked that, at the Radiumhemmet, the use of colloidal gold had been discontinued several years previously because of complications, but was currently in use. However, he said, since most patients with serous ovarian carcinoma had metastases much larger than one inch in diameter, he wondered if colloidal gold had anything to offer these patients. He also commented on the difficulties of application with a needle. He had recently instituted the use of a polyethylene catheter which was placed in two to four locations after removal of the tumour masses; the colloidal gold was injected four or five days after the surgical procedure. He added that some use had been made of colloidal yttrium which has a heavier beta irradiation than the radioactive gold.

MULLER said that he advocated decidedly the use of colloidal radioactive gold in preference to chemotherapy for all patients considered potentially curable, since the curative virtues of irradiation are proved and because of the possibility of the paraselective concentration of radiogold in and around implants and the uptake by the lymphatic vessels, advantages not possible with chemotherapy, — and since the presented 5-year results in 230 unselected cases do indicate evidence of curative progress.

As to the visceral complications of radioactive gold, he admitted that for thin patients there is some danger, although actually he had lost only one patient because of complications. Obese patients tolerated the treatment well, and, if there was no urgency, he advised his thin patients to gain weight before treatment.

He agreed with KOTTMEIER, that patients with large metastatic masses are less suited to colloidal gold therapy. He has discontinued using the gold immediately after surgical intervention because ovarian cancer patients are often debilitated. Therefore, preferably, three weeks should lapse before conventional irradiation is begun. After about 1,000 R have been given to the pelvis, the gold was administered, in a number of cases even later, up to several weeks after completion of the conventional radiation therapy. The problems involved in clinical management and administration technique of intraperitoneal colloidal radiogold are discussed in the written paper.

He did not consider "colloidal" yttrium satisfactory for use, he said, since this isotope behaves rather as a large particle suspension, and therefore does not enter easily into the lymphatic vessels. Furthermore, with yttrium there is potential danger of contamination with strontium or excessive doses of the yttrium iself, with consequent toxicity.

References

ELKINS, H. B., and KEETTEL, W. C., Radioactive gold in the treatment of ovarian carcinoma. *Amer. J. Roentgenol.* **75**, 1117 (1956).

GRAHAM, RUTH M., Diagnosis of ovarian carcinoma by cul-de-sac aspiration. (The paper of R. GRAHAM is in *this book.* pp. 122—133.)

HALPERN, B., The reticuloendothelial system and immunity. *Triangle ("Sandoz")* **6**, 174 (1964).

HELD, E., Über die Behandlung des Ovarialkarzinoms. *Gynaecologia (Basel)* **150**, 65—66 (1960).

KEPP, R., and CLEMENS, H., Ergebnisse der postoperativen Radiogoldtherape bei bösartigen Ovarialtumoren. *Strahlentherapie* **126**, 3—7 (1965).

KEETTEL, W. C., FOX, M.R., LONGNECKER, D. S., and LATOURETTE, H. B., Prophylactic use of radioactive gold in the treatment of primary ovarian cancer. *Amer. J. Obst.* **94**, 766—779 (1966).

KOTTMEIER, H. L., Classification and staging of malignant tumors in the female pelvis. *J. int. Fed. Gynaec. Obstet.* **3**, 204—210 (1965).

LATOURETTE, H. B., Personal Communication 1961.

MAURICE, P. A., and JEANRENAUD, A., Erythropoietic depression due to splenic irradiation: Experimental study of distant radiological effect. *Brit. J. Haemat.* **10**, 327 (1964).

— — FLATT, J. P., and MAUEL, J., Mécanisme de la dépression erythropoétique provoquée par irradiation du tissu lymphoide. X^th Congress Internat. Society of Haematology 1964.

MULLER, J. H., Pathologisch-anatomische Gruppierung der Malignen epithelialen Ovarialtumoren, im Lichte der Behandlungsprognose. *Mschr. Geburtsh. Gynäk.* **120**, 17—32 (1945).

— Zur Strahlentherapie der Ovarialcarcinome. *Gynaecologia (Basel)* **125**, 67—73 (1948).

— Weitere Entwicklung der Therapie von Peritonealcarzinosen bei Ovarialcarzinom mit künstlicher Radioaktivität (198-Au). *Gynaecologia (Basel)* **129**, 289—294 (1950).

MULLER, J. H., *Radioactive isotope therapy, with particular reference to the use of radiocolloids.* I.A.E.A. Review Series No. 27. Vienna 1962.

— Curative aim and results of routine intraperitoneal radiocolloid administration in the treatment of ovarian cancer. *Amer. J. Roentgenol.* **89**, 533—540 (1963).

— Le traitement du cancer des ovaires — son perfectionnement par l'administration intrapéritonéale d'or radioactif colloïdal. *Rev. franç. Gynéc.* **58**, 197—214 (1963).

— *Treatment of malignant disease with radiocolloids.* In: Nuclear medicine, chapt. 27, p. 705—737. W. H. BLAHD, Editor. McGraw-Hill Book Co. 1965.

— Remarques sur les interactions des thérapies par radiocolloïdes avec le système réticuloendothélial. *J. Radiol. Electrol.* **46**, 266—270 (1965).

— Zu den Wechselwirkungen der therapeutischen Anwendungen von Radiokolloiden mit dem Reticulo-Endothelialen System. *Gynaecologia (Basel)* **159**, 322—328 (1965).

— Vermeidung von Früh- und Spätkomplikationen bei der Intraperitonealen Applikation von kolloidalem Radiogold ^198Au. In: *Radioaktive Isotope in Klinik und Forschung, Band VIII.* Urban & Schwarzenberg 1967.

—, and ROSSIER, P. H., A new method for treatment of cancer of the lungs by means of artificial radioactivity (^63Zn and ^198Au); first experimental and clinical studies. *Acta Radiol. (Stockh.)* **35**, 449 (1951).

— WACHSMANN, F., u. SCHUSTER, G., Die Zürcher Bestrahlungsmethode des Kollumkarzinoms, unter besonderer Berücksichtigung der angewendeten zeitlichen Dosisverteilung. *Strahlentherapie* **125**, 503—523 (1964).

PERKINS, E. H., NETTESHEIM, P., and MORITA, T., Radioresistance of the engulfing and degradative capacities of peritoneal phagocytes to kiloroentgen X-ray doses. *RES-J.* Reticuloendothelial Soc. **3**, 71—82 (1966).

Intracavitary Chemotherapy in Ovarian Carcinoma

G. Brulé

Médecin de l'Institut Gustave-Roussy, Chef du Service de Chimiothérapie des Tumeurs Solides, Villejuif/Seine, France

Introduction

One of the most difficult problems which faces the physician in treating patients with ovarian carcinoma is the control of effusions, either pleural or ascitic, which frequently occur as the tumour involves serous surfaces.

These effusions usually occur late in the course of this disease and, in the majority of patients, the neoplastic effusion is not the sole manifestation of dissemination.

Nevertheless, recurrent accumulation of pleural fluid or ascites, often symptomatic and disabling, may be a most distressing complication. Frequent thoracenteses or paracenteses may result in hypoproteinemia and further fluid retention.

Unless a patient is terminal, symptomatic relief is worthwhile and should be attempted. Control of recurrent effusion, however, rarely has any effect on the natural history of the cancer.

Material and Methods of Evaluation

Several hundred cases can be collected in the literature but these are always patients who underwent other therapy and it is impossible to establish the benefit of the simple cavitary chemotherapy.

In our own institute, most patients with effusions are treated by radioisotopes and the cases which were treated by cavitary chemotherapy were those not benefited by other techniques.

The degree of response is difficult to evaluate as the tumour masses are deep-seated. All physicians have seen cases of inoperable ovarian tumours which, left untreated, survived for longer periods than would have been predicted. Therefore, the duration of survival after the initiation of the therapy is not a reliable criterion, especially in a small and uncontrolled series.

The best way to prove the value of this therapy is the suppression of serous effusion as indicated by spacing of thoracenteses or paracenteses.

Subjective signs, such as improved performance and relief from discomfort, are also parameters of drug response. Since chemotherapy of ovarian cancer is initiated in the advanced stage of the disease, when there are already large masses of tumour tissue, complete regression and cure cannot be expected.

Technique

It is not necessary to describe here the technique of thoracenteses or of paracenteses, which is well-known. Before beginning treatment, one must be sure that effusion of the pleural, peritoneal or pericardial cavity is really neoplastic. Cytologic study of the fluid should be done by numerous techniques including the Papanicolau test.

As much fluid as possible is removed and the antimitotic drug, generally in a single dose, is injected through the cannula.

Whatever compound is used, great care must be taken to ensure that the needle tip is within the cavity and that the fluid is draining freely. Leakage of the antimitotic drugs into the abdominal or chest wall causes painful indurations which take some time to heal.

After the injection, the patient's position must be frequently changed during the next two hours, to distribute the compound as evenly as possible. We do not think it is useful to aspirate the effusion on the following day.

These injections can be repeated several times, according to the speed with which the fluid re-accumulates.

Direct injection of oxygen into the pleural or peritoneal cavities might possibly increase the sensitivity of the cancer cells.

Drugs and Doses

It is difficult to choose among the great number of antimitotic drugs. Most physicians use alkylating agents, but some trials have been made with anti-pyrimidine derivatives and Quinacrine has a special place.

The main biological effect of alkylating agents is their harmful influence on proliferating cells, either normal or cancerous, as shown in depression of mitotic activity, even with low doses and concentrations.

This effect is similar to that of ionizing radiations, but there are some differences; thus for example the stages of interkinesis differ in sensitivity to ionizing radiations and alkylating agents.

The various classes of alkylating agents and even individual substances, for example some chloroethylamines, differ somewhat in their biological effect. These facts explain the numerous compounds tried in intracavitary chemotherapy.

Nitrogen mustard (HN_2) is the hydrochloride of bis (2 Chloroethyl) methyla-

mine. It was used as intracavitary chemotherapy for the first time in 1948, by D. Karnofsky in a pleural effusion.

The average dose for cavitary injection is 0.2 to 0.4 mg per kg body weight, but not exceeding a total dose of 30 mg of HN_2, freshly made up, in 20 cc. of sterile saline for pleural effusions or 50 cc. for ascitis.

Great care should be taken to avoid penetration of HN_2 into the subcutaneous cellular tissue when retrieving the cannula. To prevent a marked reaction, an isotonic solution of sodium thiosulphate is injected at the same site and ice applied for a few hours. In the absence of thio-sulphate, physiological saline can be given.

Side effects are usually minimal. Local pain, lasting from two to three days, may occur. There may be some nausea and sickness, mostly transient, but sometimes lasting for 48 or 72 hours. To prevent or lessen these effects, anti-emetics can be used, for example 25 mg chlorpromazine in tablet form or in injection before the paracenteses. Hematological toxicity is unusual with this method and these dosages.

Degranol, Mannomustine or BCM is 1,6-bis(2 chloroethylamino)-1,6-dideoxy-D-manitol dihydrochloride. The first clinical reports of this compound were made by Sellei and Eckhardt (1958).

Synthesis of BCM or Degranol was undertaken, based on the assumption that use of a sugar or sugar-like substance, as carrier of the active chloroethylamino group, might improve penetration through the cell membranes and the selectivity of action on the tumour cells.

This compound has good stability, solubility in water and marked antitumour properties.

The dosage for cavitary instillations is 100 to 200 mg per injection, which can be repeated several times in case of very rapid re-formation of the fluid. These low doses of Degranol are remarkably tolerated and very effective.

Side effects are rare; when they occur they are of the same type as those seen with HN$_2$.

Phenylalanine mustard (L. Sarcolysin, melphalan, Alkeran®, PAM) is p-bis [2 chlorethyl] amino D,L phenylalanine hydrochloride.

Synthesis of this compound was undertaken with the idea that metabolites (amino acids, in particular) may be suitable conveyors of the cytotoxic group into tumour tissue, giving higher selectivity of antitumour action. PAM is soluble in water.

For intraperitoneal injection a single dose of 40 or 60 mg is used; for intrapleural injection, the dose is 20 mg (powdered substance in ampoules dissolved in saline). Before administration of the preparation the exudate is withdrawn from the serous cavity. Then, as proposed by COSTACHEL et al. (1959), 60—100 ml of 0.5 per cent procaine solution is introduced into the cavity (or the syringe needle from the pleural cavity); the patient is placed for 10 minutes in a recumbent position and is turned as much as possible from one side to another. Finally, the solution of sarcolysin is given.

Intracavitary administration is usually done once a week but the interval may change with circumstances. Usually, 4 to 5 injections are given. Arrest of ascitic formation is not an obstacle to further injections of the compound into the peritoneal cavity. In this case, the solution should be injected, not through a trocar, but through a needle, 0.3—0.5 mm diameter.

The side effects are not negligible.

With inadequate anaesthesia, 2 to 3 hours after administration of sarcolysin, symptoms of irritation of the peritoneum may appear (abdominal pains, vomiting, rise in temperature, quickened pulse, dyspnoea). After intrapleural injection performed without adequate anaesthesia, pains may develop in the chest with nausea and sometimes vomiting. These manifestations fade gradually and disappear after 3 to 4 hours without any special measures (ABBASOV, 1960).

Depression of haemopoiesis with intracavitary administration of sarcolysin usually either does not occur or is slight, due to the binding of the substance by the exudate and tumour tissues. Thus immediate intraperitoneal injection of such a comparatively high dose as 60 mg is permitted.

Cyclophosphamide, Cytoxan® or *Endoxan* is the cyclic ester 1-bis (2 chlorethyl) amino-1-oxo-2-aza-5-oxaphosphoridin.

In the synthesis of Endoxan, German investigators began with the idea of producing compounds which would circulate in the body, first in the inactive transport form, to be transformed into the active form at the point of application. It was supposed that Cytoxan as an internal ester amide of phosphoric acid would be split by phosphatases and phosphamidases, especially in tumour tissue releasing a chemically and biologically active derivative of chlorethylamine. In fact, Endoxan is very stable in an aqueous medium, which explains the very weak activity of this compound in cavitary chemotherapy. The enzymes necessary to split the molecule of Endoxan are chiefly in the liver or in the blood stream.

Because of the minimal toxicity of this compound, one must use high dosages, 1 g or more for cavitary instillation, according to the massive course technique which is now widely used for systemic administration.

Thiophosphoramide, Thio(TEPA,TSPA) is N, N', N''-triethylene Thiophosphoramide, a crystalline substance soluble in water.

This compound, because of the intensive studies of J. BATEMAN *et al.* (1960) and J. WRIGHT *et al.*, is still the main chemotherapeutic agent for ovarian carcinoma.

The majority of workers report a positive effect of Thio-TEPA in papillary adenocarcinomas and undifferentiated cancers of the ovary.

Administration of the compound by either intramuscular, intravenous or intraperitoneal routes leads, in many patients, to retardation or arrest of the formation of ascitic fluid, with reduction in the size of the tumour nodes.

For our purpose, the important feature of Thio-TEPA is that it can be introduced into serous cavities, even into the cavity of the pericardium. Usually 20 to 30 mg per injection is given at intervals of a week, or less. Finally, a solution of Thio-TEPA can also be given directly into tumours in an amount of 6—10 mg of the substance in 4 to 20 cc. saline.

The side effects of Thio-TEPA on the gastrointestinal tract are less than for other compounds with alkylating effects. The depressed effect on hemopoieses, however, is sometimes important, especially in individuals who previously received radiation treatment. Profound leucopenia and thrombocytopenia occur sometimes only three weeks after the end of the course. For this reason it is necessary to limit the total dose of Thio-TEPA, whatever route is taken, to an amount of 100 or 120 mg per course and to watch carefully the status of the blood after treatment. Depression of thrombocytopoiesis often persists longer than the leucopoiesis; therefore, with short intervals between courses, very sharp and persistant thrombocytopenia may develop.

5-Fluorouracil (5-Fu). Among the metabolic antagonists of use in the temporary control of some forms of disseminated carcinoma, 5-Fluorouracil seems to be the only one which has been given by intracavitary administration in ovarian tumours. 5-Fu is an antimetabolite which resembles Uracil. It has been shown that this pyrimidine was incorporated into rodent tumour tissue to a greater extent than into normal tissues.

Intracavitary use of this anti-pyrimidine has been studied by SUHRLAND and WEISBERGER (1965). This compound, soluble in water, was injected at doses varying from 2 to 3 g, with an average of 2.5 g per patient.

In our own technique, we inject 1 g of 5-Fu, in combination with an alkylating agent, for example Degranol, at the dosage of 100 mg. These injections can easily be repeated once or twice a week with minimal side effects.

Quinacrine. Some years ago, the usefulness of Quinacrine (Atabrine) as a carcinostatic agent was evaluated. HIRSCHBERG and GELLHORN noted Quinacrine to be a highly effective carcinostatic agent when given intraperitoneally to mice bearing the Ehrlich ascites carcinoma. This observation prompted a study of the effect of local instillation of Quinacrine in patients with recurrent, neoplastic serous effusions containing tumour cells. The intracavitary route is the only one used since this action would only be possible if the compound were administred in a rather high concentration, which cannot be obtained by systemic administration.

After removal of a major portion of the fluid, Quinacrine, dissolved in serous fluid or in sterile physiologic saline solution, is injected.

The recommended dosage is 200 mg Quinacrine daily for five consecutive days in the treatment of pleural effusions;

for ascites, 400—1000 mg daily for two to four days is administered. Side effects are not negligible and correlate closely with the total quantity of drug received by the patient.

The injection of 1.200 mg of Atabrine into the peritoneal cavity appears to be a maximum dose; the major difficulty is the result of the inflammatory reaction produced by contact with the peritoneal surface.

This reaction brings serositis with abdominal pain, tenderness and paralytic ileus.

High temperature often occurs for several days after the initiation of therapy, and in some instances the ileus is severe enough to require several days of nasogastric intubation until adequate mobility of the gastrointestinal tract is restored.

Skin discoloration is also seen in some patients, especially those receiving more than three doses.

Toxic effects upon the central nervous system take the form of hallucinatory episodes, as well as other cerebral difficulties.

All these symptoms are transient and disappear relatively quickly, but they are severe enough to limit the use of this drug which has the great advantage of having no leucopenic or thrombocytopenic effect.

Corticoids may also be used by the intracavitary route; 50 to 70 mg of deltahydrocortisone acetate can be instilled one to six times in the pleural or peritoneal cavity after removal of the major portion of the fluid. Good results are achieved with very few side effects.

Results

Results are quite similar, according to different authors, whatever compound is used. Improvement of symptoms, no re-accumulation of fluid for periods exceeding two months, are seen in more than 50% of the cases, whatever compound is used.

LEVISON (1961) has 4 cases of ovarian adenocarcinomas which responded satisfactorily and two which failed to do so; one was an anaplastic tumour.

Twenty of the 43 patients treated by WEISBERGER et al. (1953) showed disappearance of fluid and 8 were improved with HN_2. BONTE et al. (1956) treated 40 patients, with improvement in 25.

An additional 88 patients reported by WEISBERGER (1958) showed approximately the same percentage (64) of improvements.

The results obtained with intracavitary Thio-TEPA are about the same but more difficult to interpret. Most of the patients treated by J. BATEMAN, as by ourselves at the Institut Gustave-Roussy, were treated by both systemic and intracavitary infusion. We obtained 21 improvements lasting from 2 to 18 months out of 33 patients.

Mannomustine seemed to give us some better results than the other alkylating agents and it is the routine technique we now use for all neoplastic effusions. A few months ago, we began a series of combined infusions of Degranol with 5-FU.

This technique seems very promising but it is too early to form any definite opinion.

SUHRLAND and WEISBERGER (1965) treated 55 patients with the intracavitary administration of 5-FU; 32, or 58%, were significantly improved. In this series, however, only 4 ovarian tumours out of 9 benefited from the treatment. It seems that, with this compound, the re-results are better with effusion due to metastatic carcinoma of the breast, gastrointestinal tract or kidney, than with those due to ovary adenocarcinoma.

ROCHLIN et al. (1964) treated 13 patients with ascites complicating ovary carcinoma with Atabrine. Nine improved sufficiently to have no recurrence of fluid for a minimum time of 3 months, but 3 of them died 1 to 3 months after therapy.

Of 7 patients treated with intracavitary instillation of Quinacrine, Ultmann et al. (1965) obtained 6 responses with a duration of 2, 2, 2, 4, 4 and 18 months respectively.

Discussion

The theoretical value of these agents was that they might have a direct effect on the malignant cells, rather than preventing fluid formation by causing adhesions to form. It became apparent, however, after necropsy on several patients that this was not the case. In all instances, the presence of many adhesions is similar to those cases in which successful results are obtained in the relief of malignant effusions by means of colloidal radioisotopes.

Colloidal isotope solutions such as chromic phosphate, colloidal gold (Au 198) or Yttrium 96, are expensive and results with them have been disappointing, including difficulty in handling these substances. Perhaps the most important of these problems is the radiation hazard involved to the medical and nursing personnel administering the treatment.

Levison (1961) one of the chief radiotherapists at the North Middlesex Hospital in London, concluded that the results of treating malignant effusions with Au 198 or with HN$_2$ are virtually the same. The latter would appear to have definite advantages in that no radiation hazard is involved, no protective measures are required, administration is consequently simple and can be done in a general hospital without a radiotherapy department. It is perhaps also pertinent to point out that 20 mg of HN$_2$ is 27 times cheaper than the average dose of Au 198 (100 mc).

We have seen that the use of soluble preparations is advisable, not only systemically but also by insertion into the peritoneal or pleural cavity. However, these preparations are absorbed from the peritoneal cavity into the blood stream even in the presence of ascitic fluid and tumour nodes. Therefore they might have a depressing action on hemapoiesis at almost the same doses as used for other modes of administration. Thus it is necessary to use, for the same therapeutic effect, the conpounds with the lowest toxicity. This is the main reason which prompted us to use Mannomustin instead of HN$_2$.

It has been established that PAM introduced into the peritoneal cavity with the technique described by Abbasov (1960) is hardly absorbed into the blood and apparently exerts a more potent effect on formation of ascitic fluid and on the small nodes scattered in the peritoneum. This makes it possible to use higher doses of sarcolysin to achieve a more persistent effect. However in such cases it cannot affect large tumour nodes which can be sensitive to other compounds administered by a different route.

Since intracavitary chemotherapy of ovarian cancer is initiated in the advanced stage of the disease, when there are already large masses of tumour tissue, complete regression and cure cannot be expected. However, one should strive to achieve the best possible effect. Treatment can be started both with intraperitoneal injections of the antimitotic preparations and by using other routes of administration or a combination of them. In both cases, the aim in the first course should be to achieve sharp inhibition or arrest ascitic fluid formation and reduction in the tumour nodes. If one course does not give a favourable effect, the tumour is most probably insensitive to this entire group of preparations. Then there is still an opportunity for trying some other compounds with another mechanism of action, i.e. 5-Fluorouracil or Atabrine.

If a positive result is obtained in the first course (or two), it is essential to continue treatment in one form or another; the object is to enhance or at least maintain the effect obtained and, as far as possible, prolong life in a satisfactory general condition.

To achieve this, it is possible either to repeat courses at definite intervals or to use more or less continuous maintenance treatment with low doses. Both methods have advantages and drawbacks. Repeat courses given in an institution are good in that they are given under the supervision of a specialist. However, the patient often seeks readmission, not at the start of a relapse, but when it has completely developed. As a result, the whole procedure has to be done again from the beginning. However, if chemotherapy results in the arrest of ascitic fluid formation and the tumour nodes are reduced in size, subsequent surgery may be facilitated.

Cavitary chemotherapy does not cure patients with advanced ovary carcinoma. Nevertheless, regression of tumours, inhibition or arrest of ascitic formation, can be produced in many patients with a variety of different agents. Evaluation of the increase in survival time is difficult, but it certainly was observed in some patients who responded.

The cancer chemotherapeutic drugs are usually toxic to some of the patients' normal cells and potentially lethal at doses near those where therapeutic effects are seen. Thus, thorough familiarity with these drugs on the part of the physician is a prerequisite to their use.

Summary

The subject of intracavitary chemotherapy of ovarian tumours was reviewed. After a brief outline of the techniques, the different compounds which may be useful were discussed and reports were summarized indicating that alkylating agents, antipyrimidines or quinacrine offer symptomatic relief in about 50% of the cases. These results do not differ from those obtained by isotopes. The choice of agent depends largely on the facilities available and the experience of the physician.

Discussion

RUTLEDGE said that ThioTEPA had been used at the University of Texas M.D. Anderson Hospital and Tumour Institute, but the circumstances were so varied that no accurate appraisal of its value was possible. Usually ThioTEPA or nitrogen mustard was used intraperitoneally or intrapleurally and it was the impression, he said, that when ThioTEPA was placed in a serous cavity, about one half of the dose was absorbed systemically so that the side effects might be a problem. Therefore, the systemic treatment was preferable because better control of absorption and toxic effects was possible. Experience had shown that fluid formation could be controlled by systemic administration when PAM was used.

RUTLEDGE asked if BRULÉ had had any experience with the use of a drug, given intraperitoneally, after an operation in which there was spillage or in the use of these agents in the pericardial cavity.

MULLER remarked that the French colloidal gold is of larger average particles than those from England or Switzerland and also different from the type in use in the United States. Colloidal gold, prepared along the principles developed by HENRY in France, with the preselected size of particles, seemed to have one new application in that when it is used for direct intraeavnary application, diffusion in the blood stream is not a problem. He asked if BRULÉ's remark, about the complications and results being the same with intralymphatic chemotherapy as with radioactive gold, pertained to patients with Stages I and II disease. In his own series, he said, including patients with III A disease, the percentages of five-year survivors were 64% (stages I + II) and 50% (stages I, II + IIIA).

MULLER also questioned BRULÉ's statement that chemotherapy was less expensive than gold when the cost of the care which the chemotherapy patient would require was considered. As to the intrapleural application of radioactive colloidal gold in patients with pleural carcinomatosis, he had achieved good results he said. Only one application was needed and there had been no complications.

JUNQUEIRA said that he was in general agreement with BRULÉ, although in his own and others' experience, Cytoxan had not been useful in the control of fluid. He believed ThioTEPA to be the most satisfactory drug for treatment of fluid. This compound acted slowly however; nitrogen mustard was much more rapid. ThioTEPA had been used in his institution for about five years and had been used systemically for some patients with ascites and pleural effusion. ThioTEPA and corticosteroids, usually Prednisone, had been used together with better results than when only the alkylating agent was used. In reply to a question from J. GRAHAM, JUNQUEIRA said that the principal benefit achieved by the corticosteroids was the control of small effusions, but he could not explain the way in which this benefit was achieved.

BURNS presented the results achieved with L-sarcolysin in the treatment for ascites in a group of terminal patients. Ninety-seven (67 per cent) of 144 patients responded well. In most instances, if the fluid was controlled, it was completely controlled and the patient did not require a tap for a long period of time, sometimes as long as five years.

BRULÉ, in closing, said that chemotherapy was used when other means were exhausted and therefore results were always poor. In reply to RUTLEDGE's question, he said he had had no experience with peritoneal infusion immediately after surgical intervention. He had injected ThioTEPA into the pericardium for one patient when pleural effusion and ascites were present. Some benefit had been achieved. At autopsy, the pericardium and tumour were completely fused.

He could not answer MULLER's question about the Stage I and II patients, because he had had no experience with patients with early disease. A colleague had used colloidal gold, however, for pleural effusion at one time but the practice had been discontinued because many patients had severe chest pain.

References

ABBASOV, AT., Experiences in the intracavitary administration of sarcolysin and Thio-tepa in malignant tumours of the ovaries. *Vop. Onkol.* **6**, 23—30 (1960).

ADAMS, S., Combined nitrogen mustard and hyperbasic oxygen therapy in advanced malignant disease. *Brit. Med. J.* **1963**, No 5326, 314—315.

BACK, E., Effect of oxygen tension on the sensitivity of normal and tumor tissues to alkylating agents. *J. nat. Cancer Inst.* **30**, 17—29 (1963).

BATEMAN, J. C., CARLTON, H. N., CALVERT, R. C., and LINDENBLAD, G. E., Investigation of distribution and excretion of C 14 tagged triethylenethiophosphoramide following injection by various routes. *Int. J. appl. Radiat.* **7**, 287—298 (1960).

—, and MOULTON, B., Control of neoplastic effusion by phosphoramide chemotherapy. *Arch. intern. Med.* **95**, 713—718 (1955).

BRULÉ, G., BAIRON, M., and TRUHAUT, R., Etude sur l'emploi du triethylène thiophosphoramide (Thio-Tepa) en chimiothérapie anticancéreuse. *Path. et Biol.* **11**, 742—754 (1963).

—, et THOMAS, M., La chimiothérapie locale des cancers. *Rev. franç. Étud. clin. biol.* **7**, 978—987 (1962).

COSTACHEL, O., IONESCU, N., and DEMETRIU, I. F., Substitution of the intracavity administration of radioactive isotopes with cytostatics in the treatment of cancerous exudates under novocaïne protection. *Rev. Sci. méd. (Buc.)* **4**, 23—27 (1959).

FRANZ, G., Cytostatic chemotherapy of malignancies in the gynecological field. *Med. Welt* **28**, 1445—1451 (1963).

KRAWCZYK, B., Treatment of inoperable ovarian cancer with Bayer E-39 soluble. *Zbl. Gynäk.* **85**, 792—796 (1963).

KREMENTZ, E. T., and KNODSON, L., The effect of increased oxygen tension on the tumoricidal effect of nitrogen mustard. *Surgery* **50**, 266—271 (1961).

LEVISON, V. B., Nitrogen mustard in palliation of malignant effusions. *Brit. med. J.* **1961**, No 5233, 1143—1145.

RIVENZON, A., COMISEL, V., and RIVENZON, M., Traitement de l'épithélioma ovarien ascitique OIA par oxygènopéritoine associé au cytostatique (triéthylènemélanine). *Oncologia (Basel)* **19**, 321—325 (1965).

ROCHLIN, D. B., SMART, C. R., WAGNER, D. E., and SILVA, A. R. M., The control of recurrent malignant effusions using quinacrine hydrochloride. *Surg. Gynec. Obstet.* **118**, 991—994 (1964).

SELLEI, C., and ECKHARDT, S., Clinical observations with 1,6-bis (ß-chloroethylamino) 1,6-desoxy-D-mannitol dihydrochloride (BCM) in malignant diseases. *Ann. N.Y. Acad. Sci.* **68**, 1164—1180 (1958).

SUHRLAND, L. G., and WEISBERGER, A. S., Intracavitary 5-fluorouracil in malignant effusions. *Arch. intern. Med.* **116**, 431—433 (1965).

ULTMANN, J. E., Diagnosis and treatment of neoplastic effusions. *Cancer (Philad.)* **12**, 42—50 (1962).

—, GELLHORN, A., OSNOS, M., and HIRSCHBERG, E., The effect of quinacrin on neoplastic effusions and certain of their enzymes. *Cancer (Philad.)* **16**, 283—288 (1963).

WEGHAUPT, K., Die Anwendung von „Bayer E 39" in der gynakologischen Krebsbehandlung. *Krebsarzt* **16**, 130—133 (1961).

WEISBERGER, A. S., LEVINE, B., and STORAASLI, J. P., Use of nitrogen mustard in the treatment of serous effusions of neoplastic origin. *J. Amer. med. Ass.* **159**, 1704 (1955).

WOLFF, J. P., et ICONIKOFF, L. K., La chimiothérapie des tumeurs malignes de l'ovaire, Essais et résultats du Thiotépa à l'Institut Gustave-Roussy. *Bull. Féd. Soc. Gynéc. Obstét. franç.* **15**, 315—319 (1963).

—, et TOUDOIRE, A., Tumeur maligne de l'ovaire et Thiotepa: Une voie d'introduction originale. To be published.

Chemotherapy in Ovarian Cancer

FELIX RUTLEDGE, M.D., and BEAURY BURNS, Jr., M.D.

Chief, Section of Gynecology, Department of Surgery; Associate Gynecologist, Section of Gynecology, Department of Surgery, The University of Texas M. D. Anderson Hospital and Tumour Institute, Houston, Texas, U.S.A.

Introduction

Although the sensitivity of ovarian cancer to chemotherapeutic agents has been demonstrated frequently (FRICK *et al.*, 1965; MASTERSON and NELSON, 1965; PARKER and SHINGLETON, 1962; WILTSHAW, 1965), clinicians have been slow to utilize this type of treatment for patients with advanced inoperable disease. At one time we shared this reluctance but, because there was no satisfactory therapeutic method for these patients, about 5 years ago we began gingerly to use chemotherapy for our advanced inoperable ovarian cancer patients. As our experience increased, we were impressed by the benefits obtained and the lack of toxicity attendant on the agent we were using. We have recently reviewed the case histories of patients treated with this agent to determine statistically whether our clinical impressions were valid.

Material and Methods

Drug effect was studied by review of experience with 213 patients (Table I) with advanced inoperable ovarian cancer who had one of the three common types of ovarian cancer (papillary serous, adenocarcinoma, pseudomucinous carcinoma). An additional 62 patients in our series were excluded because they did not survive long enough to receive 3 courses of the drug, the minimum required for any measurable effect. Thirteen others were also excluded because they had neoplasms of unusual or indeterminate histologic pattern.

Table I. *Carcinoma ovary — 288*

	X-ray-PAM	PAM-X-ray	PAM
Excluded	40	40	212
Insufficient drug	—7	0	—55
Special cell type	—6	—3	— 4
	33	37	143
Carcinoma cell type — retained			
Papillary serous	24	26	83
Adenocarcinoma	6	10	47
Pseudomucinous	3	1	13
	33	37	143
Study group 213			

The drug effect was evaluated according to the sequence in which it was used, i.e. irradiation and chemotherapy (33 patients), chemotherapy and irradiation (37 patients), or chemotherapy alone (143 patients). The time interval between the administration of irradiation and chemotherapy (Table II) was also examined to eliminate the possibility that the benefits attributed to the drug might actually reflect a delayed response to x-ray therapy and also because the time interval might have some influence on the tolerance of the drug.

The criteria for recovery of the bone marrow were a leukocyte count of above 3,000 mm and a platelet count of above 150,000 mm. There were few other manifestations of toxicity. Usually the drug was tolerated well and it was seldom necessary to discontinue treatment.

A measurable reduction in tumour bulk and a diminution of serous effusion were the principal criteria for evaluation of the drug effect. Combined pelvic and abdominal palpation were used to measure the mass. The frequency with which paracentesis was performed and meas-

Table II. *X-ray and PAM — 33 patients*

Method of irradiation		Recurrence sites	
		Abdomen	Lung
Whole abdomen "strip"	5	5	0
Whole abdomen "strip" added total pelvis	19	12	7
Total pelvis	7	7	0
Isotope	2	2	
Interval — irradiation to PAM — 33 patients:			
Less than 3 months		9*	
More than 3 months		24	

* Months of survival after chemotherapy when irradiation produced no regression of added growth was noted. Dead (4, 4, 4, 5, 7, 8) 4 patients died in less than 6 months from start of drug. Alive: 12, 30, 60.

The agent used in this study was L-phenylalanine mustard (PAM, L-Sarcolysin, melphalan, Alkeran®). The drug was given either intravenously or orally; the usual course was 1 mg/kg body weight. When given intravenously, the drug was dissolved in 500 ml of chilled dextrose and water and was given in a slow drip for about 8 hours. Orally, the dose was the same, and was given in 2 mg tablets to be taken in 3 or 4 daily doses for a 5-day period. The interval between courses was usually 3 or 4 weeks for both methods of administration unless bone marrow depression required a longer interval.

urements of the abdominal girth were used to evaluate the control of ascitic fluid. Patients were designated as "responders" when the tumour regressed about 50 per cent in size and/or a 50 per cent reduction of serous effusion was noted. The course of the drug was also followed by x-ray examinations and observations of the surface nodal metastases by measurement and biopsy. Laparotomy was performed in some instances.

Results

About one half of these patients showed a 50 per cent regression in the measurable size of the tumour or a 50 per cent reduction in serous effusion. The length of these remissions varied but some had a prolonged period of comfort.

Some who did not benefit by x-ray treatment responded to chemotherapy. The 9 patients who were given PAM in less that 3 months after irradiation (Table II)

Table III. *Tumour response to PAM*

Stage*	Prior X-ray therapy		No prior X-ray therapy	
	Good	Poor	Good	Poor
I A		1	1	
I B	1	1	1	
II A	2	2	7	
II B	1			
III A	26	12	38	4
III B	4	5	22	22
IV A	7	5	22	20
IV B	1		5	3
Totals	42 (62%)	26 (38%)	96 (66%)	49 (34%)

* I A: one ovary is involved. I B: both ovaries are involved. II A: ovaries removed but pelvic metastases. II B: general pelvic metastases, primary removed or not. III A: general abdominal metastases, primary removed. III B: metastases outside peritoneal cavity. IV A: inoperable, biopsy only. IV B: no operation.

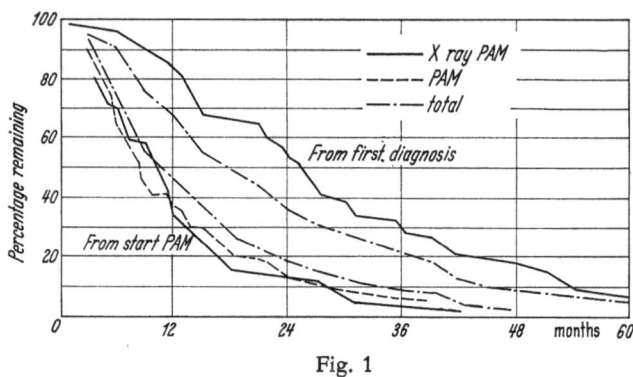

Fig. 1

Experience with patients who received x-ray therapy, whether it was given before or after admission to this institution, as compared with the non-irradiated group is shown in Table III. The group of 37 patients who received PAM and irradiation had an unusually good survival time, but these patients do represent some selection. The patients who received irradiation and PAM, in that order, generally tolerated the drug well.

showed no response to the initial irradiation. Five were benefited by PAM but 4 were dead within 6 months.

The survival curve (Fig. 1) shows that the PAM and x-ray treated patients generally behaved similarly to the patients who received only the agent. Although it is not shown on the graph, patients who received chemotherapy first and x-ray therapy second had a slightly better survival rate.

FRICK *et al.* (1965) used a superimposed survival curve to find that there was a six-months better survival in drug treated patients. If the survival time in patients treated in an era during which irradiation only was available for inoperable ovarian cancer was compared with those treated recently, when both irradiation and chemotherapy are available, we would predict from our experience that the survival rate would be improved. We made our definition of "response" more exact by insisting that it be maintained for 6 months. Using this definition, the survival time for responders and nonresponders has been plotted. For the first two years, the survival time in the responders was better but, after that period, less difference was noted between the two groups.

In advanced ovarian cancer, about 50 per cent of all patients will die within the first year and about 80 per cent will die within the first 18 months. After this time, the death rate slows; approximately 10 per cent live 3 years from the beginning of chemotherapy.

Of special interest are 13 patients who had unusually good responses. In all but one instance, the disease was histologically established; the one patient without histologic diagnosis had strong clinical evidence of ovarian carcinoma. Laparotomy was performed for these patients to determine if an inoperable tumour had become removable or to evaluate the need for additional drug therapy. In each of the patients, no tumour was found and chemotherapy was discontinued. These case histories are reviewed briefly:

Case One (M. McE. No. 39530). This 43-year-old white patient was referred to M. D. Anderson Hospital in May, 1961 with a diagnosis of papillary cystadenocarcinoma Grade III of the ovary. Eight months earlier, at another institution, subtotal hysterectomy, bilateral salpingo-oophorectomy and omentectomy had been performed and diffuse peritoneal and bowel metastases were found at that time. She had also received irradiation to a total dose of 4,000 rads. On admission to M. D. Anderson Hospital, she had a palpable pelvic mass, 8 to 10 cm in diameter, a pulmonary lesion detectable on the x-ray, an enlarged left supraclavicular node and cul-de-sac erosion by the tumour. A specimen of the cul-de-sac lesion contained papillary adenocarcinoma. Treatment with PAM was given intravenously and she received a total of 18 doses.

In April 1964, about three years after admission, exploratory laparotomy was performed and the cervical stump was removed. No gross tumour was found; a biopsy specimen showed fat necrosis but no tumour cells. The peritoneal washings contained no tumour cells. In April, 1966, she had no evidence of disease, although she has had no additional drug therapy.

Case Two (E. M. No. 41 150). This 37-year-old patient was admitted September 29, 1961. One year before admission she received intraperitoneal radioactive gold (Au 198) and x-ray therapy to the abdomen for papillary carcinoma of the ovary which had spread diffusely over the peritoneum. Abdominal and pelvic tumour masses up to 4 cm in diameter were observed to be growing. From September 1961 to July 1964, 22 courses of PAM were given. Rapid regression was noted by completion of the third course of drug. No residual carcinoma was found at laparotomy in July of 1964; omentum and peritoneal lavage specimens were negative for cancer. No additional drug has been given and no recurrence observed.

Case Three (M. S. No. 43 675). This 59-year-old patient was admitted in April, 1962, with recurrent cancer in an inguinal node. Three years previously she had undergone hysterectomy, bilateral salpingo-oophorectomy, resection of peritoneal implants, and intraperitoneal nitrogen mustard treatment for papillary serous adenocarcinoma. She was started on PAM and tolerated the drug extremely well. From May, 1962, to December, 1964, she received 35 courses, a total of 80 mg given intravenously. At laparotomy in January, 1965, no tumour was found and the peritoneal lavage was also negative for tumour cells. Chemotherapy was stopped.

Case Four (D.M. N. 44596). This 51-year-old patient was admitted in July, 1962, after left oophorectomy performed elsewhere, with a diagnosis of residual inoperable grade IV serous adenocarcinoma, ascites, metastases to the rectosigmoid, and a ruptured carcinomatous cyst. A mass, about 10 cm in diameter, was palpable in the lower abdomen and pelvis. Maximum resolution of the mass was noted after seven courses of the drug. When no further reduction in the tumour mass was detected after an additional two courses, in June, 1964, exploratory laparotomy was performed. The remaining ovary and tube were removed. Neither the excised specimen, biopsies of the omentum nor the peritoneal lavage contained tumour cells. She has been observed for an additional two years without drug and no evidence of recurrence.

Case Five (E.V. No. 45355). This patient was a 32-year-old Latin American patient who was referred to us in September, 1962, after exploratory laparotomy performed two months previously. According to the history, she had had subtotal hysterectomy and bilateral oophorectomy, but we later found that the uterus and one ovary were still intact. A diagnosis of cystadenocarcinoma, ascites and multiple small and large implants over the large and small intestines had been made. A pelvic mass, about 8 cm in diameter, was palpable on admission. She was given ten courses of PAM from September, 1962 to May, 1963. In July, 1963, laparotomy was again performed. Some necrotic areas in the peritoneal cul-de-sac were the only gross signs of residual cancer. These sites were excised and total abdominal hysterectomy and left salpingo-oophorectomy were performed. No tumour cells were found in the removed specimen except for a focus of pseudomucinous cancer in the ovary. No additional treatment was given, and no further evidence of cancer has been noted for almost three years.

Case Six (Z.S. No. 45689). This patient was 44 years old when she was referred to us in October, 1962 because of ascites. Tumour cells were present in 3,000 cc of ascitic fluid removed from the abdomen one month before admission. A large mass extended from the lower abdomen to above the umbilicus. At laparotomy in November, 1962, a semicystic ovarian tumour, about 15 to 25 cm in diameter, which had ruptured, was removed. Histological diagnosis was pseudomucinous cancer grade II. Postoperatively, the patient received 13 courses of PAM intravenously. The drug was discontinued in April, 1964. Laparotomy was performed in July, 1965. No gross cancer was found and the lavage contained no tumour cells. No additional treatment has been used and no recurrence has been noted.

Case Seven (B.O. No. 45691). This 56-year-old patient was referred in October, 1962, with a diagnosis of inoperable papillary serous cystadenocarcinoma of the ovary metastatic to the omentum. From October, 1962 to December, 1962, she received x-ray therapy,

2,900 rads to the entire abdomen and an extra 2,000 rads to the pelvis. No regression of the residual postoperative pelvic and abdominal mass was observed.

One month after the irradiation was completed, tumour growth was again noted. She was then started on PAM. From August, 1963, to August, 1965, she received 14 courses of PAM intravenously (total, 50 mg). After four courses of the drug the mass measurements decreased from 12 cm in size to 4 cm; after the seventh course, no cancer could be detected. Peritoneal washings were also negative for cancer. No additional drug has been given and the patient remains free of disease.

Case Eight (C. S. No. 50251). This patient was 56 years of age when she was referred to us, also in October, 1962, with a diagnosis made elsewhere, at laparotomy, of ascites, diffuse abdominal, peritoneal and omental metastases from adenocarcinoma grade IV of the ovary. From October, 1963 to February 7, 1964, she received four courses of PAM (50—59 mgm) in an 8-hour slow intravenous drip. A multinodular abdominal and pelvic mass, 12 cm in diameter, served as a guide to the drug action. After the second course, a 50 per cent regression in tumour size was observed. This rapid regression continued and no masses could be palpated after the fourth course was completed, three and one-half months after chemotherapy was started. At laparotomy in March, 1964, the only evidence of the once extensive ovarian cancer were a few necrotic-like lesions in the cul-de-sac. These were excised with the uterus. No tumour cells were found in a biopsy specimen of the peritoneum and the peritoneal lavage was also negative. There was no recurrence for over 2 years postoperatively without additional drug therapy. Twenty-seven months after the last course of the drug was given, however, she developed symptoms of recurrent cancer. At laparotomy, evidence of recurrent disease was found. Drug therapy was again instituted, and she is responding again to the agent.

Case Nine (L. Y. No. 47 974). This 57-year-old patient developed pleural effusion one month before admission in April, 1963. At laparotomy, at another instituion, a diagnosis of disseminated papillary adenocarcinoma was made. On admission to our institution, multiple abdominal and pelvic masses, about 20 cm in diameter, were noted. She received four courses of PAM orally between April 1963 and August 1963, with, subsequently, complete resolution of all physical signs of cancer. Laparotomy and bilateral salpingo-oophorectomy were performed in August 1963; the only gross evidence of tumour was residual necrotic implants over the visceral and parietal peritoneum. No viable tumour was found in biopsies of the multiple sites of the parietal peritoneum and the omentum. The drug was discontinued; seven months later, at a "second look" laparotomy, no evidence of cancer was found. She remained without evidence of cancer after drug was discontinued until July 1966, 38 months after the agent was discontinued. At that time, evidence of cancer was found at laparotomy. She is again responding to the agent.

Case Ten (M. M. No. 52 220). This 63-year-old patient was admitted in April 1964 with a diagnosis of generalized abdominal metastases from papillary serous adenocarcinoma of the ovary. The diagnosis was made by laparotomy at another institution. At the same time, omentectomy had been performed and a colostomy established. The pathologic report on the omentum was "positive for tumour cells". A biopsy of the cervix contained cancer in the lymph vessels. From April 1964 to May 1965 she received 12 courses, one each month, of oral PAM. Response was slow but complete resolution of the palpable abdominal and pelvic masses was noted after 10 months. In June 1965 abdominal exploration, bilateral salpingo-oophorectomy and closure of the colostomy were performed. No gross evidence of cancer was seen; the excised ovaries and the peritoneal lavage contained no tumour cells. No sign of recurrence has developed in the months since the drug was discontinued.

Case Eleven (O. H. No. 55368). This 34-year-old patient was referred to us in January 1965 after operation one month earlier for bilateral papillary serous adenocarcinoma grade II of the ovary; the masses were adherent and were incompletely excised, and there was spillage from the tumour.

On admission, a 8 cm nodular mass was palpable in the cul-de-sac. Intravenous PAM was begun in January 1965 as a preirradiation measure. The pelvic mass slowly regressed but was not completely resolved after six courses. In July 1965, laparotomy was again performed and a 4 cm necrotic tumour mass which showed microscopic evidence of destroyed cancer was found in the cul-de-sac. Peritoneal lavage did not contain any tumour cells. With no additional therapy, she has been free of any physical evidence of cancer.

Case Twelve (E. H. No. 59093). This 57-year-old patient was admitted in October 1965 with large abdominal ascites, pleural effusion and extensive pelvic and abdominal tumour masses. She was too ill and the tumour too extensive for exploration. From October 1965 to February 1966, she received 5 courses of PAM orally and exhibited rapid improvement. In February 1966, she underwent total abdominal hysterectomy and bilateral salpingo-oophorectomy. No sign of cancer was found in the abdomen. The specimen and the peritoneal lavage contained no cancer cells.

The objection can be made that for this patient, there was no pre-treatment biopsy obtained, but the large tumour masses, ascites, and pleural effusion, as well as the rapid regression, support the clinical diagnosis.

Case Thirteen (S. S. No. 58198). Two months before this 43-year-old patient was admitted in August 1965, serous carcinoma was incompletely removed by total abdominal hysterectomy and bilateral salpingo-oophorectomy. Metastases to the pelvic peritoneum and the omentum remained. Only 4 x-ray treatments to the pelvis were given before treatment was interrupted because of an intestinal obstruction caused by a 15 cm in diameter neoplastic mass filling the pelvis. PAM was started in August 1965 and by December no tumour could be found by abdominal and pelvic examination. In January 1966, laparotomy was performed and no gross or microscopic disease on peritoneal lavage was found. Drug was discontinued and the patient remains free of disease.

Discussion

In our analysis we sought the answers to these 5 questions:

1. Should chemotherapy become standard therapy in the late stages of ovarian cancer? In some instances this question is academic, because many patients are either too ill to tolerate irradiation, have such extensive tumour that, even though it is localized, irradiation is not feasible, or have ascites. Many such patients in our series were benefited by chemotherapy. About one half of the patients with the three common cell types of ovarian cancer will benefit by a reduction in tumour bulk or control of serous effusion. The time of remission will vary but some will experience a prolonged remission. Toxicity is minimal even when the patient is extremely ill or is non-responsive. Although there is no way to determine which patients will respond, the fact that many will benefit and those who do not will not be injured, justifies a trial of the agent for all patients.

3. Would reliance solely on the drug without irradiation be justified? In the early days of our experience, when a patient responded to chemotherapy sufficiently so that she was able to tolerate radiation therapy, we felt obligated to try this latter type of treatment. In time, however, we were more and more inclined to keep the patient who was improving on chemotherapy on the drug rather than change the type of treatment.

4. Should laparotomy be used more often, when a patient has an unusually good response, to determine if the drug should be discontinued? We were slow to concede that a

Table IV. *Laparotomy following PAM — 41*

	Patients	Finding		
		Gross *	Carcinoma	
			Micro.	Neg.
Purpose				
Excise tumour	11	12		
Need to continue treatment	28		15	12
Relieve intestinal obstruction	2	2		

* Gross tumour was visible though remarkably reduced from its original size.

2. Can x-ray treatment be potentiated by pre-irradiation drug therapy? The 37 patients who received PAM first and irradiation second had an unusually good survival, but these patients do represent some selection in that they were "responders". Some were too ill initially to receive irradiation but responded so well to the drug that they were able later to have irradiation treatment. Only occasionally was the depression of the bone marrow so severe that irradiation could not be given. It is also noteworthy that the prior effect of irradiation does not exclude the use of chemotherapy. Many patients received high dose irradiation but they tolerated the drug as well as those who had not had previous irradiation.

good response to the drug was reason for laparotomy. A second laparotomy was performed in some instances to determine if what was once inoperable disease could be removed and in other cases to relieve intestinal obstruction. Later in the series, we performed laparotomy to assist us in deciding whether the drug therapy should be discontinued. We found that in many instances this was the only way to avoid errors in appraisal of the disease status (Table IV). As long as the pelvic or abdominal mass was palpable, errors in assessing the state of the disease were limited to mistaking a benign intra-abdominal tumour for a neoplastic mass. But this type of appraisal is no longer helpful when the mass is reduced by the drug. Many ovarian masses are fluid-filled cysts and these can collapse during initial treatment. This does not represent destruction of cancer. Laparotomy may be the only way in which the extent of the disease can be determined.

5. Is chemotherapy capable of totally eradicating advanced ovarian cancer? This question still remains unanswered, but the experience with these 13 patients who had unusualy responses is certainly encouraging. Although two have since had recurrences, they are again responding to the agent and it may be possible that we discontinued the drug too soon. However even total clinical regression, no evidence of gross disease at laparotomy, and even the absence of cancer cells in the washings of the peritoneal cavity, are not conclusive evidence that all metastases have been destroyed. Disease may still remain in the pelvic or aortic lymph nodes; these were not systematically biopsied. Cancerous foci may well remain in other sites. This is another question which will have to be answered by more experience, because

the factors of host resistance and susceptible tumour types cannot be discounted.

Summary

Experience with 213 advanced ovarian cancer patients with one of the three common types of ovarian cancer has shown that L-phenylalanine mustard, used either alone or in combination with irradiation, is useful in this disease. About 50 per cent of the patients were benefited by control of ascites, reduction in tumour mass and symptomatic relief. Increased survival because of drug effect is difficult to establish statistically, but evidence indicates that survival time is increased in those patients who do respond. The case histories of 13 patients who experienced an unusual response, in that clinical evidence of the disease disappeared and no gross evidence was found at laparotomy, were presented. Two for whom the disease later recurred, 26 and 38 months respectively after the agent was discontinued, have again responded to the agent.

Discussion

Brulé inquired if Rutledge was sure the compound remained stable in aqueous solution during intravenous administration over a period of eight hours, because most alkylating agents would quickly lose much of their effectiveness when they were in aqueous solution for more than an hour. He also asked if patients had digestive disorders with the large doses that were given in this series. In his experience with sarcolysin or phenylalanine, mustard gastric intolerance was such that it was impossible to give more than 10 or 15 mg in one day and additional doses had to be postponed for three or four days.

He agreed, Brulé said, that chemotherapy should be the first treatment in

advanced ovarian carcinoma instead of radiotherapy. He was surprised that there was less gastrointestinal disturbance with chemotherapy than with irradiation because at his own institution most patients who received irradiation had only slight difficulty.

Two important points in Rutledge's series, he said, were that the same results were obtained whether the compound was given intravenously or orally and that chemotherapy does not preclude subsequent x-ray therapy if the disease does change. For some time, it has been customary to give chemotherapy first in disseminated diseases, such as the lymphomas and Hodgkin's disease, and then administer irradiation to the retroperitoneal nodes. However, this plan was not advisable for some diseases, such as one type of embryonal tumour of the testis. It was necessary to know which treatment should be used for a particular disease. Seminoma, for example, responds well to irradiation, even when lung or hepatic metastases are present, but Müllerian carcinoma or choriocarcinoma do not respond to irradiation but will sometimes respond to chemotherapy.

Once chemotherapy is begun, said BRULÉ, treatment should not be discontinued unless there is evidence of complete regression such as was shown in the group of 13 patients. Even for two of these patients, he pointed out, the drug was discontinued too soon in the belief that healing was complete. Relapses occur much more rapidly and frequently after chemotherapy is discontinued than after irradiation is stopped. Therefore, toxicity should not be induced too quickly, although results will be less dramatic. The dose should be calculated so that after an "attack" treatment which causes minor toxicity, chemotherapy of another type, one which can be used over a long period of time, can be instituted.

The maintenance treatment, as described by RUTLEDGE, was attractive because the patient need be seen only once a month. Some types of treatment require that the patient be seen once a week, which creates a problem when she lives at some distance from the hospital. It was difficult to understand however, BUBLÉ said, how an alkylating agent which is unstable and disappears rapidly can be effective when it is given only once a month.

BRULÉ said he used a combined treatment, with a metabolite such as 5-fluorouracil, for example, and one alkylating agent for a maintenance treatment. For a patient who weighs about 60 kilo-

grams, one gram can be given in a slow drip infusion of about four hours' duration; thus, as much as 25 grams of effective treatment can be given. Treatment can be given for 20 or 25 days without toxicity. When the first sign of toxicity, usually diarrhea, develops, treatment is discontinued and in about a week or 10 days the diarrhea disappears. Then, maintenance treatment with infusion is given each week or three times a month for as long as the patient can tolerate it. Since one of the technical problems is to find the vein, at the beginning of chemotherapy, a by-pass catheter, such as is used for renal lavage, is put in place. An "attack" course of 5-FU plus 100 mg of ThioTEPA is given. Hematologic disturbance sometimes occurs late, after the attack treatment is given, so that the maintenance treatment is delayed for a month. On maintenance treatment, the patient receives one gram of 5-FU and 10 mg of ThioTEPA once a week. As to when to stop treatment, he did not know, BRULÉ said. Some patients have been on this regimen for more than a year, but he had not been able to persuade the surgeons that a "second look" operation was needed.

KOTTMEIER said that at the Radiumhemmet, since 1960, only ThioTEPA had been used for ovarian carcinoma. From 1960 to 1962, a study at random was made of (1) patients who received chemotherapy in addition to surgical intervention, (2) those with metastases limited to the pelvis and (3) those with nonresectable metastases above the pelvis. Some patients in the first two groups received radiation and chemotherapy; some received only ThioTEPA, and some were treated only by irradiation. For these patients, ThioTEPA was given only until a moderate degree of bone marrow toxicity was induced, and was always discontinued when the white cell count dropped below 1,500. The patients with nonresectable metastases above the pelvis, however, were given the compound until severe toxicity developed, even when the white cell count was below 500.

Based on experience with this latter group of patients, he and his colleagues thought that the combination of irradiation and chemotherapy was advantageous when irradiation was given first because a hyperplasia of the major megakaryocytes developed in the bone marrow 10 to 14 days after irradiation was started. In serous carcinoma with extensive metastases, however, since the randomized series was done, only ThioTEPA has been used. Eleven patients who have been followed for more than 11 months have received between 730 and 1,260 mg of ThioTEPA intravenously. One patient died from bone marrow hypoplasia; two have died of cancer; eight patients are in satisfactory condition. (For more complete information, see KOTTMEIER, H.L.: Proposals for the Standardization of the Combined Treatment of Ovarian Cancer.)

From this experience, KOTTMEIER said he had three questions for RUTLEDGE: 1. Was it necessary to give the compound to the point of severe toxicity? 2. Was it important when there was no correlation between the findings in the peripheral blood and the bone marrow? 3. Were there severe late reactions such as have been reported to occur three to four weeks after treatment with other compounds?

GENTIL said that he and his colleagues routinely used chemotherapy at the time of any operation for cancer. They preferred ThioTEPA and tried to administer the compound by different routes. Routinely, nitrogen mustard was left in the peritoneal cavity after operation for ovarian cancer. This practice

developed because, when as often happens in the management of cancer a second or third operation was necessary, no adhesions were found if a small dose of nitrogen mustard had been left in the cavity.

In some instances, when a patient had had ThioTEPA, and later some fluid was removed, the cancer cells were entirely destroyed by the action of the compound. This did not occur in a control group. Usually 1 mg of ThioTEPA per kilogram of body weight was given as a total dose and, during the operation, only one half was given; the other part was given during the postoperative period, as the patient's condition dictated.

In his opinion, GENTIL said, chemotherapy and irradiation should be used simultaneously, but he was interested in RUTLEDGE's evidence that chemotherapy should be given initially and in KOTTMEIER's work that showed there was an advantage in beginning chemotherapy on the fourteenth day after irradiation was begun. However, if chemotherapy is given after irradiation, the fibrosis and the changes in the tumour bed caused by the irradiation obviously mean that there will be less blood to transport the chemotherapeutic agent. Therefore, the results of chemotherapy after irradiation will not be as satisfactory.

RUTLEDGE said that the opinion was that the drug continued to be stable during intravenous administration for eight hours, because the products could be totally recovered from the urine and because the bone marrow was depressed about the same degree as when the oral route was used. As to how long the drug had been given, one patient received 35 courses over a period of about three years, he said. The interval between courses of the drug was determined largely by the bone marrow response. The dose was the same, whether the route was oral or intravenous. Some nausea did occur, particularly after the drug was discontinued, but yielded to medication. Orally, the drug is given three times a day over a five-day period, with appropriate antiemetic therapy, and tolerance is good. Patients who are treated at the University of Texas M. D. Anderson Hospital and Tumour Institute often have to travel some distance. Therefore, a patient is sometimes given a supply of pills for one or two courses, and the family physician is asked to check the blood count and advise patient to start a course of medication.

ThioTEPA was used at this institution at one time for a period of two years, but PAM was considered less toxic and as effective. The drug has not been used in close sequence with x-ray therapy at M. D. Anderson Hospital, because with the method of irradiating large areas of abdomen used at this institution, drug therapy cannot be re-instituted after irradiation because of bone marrow damage.

The danger in long-continued use of the drug was one reason for performing second or third laparotomy, but when it is safe to discontinue the drug is not known. There must be some time when irreparable damage to the bone marrow occurs, although this is not common. If more patients lived longer, more might have this type of bone marrow damage.

BURNS said that nodal metastases from advanced ovarian carcinoma were particularly sensitive to L-sarcolysin. He agreed that a study at random of a series of patients was important but since an appreciable number of patients benefited, he and his colleagues did not feel that the treatment could be withheld from any. He suggested that a study at random would be useful in "spill" patients and in those with late disease who have responded to chemotherapy. For example, a randomized series using radioactive gold or external irradiation could be made of patients who responded and were explored.

In this series patients who exhibited marrow toxicity have been charted by response and nonresponse. The non-responders were those who did not exhibit marrow toxicity so that the interval between drug doses in those who responded increased as more drug was given. If, after three courses of the drug, given at a rate of one mg per kg, marrow toxicity was not exhibited, the dose was increased in an effort to induce response. Patients considered nonresponders were those who did not show a 50 per cent decrease in pelvic tumour parameter, but there were some patients who, although they showed no increase, did not show a decrease. Many of these lived for three years at least so that even though the patient's disease was not completely controlled, she benefited.

One patient died of marrow depression; other than this there was no severe toxicity. The bone marrow was not routinely examined, except for those patients who had considerable marrow toxicity. No late reactions to the drug were noted, although one patient who received about nine courses became sensitive and was changed to Chlorambucil. It has not been the practice, BURNS said, to use ThioTEPA at the time of operation, because use of this drug would delay the administration of L-sarcolysin.

References

Burns jr., B. C., Rutledge, F., and Gallager, H. S., Phenylalanine mustard in the palliative management of carcinoma of the ovary. *Obstet. and Gynec.* **22**, 30—37 (1963).

Frick II, H. C., Atchoo, N., Adamson jr., K., and Taylor, H. C., The efficacy of chemotherapeutic agents in the management of gynecologic cancer. *Amer. J. Obstet. Gynec.* **93**, 1112—1121 (1965).

Masterson, J. G., and Nelson, J. H., The role of chemotherapy in the treatment of gynecologic malignancy. *Amer. J. Obstet. Gynec.* **93**, 1102—1111 (1965).

Parker, R. T., and Shingleton, W. W., Chemotherapy in genital cancer: Systemic therapy and regional perfusion. *Amer. J. Obstet. Gynec.* **83**, 981—1003 (1962).

Wiltshaw, E. J., Chlorambucil in the treatment of primary adenocarcinoma of the ovary. *J. Obstet. Gynaec. Brit. Emp.* **72**, 586—602 (1965).

Systemic Chemotherapy in the Treatment of Ovarian Cancer

Prof. L. A. NOVIKOVA *

Head of Department of Gynecology, Institut Experimentalnoy i Klinicheskoy Onkologii, Academia Meditsinkikh Nauk, Moscow, U.S.S.R.

Introduction

Until recently, malignant ovarian tumours were diagnosed, in the majority of cases, in the late stages of disease. Hence their treatment has become a difficult and thankless task.

Under these conditions the addition of chemotherapy to other therapeutic measures for malignant ovarian tumours becomes an important achievement of modern medical science. However, this branch of therapy still requires much investigation before the desired effect can be completely achieved.

Along with the development of chemotherapy as a whole, the arsenal of medicinal agents for malignant ovarian tumours has gradually increased. We shall describe here only the more popular drugs used for treatment of malignant ovarian tumours.

Among the ethyleneamines are thiophosphamide (Thio-TEF, Thio-TEPA, TSPA), triethyleneamine (TEM, Tretamine), benzotef, benzodet, ethimidine E-39, trenimon etc. Among the chlorethylamines the following were found useful: sarcolysin (melphalan, phenylalanine mustard, PAM, sarcochloran), chlorambucyl (chlorbutin, leukeran), en-

doxan (cyclophosphan, B 518, Cytoxan, cyclophosphamide) etc.

Among the antimetabolites (much less used in this disease) 5-fluorouracil was found effective in some ovarian tumours, although methotrexate has failed (MUIR, 1962).

The primary therapeutic effect with each of these drugs is mostly achieved in ascitic forms of tumours and results in the drying of serous cavities (abdominal and pleural), decrease of tumour masses, which sometimes apparently disappear, with a corresponding increase of the general well-being and their rehabilitation. Each drug produces some side effects, but they usually affect leucopoiesis to a lesser or greater extent, and partially thrombocytopoiesis. This complication generally forces reduction of the doses. They often produce therapeutic effects which are, however, insufficient for total arrest of the disease. Even 5-fluorouracil, causing first, in the majority of cases, gastrointestinal reactions (herpes, stomatitis, nausea, vomiting), depresses leucopoiesis at the same time.

Since 1958, about 400 patients with malignant ovarian tumours have been treated at the Institute of Experimental and Clinical Oncology, Academy of Medical Sciences of the USSR. Various drugs were used and the results reported in the medical press. (BLOKHINA, 1958;

---

* Professor NOVIKOVA was unable to attend the meeting. Her paper, which was precirculated to all participants, is included in these proceedings for the record.

ABBASOV, 1960; NOVIKOVA *et al.*, 1962 to 1964; KOLIADINA, 1965, etc.) Among the many drugs used over the last years in the treatment of malignant ovarian tumours, the following four were mainly administered: Thio-TEPA, sarcolysin, endoxan, and the antiblastic antibiotic chrysomalline, which was formerly tried under the number 2703.

Thio-TEPA is one of the first drugs found effective in the treatment of malignant ovarian tumours. Usually a course of treatment consists of intracavitary administration of the drug and systemic administration, either intramuscularly or intravenously.

Single dose of the drug varies, depending on the condition of the patient, from 10—20 mg every other day to a total dose 200—300 mg. According to our observations and those of NE-CHAEVA (1966) an initial effect appears in approximately 73—75% of patients.

The main defect of the drug is its action on leucopoiesis. Leucopenia (below 3,500) generally appears after administration of 150—200 mg of the drug, and, in certain cases, even after smaller doses. In some instances we were forced to stop the treatment after administration of 120 mg and even 80 mg of the drug. In one case agranulocytosis developed after 140 mg and led to a lethal outcome. Other authors saw similar results. A. N. KOSAREVA reported severe leucopenia (550—350 per ml) in 6 patients; in one case the dose of the drug did not exceed 150 mg. Two patients died from agranulocytosis. This author remarked that especially severe leucopenia develops with the accelerated method of treatment (10—20 mg daily).

The drug has a cumulative action. Severe leucopenia and bone marrow aplasia can develop within 1 to 2 weeks after the end of treatment.

Dl-sarcolysin produces even more marked toxic effect on hemopoiesis and provokes pronounced reactions of the gastric tract (nausea, vomiting).

Reactions appear even after intracavitary administration, though this method of administration is called "local". Depression of leucopoiesis is likewise seen with this method though it appears more slowly than after direct administration of the drug into the bloodstream.

One patient, after intravenous administration of 120 mg of sarcolysin, showed considerable decrease of an ovarian tumour (dysgerminoma), which occupied all the lower half of the abdominal cavity and the pelvis with compression of the bladder and the rectum. Functions of these organs reverted to normal; however, the fall of leucocytes (down to 750 per ml) forced us to interrupt treatment and the tumour again progressed rapidly.

ABBASOV (1960) saw effects from sarcolysin mainly after intracavitary administration (40—50 mg once a week) with a total dose per course of 150—250 mg. He found that, at times, sarcolysin produced effects where Thio-TEPA had failed. However, further studies at our Institute showed that changing the pattern of administration of this drug affects the results as well (A. M. GARIN *et al.*, 1965). Large single doses of sarcolysin (1.0 to 2.5 mg per kg of body weight) gave an objective effect in 2 out of 4 patients with extensive ovarian cancer. However, repetition of high single doses of sarcolysin in the majority of patients with tumours of various sites was found to be impractical due to complications. One patient with ovarian cancer after a single administration of sarcolysin in the dose of 160 mg (2 mg per kg of body weight) died on the twenty-eightth day from agranulocytosis. (This was the only lethal complication in 40 cases receiving similar doses).

Endoxan can also be administered locally (into the cavity) or systemically. In the latter method the dose would be 200—400 mg daily with a total dose of 8—10 gm.

Initial results in the treatment of ovarian tumours with Endoxan and Thio-TEPA are practically the same. Duration of remissions depends on the dose of Endoxan used: the greater the dose, the longer the remission. Remissions lasting from 1 year to 1 year 8 months were seen in patients who received the total dose of 7—10 g (KOLIADINA, 1965).

Side effects differ somewhat. Endoxan exerts less effect on leucopoiesis and practically none on thrombocytopoiesis, but it produced alopecia. Three patients had jaundice though the role of Endoxan in this was not clear. GARIN et al. (1965) tried high single doses of Endoxan (20—50 mg per kg of body weight and over in single doses of 1 to 2,5 g) in various malignant tumours. These authors saw, however, that large single doses cannot shorten the course of treatment and do not help to increase total dose of the drug per course. Toxicity with this method is not decreased, though it seems that its efficacy is enhanced when used in high doses, but it must be stressed that the use of high single doses demands good hematological findings initially.

Advantages of high single doses of any drug are as follows: (1) the possibility of testing tumour sensitivity to the drug after the first dose, which permits changing the plan of treatment if no effect is obtained and (2) the possibility of helping rapidly the patient who is severely ill. Administration of high single doses is especially indicated in recurring exudates in the pleural and abdominal cavities. We saw good effects in a number of cases after one drug or another, but usually after their administration, particularly, into the cavities.

As the use of a single drug is limited by the reactions it produces, which forces discontinuance of treatment, it is tempting to increase therapeutic effect by continuing treatment with the aid of other drugs. Naturally, the second drug should not produce reactions of the same type. Antiblastic antibiotic chrysomalline appeared to be such a drug. We shall dwell on this subject at some length as this drug has only recently received clinical approbation and authorization for clinical use.

Actinomycins occupy the main place among the antiblastic antibiotics. They are all chemically related to each other. They have a phenaxolon chromophore group and a polypeptid chain with 8 to 10 aminoacids. Different actinomycins differ in the composition and orientation of aminoacids in the polypeptid chain.

Material and Methods

Antiblastic antibiotic chrysomalline was isolated from the culture of Actinomyces chrysomallus. It is a mixture of three ingredients qualitatively analogous to actinomycin C1 (similar to actinomycin D) C 2 and C 3 (C_1-20%, C_2-30%, C_3-50%). (MENSHIKOV et al., 1964.) It was isolated from soil and studied by the Institute of Microbiology of the Academy of Sciences of USSR, in the laboratory headed by N. A. KRASILNIKOV. Isolation and chemical purification of the drug were carried out at the Institute of Experimental and Clinical Oncology, Academy of Medical Sciences of USSR, in the laboratory of Professor G. P. MENSHIKOV; its antiblastic activity was shown by the laboratory of Professor I. I. MAEVSKY and experimental testing and clinical study of the drug were carried out at the chemotherapy department under the direction of Professor V. I. AST-RAKHAN (R. N. KUCHKAREV, 1963).

Special observations of the use of this antibiotic in the treatment of malignant ovarian tumours were made in the gynecological department of this Institute (L. A. NOVIKOVA, P. I. KOLIADINA 1964).

The drug is used through intravenous administration. Infiltrates develop if chrysomalline is injected subcutaneously or in the muscle. Prior to administration, 500—1,000 gamma of the drug are dissolved in 0.5 ml of ethyl alcohol with subsequent addition of 8—10 ml of saline. It is injected slowly and given either in doses of 500 gamma every other day, or 1,000 gamma every two days. The desired total dose per course is 8,000 to 10,000 gamma. If well tolerated, an even greater total dose could be given.

When exudates are present in the abdominal and pleural cavities, the drug can be introduced into these and other cavities in the same doses.

Side effects after administration of chrysomalline appear, generally in the gastrointestinal tract, 3 to 4 hours after injections or on the next day. The majority of patients lose appetite and about one-half of them complain of nausea and vomiting, sometimes of abdominal pains. Rarely (2 cases out of 76) we saw allergic reactions: pruritus, joint pain, urticaria. After a variable total dose (usually not less than 3,500 gamma) some patients develop stomatitis, sometimes diarrhoea, which requires suspension of treatment until disappearance of reaction. Roughly 15—20% of patients tolerate the drug without side effects.

Chrysomalline is good because it exerts but slight effect on haemopoiesis. This fact permits its use when leucopenia and thrombocytopenia are produced by other alkylating agents. We gave chrysomalline with 2,000, 2,600 and 2,800 leucocytes per ml. During treatment leucocytes were correspondingly 3,200, 7,300 and 6,600. Some patients had slow ESR. These qualities of chrysomalline permit its use together with, or following, alkylating drugs.

Results

We used chrysomalline for 76 patients with malignant ovarian tumours, 47 of whom had exudates in cavities: 25 only in the abdominal cavity, 21 in the abdominal and pleural cavities, and one had only a pleural exudate. After chrysomalline treatment, entire disappearance of abdominal exudates was seen in 15 patients, and in the pleural cavity in 10 cases. The majority of patients had decrease of exudates; in 11 cases there was no effect. The exudate disappeared not only in those patients who received the drug into a cavity (i.e. with evacuation of most of the fluid), but also in those who received it intravenously. Increase of diuresis was recorded. Sometimes the quantity of urine output doubled as compared to the daily fluid intake.

Effect on the tumour was perceptible in almost one-half of the patients; in the remainder, one-half showed stabilisation of the disease and the others its progression.

For various reasons, mainly due to marked reactions, in 11 patients the dose of the drug was decreased to below 4,000 gamma, i.e. a clearly insufficient dose for obtaining the initial effect.

Chrysomalline can be introduced by suppositories. To have a significant blood level of the drug we gave it in suppositories, 1,000 gamma twice daily every day. The total average dose was 20,000 gamma.

After having studied isolated administration of chrysomalline, we made it a rule to use a combination of this drug with drugs of the alkylating series, more often with Endoxan.

We use chemotherapy as a part of the combined method of treatment. If the tumour masses are not particularly large, we start chemotherapy before surgery, introduce the drug into abdominal cavity during the operation, and resume intravenous or subcutaneous injections a few days after operation.

Table I shows the results of 1 to 3 years of follow-up observations and histological types of the tumours; in 177 patients, eight patients had had no histological confirmation of disease; 7 of them died during the first year and one died in the second year after the beginning of treatment.

Of 60 patients treated over three years ago, 20 are alive. When 4 patients in I—II stages of disease are excluded, of 62 treated cases in stages III—IV, over 16 are alive after 3 years and more. Fifteen of them had a papillary type of cancer. This is the most common form of ovarian cancer and the most sensitive to chemotherapy.

In patients with ovarian tumours with a more favourable course, we are

Table I. *Immediate results of combined treatment of patients with ovarian malignant tumours*

Histological structure of tumour	Stage of disease	Date of observation					
		1 year and over		2 years and over		3 years and over	
		Treated	Alive	Treated	Alive	Treated	Alive
Papillary cancer	I—II	6	6	5	5	4	4
	III—IV	71	41	59	25	42	15
	Total	77	47	64	30	46	19
Solid cancer	I—II	1	1	1	1		
	III—IV	17	8	16	4	11	0
	Total	18	9	17	5	11	0
Adenocarcinoma	I—II	1	1	1	1	—	—
	III—IV	12	10	11	4	6	1
	Total	13	11	12	5	6	1
Granulosocellular	I—II	1	1	—	—	—	—
	III—IV	3	3	3	2	1	0
	Total	4	4	3	2	1	0
Dysgerminoma	III—IV	2	1	1	0	—	—
Pseudomucinoso cancer	III—IV	2	1	2	1	—	—
Non-differentiated cancer	III—IV	1	0	1	0	1	0
Total	I—II	9	9	7	7	4	4
	III—IV	108	64	93	36	61	16
		117	73	100	43	65	20

16*

convinced that the success depends on the whole complex of measures, including surgery. But it is quite obvious that chemotherapy plays a special role in the prolongation of life in patients with extensive forms of disease. Of importance is the persistent use of the drugs, which represents a severe obligation for doctor and patient. Throughout the course of chemotherapy, an entire arsenal of measures directed at the general improvement of the patient's condition and at the stimulation of haemopoiesis, especially leucopiesis, must be brought into action.

As an example, we can refer to two patients who, for more than 4 years, have received periodically chemotherapeutic treatment at intervals, with various drugs. Both, prior to admission to our Institute, had had exploratory laparotomies (histological structure of tumour in both cases was papillary cancer). One of them after two courses of Thio-TEPA (400 mg) and one course of sarcolysin (130 mg) was operated upon and treated with x-ray followed by a number of chemotherapeutic courses. In all she received 32 g Endoxan (7 courses), 14,000 gamma chrysomalline (2 courses), 800 mg Thio-TEPA (4 courses), 130 mg sarcolysin (1 course). The other patient had chemotherapy alone. She received 530 mg Thio-TEPA (2 courses), 44 g Endoxan (6 courses), 10,000 gamma chrysomalline (1 course).

Our conclusion is that it is more logical to use average doses of the drugs and for a long time. Repeated courses are given when necessary at intervals, but these intervals, especially during the first year, should not be too long. The drugs should be given alternately.

If the patient is in good general condition, to test her response to the drug, a single large dose may be given when the blood picture is favourable.

Our experience today does not permit us to say which drug is the best and would be efficient for all patients with ovarian tumours. The same drug will give different results even in a tumour of the same histological structure, and the tolerance to the drug varies widely from case to case.

The way of administration of the drug depends on the type of disease. After paracentesis or thoracentesis, it is reasonable to introduce the drug into the cavity. When this is not necessary, there is no point in injecting it into the cavity.

Along with the search for other drugs effective in ovarian tumours, we are looking for drugs and methods which will raise the immunological properties of the body, while fighting the cancerous disease.

Summary

The literature and personal observations (about 400 cases) suggest that chemotherapy of malignant tumours of the ovaries can be conducted with more or less success by various medicinal preparations. Almost all agents are either used systemically to produce "general effect" or introduced into cavities to produce "local action". However, both ways of administration produce similar reactions of the body and, obviously, locally introduced drugs cause a local as well as a general effect, though at a slower rate.

Weak patients with ovarian tumours require courses of "average doses", but there may be indications for massive single or double administrations of one drug or another.

The main defect in the modern chemotherapy of ovarian tumours is the relatively early appearance of toxic effects on the body, which requires discontinuance of treatment. It appears desirable to use a chain combination of various drugs without similar side effects.

Experience with an antiblastic antibiotic chrysomalline (which does not affect leucopoiesis) with alkylating compounds is described.

Early results of combined therapy are presented.

Résumé

Les données de la littérature et les observations personnelles (environ 400) suggèrent que la chimiothérapie des tumeurs malignes des ovaires peut être pratiquée avec plus ou moins de succès par des préparations médicinales variées. Presque tous les agents médicamenteux sont employés à produire ou bien «l'effet général» ou bien, introduits localement, «l'effet local». Cependant, les deux moyens d'administration du médicament produisent des réactions semblables dans l'organisme, et apparemment les médicaments introduits localement donnent l'effet local tout aussi bien que l'effet général, bien que plus lentement.

Les malades faibles avec des tumeurs ovariennes demandent des séries de «doses moyennes» de drogues, mais on peut avoir des indications pour une seule dose massive ou une dose répétée de tel ou tel médicament.

Le défaut principal de la chimiothérapie moderne des tumeurs ovariennes est l'apparition assez rapide des effets toxiques, ce qui demande l'arrêt du traitement. Il paraît désirable d'employer une combinaison «en chaîne» de médicaments variés qui ne donnent pas des effets secondaires semblables.

L'expérience avec un antibiotique antiblastique chrysomalline (qui n'agit pas sur la leucopoïèse) avec des composés alkylés est décrite.

Les résultats immédiats de la thérapeutique combinée sont présentés.

References

ABBASOV, A. T., Experience with intracavitary use of sarcolysin and thiotepa in malignant tumours of the ovaries. *Vop. Onkol.* **6** (4), 23—30 (1960).

BLOKHINA, N. G., Preliminary results of the clinical study of Thiotepa in certain malignant tumours. In: *Questions of chemotherapy of malignant tumours*, p. 427—432. Moscow 1960.

GARIN, A. M., ASTRAKHAN, V. I., BYCHKOV, M. B., LARIONOV, L. F., and PEREVODCHIKOVA, N. I., On the clinical use of high single doses of sarcolysin and endoxan (cyclophosphane). *Vop. Onkol.* **10**, 3—9 (1965).

KOLIADINA, P. I., The role of cyclophosphane in combined treatment of patients with malignant ovarian newgrowths. In: *Cyclophosphane*, p. 169—171. Riga: Zinantne Publ. 1965.

KOSAREVA, A. N., Immediate results of treatment with thiotepa of patients with gynecological cancer. *Vop. Onkol.* **7**, 94—99 (1961).

KURCHKAREV, R. N., Preliminary results with the clinical use of antibiotic 2703. *Vop. Onkol.* **1**, 90—94 (1963).

MENSHIKOV, G. P., KUCHERIAVENKO, L. P., and DENISOVA, S. I., On aminoacid composition of actinomycins of "antibiotic No 2703". *Antibiotiki* **4**, 309—311 (1964).

NECHAEVA, I. D., *Tumours of the ovaries*. Leningrad: "Meditsina" publ. 1960.

MUIR, A. C., Methotrexate in neoplastic disease of the female genital tract. In: *Methotrexate in the treatment of cancer*. Bristol 1962.

NOVIKOVA, L. A., Chemotherapy of malignant ovarian newgrowths. *Akush. Ginek.* **3**, 88—92 (1962).

—, and KOLIADINA, P. I., Preliminary results with antibiotic chrysomalline in combined treatment of patients with malignant ovarian newgrowths. *Vestn. Akad. med. Nauk* **11**, 67—69 (1964).

— KOLIADINA, P. I., and MUSINA, T. M., Chemotherapy of malignant newgrowths of female genitalia. *Akush. i Ginek.* **4**, 6—13 (1964).

Total Treatment of Ovarian Cancer. Justification and Importance of the Combination of the Various Therapeutic Methods

Antonio Carlos Campos Junqueira, M. D.

Chefe do Serviço de Experimentação Clínica em Rádio e Quimioterapia do Instituto Central do Câncer — Hospital A. C. Camargo. São Paulo — Brasil
Membro da Comissão de Cancerologia e Chefe do Setor de Quimioterapia do Hospital do Servidor Público. São Paulo — Brasil
Assistente do Departamento de Farmacologia da Faculdade de Medicina da Universidade de São Paulo

Introduction

When an attempt is made to establish the best procedures regarding several aspects of ovarian cancer, the facts must be faced with objectivity, never forgetting new developments, still not entirely demonstrated, but which show possibilities.

If we intend to improve the results of the treatment — at present around 20 per cent survival for 5 years, in all cases — it is necessary that: a) therapeutic methods, presently at hand, be exploited in the best possible way, in an association in which the advantages will overcome the limitations of each one separately; b) several procedures be tried in diagnosis presently and treatment, if satisfactory, should be used in practice; c) new resources should be found to improve early diagnosis, to aid in understanding and predicting the behaviour of the several types of tumours and to make the therapeutic weapons more effective. It is also important that we look at all these possibilities with an optimistic and hopeful mind.

In this presentation, several aspects related to the first item mentioned will be discussed.

The ovarian tumours present several aspects of great interest to the oncologist due to the many histopathologic varieties, difficulties in early diagnosis, differences in the natural history, possibilities of propagation by several ways, and the various difficulties they present in treatment (Gray, 1964).

Early diagnosis, with the resources we have at hand presently, is practically impossible or represents an accidental finding. The symptoms are not characteristic and only late in the disease are they intense enough to justify diagnostic procedures.

The great variety of histologic types, which can be recognized only after surgery, is another factor which makes the planning of the treatment more difficult and thus contributes to the unfavourable results obtained. Radiotherapy and chemotherapy are not generally used before surgery. If the histologic type of the tumour and its possible sensitivity to both forms of treatment are not known, neither x-ray therapy nor the drugs could be used properly.

The several ways of dissemination also create difficulties. The most common ways — through invasion by continuity or by implants in the peritoneal surface — are frequently accompanied by lymphatic invasion. Distant metastases, produced by the cancer cells circulating in the blood, are less frequent.

All these factors create difficulties in treatment. For these reasons we think that, as in other fields of oncology, the combination, the working together of the different therapeutic weapons — if properly done — can be of great use (JUNQUEIRA, 1963).

Before proposing a therapeutic plan, we shall discuss briefly the limitations and advantages of surgery, radiotherapy and chemotherapy.

Surgery. This type of treatment is at present the diagnostic and therapeutic procedure that offers the best possibilities. The early cases, mainly with tumours of low grade malignancy, with less tendency to metastasize have, with surgery, the best possibility of cure. Unfortunately, in view of the difficulty of early diagnosis, generally when the patient is operated upon a great tumour is found, with invasion of other organs or tissues, peritoneal implants, metastatic lymph nodes and ascites. In the case of cystic tumours, the cyst is easily ruptured and the material contaminates the cavity. The surgical procedure is seldom conducted in satisfactory conditions. Even the most careful and experienced surgeon cannot eliminate all the cancerous foci. To make matters worse, handling of the viscera during the operation favours the propagation of tumour cells by the blood or in the abdominal cavity. All these factors and the surgical stress, reducing the host defenses, tend to increase the possibility of recurrence or metastatic spread. The behaviour of the tumour will depend mostly on the histopathologic type and the tumour — host equilibrium.

The mucinous types, when properly resected, usually do not metastasize to distant areas. They offer good possibility of cure in the early cases, when the tumour capsule is not broken and the abdominal cavity contaminated by the tumour cells. The serous tumours are more malignant. The capacity to metastasize increases in the more anaplastic tumours. Every effort should be made, in cystic tumours, to keep the capsule intact. When it is broken and the material spread in the peritoneal cavity, recurrence is to be expected.

The dysgerminomas, because of the early invasion of lymphatics and other structures, can be cured by surgery alone only in occasional cases.

The theca-cell tumours, usually with a more benign course present good opportunities for surgery. The granulosa-cell tumours, sometimes having a very malignant course with frequent recurrences, and other times a more benign and slow one, have a prognosis related to this behaviour.

Radiotherapy. The possibilities of radiation are smaller than those of surgery mainly on account of two factors:

1. Great difference in the radiosensitivity among the several histologic types. The more frequently-found tumours — papillary and mucinous — have a poor sensitivity to the different forms of radiation. The dysgerminomas usually are sensitive while the granulosa-cell tumours sometimes have a limited sensitivity.

Even when there is good radiosensitivity the possibility of cure, with radiation only, is not to be expected.

2. The necessity of reaching a high dose in a great volume of tissues — the entire pelvis and, frequently, the abdomen — is responsible for the use of special techniques, usually with supervoltage, and causes, in the majority of cases,

several local and systemic reactions. Sometimes the treatment cannot be properly conducted on account of these reactions.

The use of radioactive isotopes — principally radioactive gold — in the peritoneal cavity offers good possibilities as an adjuvant to surgery, when there are superficial tumour implants either residual or recurrent (HOLBROOK, 1964). This type of radiation, not too penetrating, but with a satisfactory distribution all through the peritoneal cavity, is very useful in these situations.

It is also important to remember the possibility of late reactions and sequelae — due to high doses of radiation — such as enterites, cystites, rectites, fibrosis and necrosis.

Chemotherapy. The main purpose of chemotherapy must be to co-operate with surgery and radiotherapy to reduce the possibility of recurrences and/or metastases (JUNQUEIRA, 1963). In some cases, when for any reason surgery is not indicated, chemotherapy can be used with radiotherapy to enhance its effect by addition or by a synergistic mechanism. In the advanced cases this kind of treatment has great usefulness. The ovarian tumours are, in general, very sensitive to several drugs now being used. Chemotherapy has limitations, however, among which the two most important are:

1. Absence of a specific activity against the tumour cell, which is the principal barrier to the use of chemotherapy. We do not have, at present, any drug active only against the tumour cell; all the drugs used are toxic also to the normal cells of the body. This fact limits the doses to those which the body can tolerate, always insufficient to destroy the tumour cells. For this reason, at present, chemotherapy can only be considered as an adjuvant to surgery and radiotherapy or as a palliative.

2. The difference in sensitivity that exists among the various types of tumour and also among the different tissues and organs of the body. Usually the chemosensitivity of a tissue is directly proportionate to its mitotic activity, metabolism and is indirectly proportionate to its differentiation. This explains the great sensitivity of the hematopoietic organs, lymphatic tissues and epithelium of the digestive tract — mainly the intestines — the first ones to be affected by the drug toxicity. The hematopoietic organs and the epithelium of the digestive tract are the two main barriers to the use of high doses of chemotherapy. A high degree of damage to these structures is not compatible with life. With the present drugs, a sufficient dose can not be given to destroy the total cancer cell population and thus cure the patient. We can achieve the destruction of 40, 60 or more, per cent of the cancer cell population, according to its sensitivity and the degree of the patient's tolerance.

3. Technical problems which also limit the use of chemotherapy. It is practically impossible to obtain a sufficient concentration of the drug in the entire region affected by the tumour and keep this concentration limited to this region, thus reducing the general toxicity and side effects.

Ovarian cancers, however, are among the most responsive tumours (FREI, 1966). Frequently in the cases submitted to chemotherapy, the disappearence of voluminous abdominal masses, ascites or metastatic nodes is observed for long periods of 3, 5 and, sometimes, more years. This indicates that this kind of tumour cell is sensitive to the drugs, mainly to those belonging to the group of the alkylating agents. For this reason the ovarian tumours are, perhaps, the best suited among the solid tumours, for the use of chemotherapy as an adjuvant to surgery and radiation. Tumour cells or small nodes that remain after surgery will be affected by the drugs. As chemotherapy is much more efficient in the presence of small nodes or masses than when there are several voluminous tumours, this is the situation where it is supposed to be more useful. If this type of treatment has already proved its value on the advanced cases it should, now, be used on the early ones, as an adjuvant therapy.

An interesting possibility, which should be tried in some services which have the facilities for it, is the test of the activity of the various drugs on the tumour cells. During the surgical procedure, fragments of the tumour could be taken and used to test the drugs. It should then, be possible, to select the one which showed more anti-tumour activity, in a particular case.

Material and Methods

In our series, 48 cases could be properly studied. When they came for treatment, with two exceptions, all had already been treated, as shown in Table I.

The situation at the beginning of treatment, as shown in Table II, was, in the majority of cases, characterized by abdominal masses and ascites. Distant metastases were rare.

The histopathologic classification is shown in Table III. The majority were

adenocarcinoma (11) and the several forms of papillary tumours (24). There were 17 cases of cystic tumours. In 4 cases, we had only a clinical diagnosis.

The drugs used in the treatment are shown in Table IV. They were used alone or in combination. By series of treatment we mean the period of time during which the patient received the drug until it had to be stopped on account of toxicity or another factor. The next period counts as another series. The same patient usually received several series of treatment. In some cases we tried to combine the drugs, simultaneously or consecutively, with the purpose of increasing the period of remission. When resistance was esta-

Table I. *Advanced ovarian tumours — 48 cases. Previous treatment*

Surgery	27 cases
Surgery + irradiation (TeCo)	9 cases
Laparotomy	2 cases
Surgery + chemotherapy	5 cases
Chemotherapy	2 cases
Irradiation (TeCo)	1 case
Untreated	2 cases

Table II. *Advanced ovarian tumours — 48 cases. Situation at the beginning of chemotherapy*

Abdominal masses	26 cases
Ascites	17 cases
Pleural effusion	4 cases
Pulmonary metastases	2 cases
Liver metastases (nodes)	2 cases

Table III. *Advanced ovarian tumours — 48 cases. Hystopathological classification*

Adeno-carcinoma	11 cases	
Papillary-adeno-carcinoma	18 cases	
Serous papillary adeno-carcinoma	3 cases	24 papillary
Mucinous papillary adeno-carcinoma	3 cases	tumours
Serous adeno-carcinoma	1 case	
Mucinous adeno-carcinoma	1 case	
Undifferentiated carcinoma	5 cases	
Granulosa-cell tumours	2 cases	
Tumours	4 cases	
Total	48 cases	
Cystic tumours	17 cases	

Table IV. *Advanced ovarian tumours — 48 cases. Drugs used in the treatment*

Alone	Series	Associated	Series
Thio-TEPA	37	Cytoxan + Thio-TEPA	3
Cytoxan	22	Thio-TEPA + Methotrexate	3
Leukeran	13	Thio-TEPA + Leukeran	2
Azetepa	7	Cytoxan + Thio-TEPA + Azetepa	2
HN$_2$	6	Thio-TEPA + Cytoxan + 5-FU	1
5-FU	3	Thio-TEPA + TEM	1
Methotrexate	2	Cytoxan + Methotrexate	1
TEM	1		
Vincaleukoblastine	1		

Table V. *Advanced ovarian tumours — 48 cases. Results of treatment. Classification of results*

9 cases:	No alteration in the evolution of the disease or a slight improvement.
18 cases:	Subjective and objective improvement for more than 1 month.
6 cases:	Disappearence of symptoms and evidence of the disease for more than 3 months.
15 cases:	Disappearence of symptoms and evidence of the disease for more than 6 months.

Table VI. *Advanced ovarian tumours — 48 cases Survival from the beginning of treatment*

Up to	6 months	23 cases (1 still alive)
Up to	1 year	10 cases (2 still alive)
Up to	2 years	8 cases (3 still alive)
Up to	3 years	2 cases (2 still alive)
Up to	5 years	2 cases (2 still alive)
More than	5 years	3 cases (3 still alive)

blished, we changed to another drug. In our opinion the most useful drug is Thio-TEPA followed by Cytoxan. Leukeran® is good for maintenance therapy (WILTSHAW, 1965).

Results

The results of treatment and the survival rate are shown in Tables V and VI. Fifteen cases had disappearence of symptoms and evidence of disease for more than 6 months out of a group of 25 which survived more than 6 months.

Several of these patients are still alive. Three cases are in the sixth year, 2 of which — a patient with a serous papillary adenocarcinoma and one with a granulosa-cell tumour — are entirely free of disease.

In our experience the papillary tumours were the ones which had most benefit from treatment and, of these, the serous are more sensitive than the mucinous types. The cystic tumours, when the capsule ruptured during the surgical procedure, had a very poor prognosis. Ascites, in some cases, disappeared with the use of Thio-TEPA or HN$_2$ and corticosteroids instilled in the peritoneal cavity.

Comments

Combination of the Therapeutic Weapons. In the planning of the total treatment — combining surgery, radiotherapy and chemotherapy — it is important that the benefits outweigh the disadvantages. This is not easy.

The treatment should be started by surgery complemented by chemotherapy. The drugs should be administered at the time of the operation, to act on the surgical field as well as on the tumour cells in the blood, whose number is increased during surgery. This implies a reduction of the dose. High doses, increasing the surgical stress and creating the possibility of hemorrhage and infection, would be disadvantageous. Smaller doses should, then, be administered with the purpose of producing a certain damage on the tumour cells. This damage would facilitate the work of the defensive mechanism of the body. After 10 to 20 days, according to the patient's condition and the extent of the surgical procedure, the drugs should be started again, this time with the histologic type of the tumour known. Considering the doubling time of the tumour cells as one month, we would have, at the most, a twofold increase in the number of tumour cells.

The treatment should proceed until toxicity signs appear. However, as the ovarian tumours are usually sensitive to several drugs and the combination of two or more drugs has proved to be more efficient against leukaemia and lymphoma, a combination of drugs should be considered for trials in the situation under discussion (FREI, 1966).

After surgery, with knowledge of the situation in the abdominal cavity — the localization of the tumour or tumour masses, the structures and lymphatics invaded, the places where the surgical procedure could be considered inadequate — and of the histologic type of the tumour, radiation can be properly planned. Here we have a great difficulty in the combined treatment. In the majority of cases it is impossible to submit the patient simultaneously to radiotherapy and to chemotherapy with adequate doses (JUNQUEIRA, 1961). The toxicity would be too severe. There are, then, three possibilities: to reduce the doses of one form of treatment, to reduce the doses of both, or to use them one after the other. In our opinion, the latter is the better choice. The simultaneous treatment, with reduced doses, can have the following disadvantages, related to the degree of the tumour

sensitivity and patient's tolerance: a) reducing the dose of both forms of treatment would risk the loss of the benefits that one of the treatments, properly conducted, could bring; b) even with reduced doses of both, the possibility of toxicity is greater than when using only one. The possibility of a synergistic effect betwen radiotherapy and chemotherapy is still under discussion and we do not yet have a definite opinion on it; c) reducing the dose of one of the treatments, we could choose to reduce precisely the one that in this particular case would be the more efficient.

By using one form of treatment subsequently to the other, it is possible to obtain the maximum benefits that each one can give, with less risk of severe toxicity. The delay brought by this sequence is not great and, we believe, well justified. Which, then, should be the first treatment used after surgery? We believe that the selection must depend on the conditions of each case, considering the radicality and extent of the surgical procedure, the histopathologic type of the tumour and the clinical situation of the patient. However, generally, chemotherapy must precede radiotherapy.

Planning the Treatment

The surgical act must be performed by an experienced surgeon, as the first therapeutic step. Only when there is a strong reason should operation be postponed. The extent of the surgery depends on the surgeon's judgment. Every effort should be made to avoid the rupture of cystic tumours. Chemotherapy should be started during the operation, using preferentially the alkylating agents, of which, in our opinion, Thio-TEPA is the most indicated. The agent should be diluted in saline solution and given by intravenous drip. The dose should be around 0.4 to lmgr per kg of body weight. The factors to be considered when choosing the dose are mainly age, weight, clinical conditions and blood status. Before closing the incision, it is convenient to leave in the cavity a certain amount of Thio-TEPA— around 20 to 30 mgr — or, as is usually done by our surgeons, a solution of sodium hypoclorite, with pH-9. This substance has proved to be efficient in the prevention of wound recurrences and has no general toxicity. In cases of ruptured cystic tumours Thio-TEPA, diluted in sufficient amount of saline to reach the entire peritoneal cavity, should be used.

The next step in the treatment depends on the surgical findings and histologic type of the tumour. When tests on the tumour sensitivity to the drugs are done — using tumour fragments or tumour culture — and show a good response, this should be taken into consideration in the planning of the future treatment.

The *mucinous* tumours are, usually, radio- and chemoresistants. When the surgical procedure is performed satisfactorily and there is no evidence of tumour left, radiotherapy should not be used (PARSONS, 1961). After 10 to 20 days, chemotherapy should be given using Thio-TEPA, 20 mg each 3 days, until the appearance of toxicity. The same applies to ruptured cystic tumours. But, in these cases, we believe it best to submit the patient also to radiotherapy, after recovery from the drug toxicity. Around 3,000 rads, in three weeks, are given to the whole abdominal cavity.

The *adenocarcinomas, serous and papillary* tumours have a limited sensitivity to radiotherapy and a good sensitivity to chemotherapy, the most responsive being the papillary. After radical surgery,

patients with these tumours should be submitted to chemotherapy and, after an interval sufficient for recovery, to radiotherapy. The same technics already mentioned can be used here, but the necessity of submitting the entire abdominal cavity to radiation may be questioned. It may be more advantageous to limit the radiation to the pelvis and increase the dose to around 4,000 rads in four to five weeks.

When the tumour cannot be removed completely, an additional dose of around 2,000 rads, in two weeks, should be delivered to the area of the residual tumour.

Dysgerminomas are the more sensitive tumours to radiotherapy and chemotherapy. After surgery — radical or not— the patient should be submitted to chemotherapy and, later, to radiotherapy. The same doses should be used.

We do not have a definite opinion on the best way to treat *granulosa-cell* and *theca-cell* tumours. Our experience is too limited.

All the situations discussed belonged to early cases. We believe that they should be submitted to repeated series of chemotherapy during the first 3 years, at intervals of approximately 6 months, even when there is no evidence of disease. The drugs to be used would be Thio-TEPA, Cytoxan R, 5-Fluoruracil, or others, according to the experience of the service.

For patients with tumours too advanced to be submitted to a radical treatment, we have two possibilities: a) If, clinically, there is the possibility of a partial removal of the tumour, she should undergo operation which will permit the histologic classification of the tumour and facilitate the work of the subsequent radiotherapy and chemotherapy. b) When partial removal of the tumour is not considered feasible or the bad condition of the patient does not encourage this procedure she should, be submitted to intensive chemotherapy. We prefer Cytoxan, in doses around 500—600 mg a day, during 4 to 8 days, or 5-Fluoruracil in the usual dose of 10—15 mg per kg a day, during 5 to 7 days. Afterwards, this treatment could be followed by the use of Thio-TEPA or Leukeran R. Depending on the results of chemotherapy, the case could be reviewed regarding the possibility of surgical treatment or radiotherapy.

Conclusions

This combined treatment should be used only in cancer institutes or services, fully prepared to do this kind of treatment in view of the difficulties and risks that it presents, the necessity of a staff with good experience in the various fields of oncology, the indispensable facilities and equipment and, above all, the good understanding and disposition to work as a team of those who administer the treatment.

As a clinical investigation, combined treatment must be done under strict control and all its details, as well as the results, properly studied in order to enable improvement in the treatment of ovarian cancer.

Summary

The results of treatment of ovarian cancer, as a rule, are very poor on account of the following factors: difficulties in early diagnosis, several histopathologic types, differences in the natural evolution, several ways of metastatic propagation and limitations of the therapeutic weapons. Surgery, the best diagnostic and therapeutic procedure, as well as radiotherapy and chemotherapy, have many limitations which are discussed. The combination of the different forms of treatment presents several problems but may be a way to improve the results. The details regarding the best way to use this combination according to the histologic type of the tumour are discussed and a proposal for this kind of total treatment is presented.

Résumé

Les résultats du traitement du cancer de l'ovaire sont en général décerants. Cela est dû aux facteurs suivants: difficulté du diagnostic précoce, variété des types histopathologiques, différences dans l'évolution et dans les formes de propagation métastatique et limitation des ressources thérapeutiques.

La chirurgie, qui est le meilleur moyen diagnostique et thérapeutique, ainsi que la radiothérapie et la chimiothérapie présentent des limitations qui sont discutées dans cet ouvrage. La combinaison des divers traitements présente certains problèmes et difficultés mais peut être une forme d'amélioration des résultats obtenus actuellement.

Les détails relatifs à la meilleure façon de faire cette combinaison, en tenant compte du type histologique de la tumeur, sont discutés dans cet ouvrage et une proposition est présentée pour le traitement global du cancer de l'ovaire.

Discussion

J. GRAHAM said that this paper emphasized the need, already expressed by FLETCHER, for a cooperative study to be made of the various types of treatment in ovarian cancer. There seemed to be general agreement that Stage I cases should be treated surgically. KOTTMEIER had shown that Stage II A cases can be treated effectively by bilateral salpingo-oophorectomy and intracavitary radium in the retained uterus. Possibly, also, these patients can be

successfully treated by total hysterectomy and bilateral salpingo-oophorectomy.
Less agreement existed about the proper
treatment for patients with Stage II B
and Stage III disease, but if the tumour
was a discrete mass which could be
entirely resected, then removal was considered worthwhile. When the disease is
a non-discrete mass, the unresolved
questions pertain to the usefulness of
preoperative irradiation, the proper doses, and whether part of the tumour
should be removed when not all of it
can be resected. Other unanswered
questions in the management of ovarian
cancer were whether chemotherapy
should be used, what agent, the dosage,
and the sequence in regard to radiotherapy for a patient with advanced
disease, upper abdominal involvement
and distant metastases.

From discussions at this conference
GRAHAM had the impression that patients with Stages II B, III, and IV
disease follow about the same course no
matter what treatment is used. In four
series of patients treated by different
methods at Roswell Park Memorial Institute, the results were similar. The
over-all five-year survival rate was eight
per cent, which is similar to that reported
by JUNQUEIRA and others. Although
he thought patients benefited by treatment, he did not think that the natural
history was changed to any great extent
and, actually, he thought there was some
danger in treatment by either irradiation
or chemotherapy. He quoted RICHARD-
SON's data which showed that there was a
temporary improvement in the survival
rate of patients who had more than
50 per cent of the tumour removed, as
opposed to those who had less than
50 per cent removed when they were
subjected to reexploration. At the end of
two years, however, the difference was
minor. He also showed data compiled by

R. GRAHAM on the survival of cases
according to how much of the tumour
was removed. These patients were referred after laparotomy and a repeat laparotomy was performed before treatment
was begun. These data showed a correlation in the six months' and one-year
survival rates with the amount of tumour removed. In one group of patients
who had not had repeat laparotomy,
however, the six-months survival rate
was better than for those who had
biopsy only. Actually, in comparison,
the survival rate for those patients who
had repeat laparotomy and partial removal of the tumour mass did not improve
until at least 90 per cent of the tumour
was removed.

He also showed some data which
supported the contention that chemotherapy was more efficacious when given
before radiation. He pointed out that if,
as KOTTMEIER had suggested, chemotherapy acts in a similar manner to radiotherapy, the second treatment modality
would naturally be less effective than the
first. He had heard nothing at this conference to indicate that any one type of
treatment was superior to another, he
said, but he deplored the use of increa-
singly high doses of irradiation. A large
dose might provide some temporary advantage but it made difficulties in the
future management of the patient. He
did not think that there was any evidence
to support the advantage of the larger
doses. He supported this remark with
data on patients with Stages III and IV
disease who were treated with different
doses of radiation.

GRAHAM suggested that, in addition
to a cooperative study, a registry or central secretariat might be developed for
several clinics. The case histories and a
section of the tumour for patients with
Stages II B, III, and IV disease, who survived for more than two years without

evidence of disease, could be sent to this registry. The histologic type could be determined by an expert and the abstract sent to all participants. Thus, a more effective management pattern might be recognized sooner.

DAVIDSOHN remarked that damage to the hematopoietic system as the result of either chemotherapy or radiotherapy was a frequent problem. The most common complications were leukopenia and thrombocytopenia. It is not commonly recognized, he said, that whole blood transfusions are not helpful in the management of these complications. Actually, whole blood transfusions can be harmful; patients can develop manifestations of heart failure. The proper treatment for granulocytopenia is the transfusion of leukocytes and for thrombocytopenia, the preferred treatment is the transfusion of platelet concentrates. By the use of leukophoresis, a donor can give more than one unit a week, because he is not deprived of his red blood cells.

In acute aplasia, such as described by KOTTMEIER, in which there are either no changes or minimal ones in the peripheral blood, but there are alterations in the bone marrow, blood transfusions are not helpful, because the blood cells survive long enough for these patients not to have anemia. After a period of time, however, they have thrombocytopenia and granulocytopenia. Ideally, the proper treatment for these patients is marrow transfusions, DAVIDSOHN said, but unfortunately there is no completely reliable way of identifying a compatible donor. The known blood group factors can be determined before transfusion, of course, but others which affect the fate of such a transplantation cannot be determined. It was necessary, therefore, to try transfusions of bone marrow, granulocyte concentrates, and platelet

concentrates in an attempt to overcome the state of acute aplasia or hypoplasia.

DAVIDSOHN proposed that a supply of bone marrow and whole blood be obtained from the patient himself, before chemotherapy. The bone marrow would be frozen for use when necessary.

BRULÉ said that for two years at the Gustave Roussy Institute, it had been the practice to obtain bone marrow from the patient before he had any chemotherapy and freeze it. Experience had been disappointing, however, because although this point has not been examined statistically as yet, the impression was that the bone marrow did not recover any quicker after injection of the frozen marrow than when it was simply permitted to recover by itself.

Tests for antitumour activity on a portion of tumour tissue, such as JUNQUEIRA suggested, had also been done at the Gustave Roussy Institute for three or four years. The tumour tissue was cultured and tested against six different compounds. The compound which was always the most efficient was 5-FU, but unfortunately the laboratory and clinical findings did not always correspond.

He agreed with GRAHAM, BRULÉ said, that it would be a long time before the value of systemic chemotherapy after surgery would be known. Administration of the compound, if limited to a few days at the time of surgery, might be useful but to continue the drug for several years afterwards, if there were no indications, would be futile and possibly dangerous.

MULLER said that he thought a mucinous carcinoma which produced mucin only in some areas would react well to irradiation, but a tumour which produced large amounts of mucin would be less sensitive to irradiation. He was concerned that in a cooperative series, such as suggested by GRAHAM, some points already established would be re-examined. For example, he had a series of patients who did not receive radioactive gold but who were treated by other comparable methods. Comparison of this series with those who received the gold showed that the survival rate was increased substantially with the gold. This type of comparison has also been made in another institution with the same results.

JUNQUEIRA said that it was difficult to make a comprehensive plan for the treatment of ovarian cancer. Since only about 20 per cent of all ovarian cancer patients survived five years, however, probably 80 per cent of the remainder had tumour left even when grossly it all appeared to have been removed. Thus, he thought that in ovarian cancer, maintenance treatment might be indicated such as is used in breast carcinoma and in Wilms's tumour.

References

FREI III, E., Selected considerations regarding chemotherapy as adjuvant in cancer treatment. *Cancer Chemother. Rep.* **50**, No 1—2, (1966).

GRAY, L. A., and BARNES, M. L., Carcinoma of the ovary. Report of 106 cases. Pathology, clinical course, treatment. *Ann. Surg.* **159**, 279—290 (1964).

HOLBROOK, M. A., WELCH, J. S., and CHILDS, D. S., Adjuvant use of radioactive colloids in the treatment of carcinoma of ovary. *Radiology* **83**, 888—891 (1964).

JUNQUEIRA, A. C. C., A associação radioterapia-quimioterapia no tratamento do câncer. *Rev. Bras. Cirurg.* **42**, 303—309 (1961).

— Quimioterapia anti-neoplásica. Finalidade de seu emprêgo em associação com a cirurgia e radioterapia. *Rev. Paul. Med.* **62**, 480—490 (1963).

PARSONS, L., Ovarian tumors. *Clin. Obstet. Gynec.* **4**, No 3 (1961).

WILTSHAW, E., Chlorambucil in the treatment of primary adeno-carcinoma of the ovary. *J. Obstet. Gynaec. Brit. Cwlth* **72**, 586—602 (1965).

Proposals for the Standardization
of the Combined Treatment of Ovarian Cancer

H. L. KOTTMEIER, M.D.

Professor of Gynecology, Radiumhemmet, Stockholm, Sweden

Introduction

Malignant neoplasms of the ovary are rather common. In 1958, for instance, 890 new cases of invasive carcinoma of the cervix, and 765 of ovarian cancer were diagnosed in Sweden. We all share the opinion that, in general, the prognosis is poor. Unfortunately, symptoms of ovarian carcinoma are often absent and these neoplasms are frequently not discovered until the growth has extended to surrounding organs or has metastasized. The treatment becomes progressively less effective with increasing anatomic extent of the disease.

Early Diagnosis. The necessity of an early diagnosis is obvious. Symptoms are not characteristic. Many patients have had vague symptoms of abdominal discomfort or cystitis. Postmenopausal bleeding may occasionally indicate a malignant neoplasm of the ovary. Laparoscopy has proved to be of value in many cases and can afford an early diagnosis. The routine use of cul-de-sac aspiration may result in the detection of occult ovarian carcinomas (GRAHAM *et al.*, 1964). WESTIN, as well as physicians at the Radiumhemmet, have tried the aspiration method in many cases. However, we have not been successful in identifying malignant cells in the cul-de-sac aspiration except in cases of ascitic fluid.

Palpation of a mass in the pelvis does not always permit a final diagnosis. Hysterosalpingography, arteriography and needle biopsy may help in the diagnosis, but sometimes a laparotomy is necessary. Microscopic examination of the growth removed or of biopsies taken is required to establish the nature of the growth.

True Ovarian Carcinoma. Further discussion will be limited to the therapy of true carcinoma which is the most common malignant neoplasm of the ovary. As far as treatment of dysgerminomas, other germ cell tumours, functioning ovarian tumours and teratomas are concerned, I refer to publications by TEILUM, HERTIG, and GONE (1961), MORRIS and SCULLY (1958), GRICOUROFF, KOTTMEIER and others. A few remarks will be made later regarding carcinomas of low potential malignancy.

Explorative laparotomy facilitates determination of the borders of the growth by direct inspection and palpation and should be carried out whenever there is the slightest suspicion of an ovarian tumour. Some years ago the gynecologists considered it appropriate to use conservative treatment in patients with physiologic enlargements or cysts of the ovary. It is often difficult to decide whether an enlargement is a physiologic one or whether it is due to a neoplasm. Today, laparotomy is a safe procedure and it is wise to perform this operation on the slightest suspicion of an ovarian neoplasm.

Surgery. On laparotomy the surgeon should outline in detail the extension of the growth and take several, rather large biopsies from areas which, on inspection, seem to be suspicious. The anatomical extent of the carcinoma is of importance in further planning the therapy. Experience has proved that serous carcinomas grow fast and give rise to extensive metastases at an early stage, while mucinous types are confined to the ovary for a long time. Endometrioid carcinomas tend to be multicentric but remain confined to the true pelvis for a long period of time. In our series metastases above the pelvis were diagnosed in 147 of 276 cases of serous carcinoma (53.3 per cent), in 9 of 51 cases of mucinous carcinoma (17.6 per cent) and in 29 of 168 cases of endometrioid carcinoma (17.2 per cent). The carcinoma was limited to the ovaries and uterus in 55 of 276 cases of serous neoplasm (19.9 per cent), in 30 of 51 cases of mucinous neoplasm (58.8 per cent) and in 58 of 168 cases of endometrioid neoplasm (34.5 per cent).

It should be stressed, though, that the excision of an ovarian carcinoma should be as extensive as possible. Every effort should be made to keep the capsule intact. Even if the tumour is unilateral, removal of the opposite ovary is advisable. In young patients and in those who want to have children a unilateral oophorectomy may be considered. If, however, microscopic examination of the removed tumour reveals a serous type, reoperation is indicated as the normal-appearing ovary may frequently harbor microscopic metastases.

An extended operation including, for instance, resection of the small or large bowel, is indicated at least in carcinomas that are probably of the mucinous type.

At a later stage, these neoplasms give rise to metastases and are apparently radio-resistant. Whether this management is advisable in serous and endometrioid carcinomas could be discussed seriously. It is our experience that extensive surgery in such neoplasms smears cancer cells all over the peritoneum, opens lymphatic and blood vessels and tends to disseminate cancer cells. The removal of serous or endometrioid carcinomas firmly fixed to surrounding tissue destroys the defensive reaction of the body. Recurrences appear rapidly and do not usually respond to radiation or to any other therapy. Although, at present we cannot prove its value, it seems logical to try radiotherapy prior to excisional surgery. Consequently, the operation should be restricted to an exploration. Biopsies should be taken. Irradiation should be administered to the area outlined during surgery. The adequate dose is about 4,000 rad. delivered in 5 to 6 weeks. Re-operation should be carried out 10 to 14 days after completion of radiotherapy.

Most gynecologists prefer to perform a panhysterectomy in addition to oophorectomy because of the possibility of transtubal metastases to the endometrium. Personally, I am not convinced that generally a hysterectomy is to be recommended. Intrauterine application of radioactive sources makes possible the treatment to the cul-de-sac. Metastases or pelvic recurrences appear first in the cul-de-sac. A heavy dose of radiation can be given to this area if external irradiation is combined with intrauterine radium (Fig. 1). Insertion of radium into the vagina is of no value. Resection of the omentum has been recommended whenever a surgical procedure for ovarian cancer is performed. Metastases to the omentum are diagnosed in many cases. At the Radium-hemmet we have not been convinced that prophylactic omentectomy is of value. In cases of metastases to the omentum a resection lessens the degree of accumulation of ascites. Yet the removal of the omentum should not be done by cutting through carcinomatous tissue.

Application of Radioactive Sources. Intraperitoneal examination and/or removal of an ovarian carcinoma will spread

many other Institutes — have substituted the isotope by chemotherapeutic agents such as Nitrogen mustard, Thio-TEPA, Cytoxan, etc. The effect of intraabdominal radioactive sources or chemotherapeutic agents has, so far, not been as satisfactory as we had expected.

Radiation therapy. The survival rate in true ovarian carcinoma is dependent

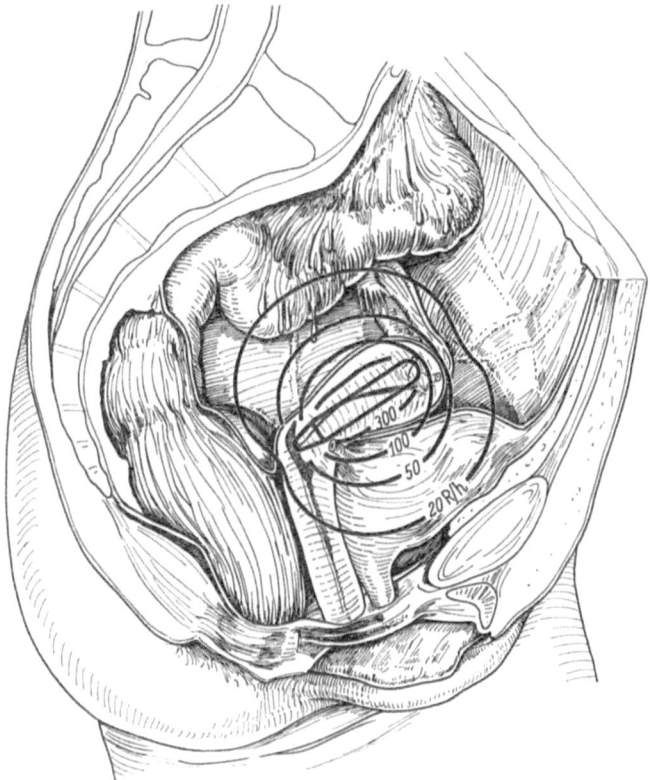

Fig. 1. Isodose-curves around an intrauterine radium-tube. 150 mg RaEl

cancer cells to various parts of the peritoneal cavity. It is probable that such superficial peritoneal transplants are eradicated by the intraperitoneal application of colloidal radioactive sources. MÜLLER has for years applied radioactive gold intraperitoneally after surgery. His results support the value of this method. The Radiumhemmet — and

on the anatomical extent of the carcinoma. Serous carcinomas tend to metastasize above the pelvis and to distant sites, while endometrioid carcinomas are often limited to the pelvis. Radiation should start as soon as possible after surgery if examination has proved that the cancer is incompletely removed but is limited to the true pelvis. Many authors have reported an increase in survival when radiotherapy is given postoperatively. At the Radiumhemmet a five-year survival rate of 17.1 per cent has been reached in 35 cases of serous, and 50 per cent in 24 cases of endometrioid carci-

Irradiation of the pelvis can be achieved more efficiently with supervoltage radiation than with conventional roentgen therapy. Because our experience indicates that endometrioid carcinomas possibly respond better to irradiation

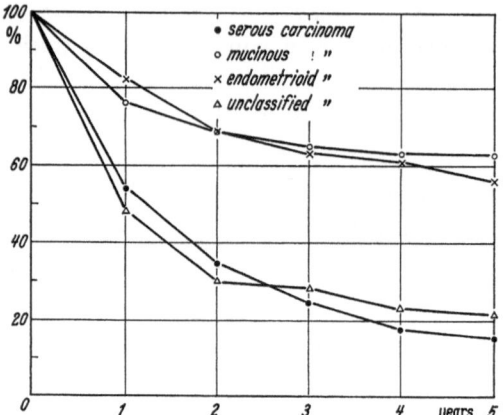

Fig. 2. Comparison of survival rates in different types of ovarian carcinoma (Ic, IIc, IIIc, IVc)

Table I. *Five-year survivals in ovarian carcinomas*

Type of carcinoma	No. of cases treated	Living after				
		1 year	2 years	3 years	4 years	5 years
Serous	276	149	95	68	48	41
Mucinous	51	39	35	33	32	32
Endometrioid	168	138	115	106	102	93
Unclassified	60	29	18	17	14	13

Table I gives the survivals in 555 cases of ovarian carcinoma treated 5 years ago or earlier.

noma with non-resectable metastases in the true pelvis. The corresponding three-year survival rates are 23.6 per cent in 55 cases of serous, and 50 per cent in 50 cases of endometrioid carcinoma. These figures suggest that endometrioid carcinomas do respond better to irradiation than serous ones.

In these patients, conventional x-ray therapy with a half value layer of 1 to 2 mmCu has been administered through two large opposing fields in addition to intrauterine application of radium.

than serous carcinomas, cases of serous and endometrioid neoplasms with extension to tissues in the true pelvis are at present receiving cobalt beam therapy with a dose of 4,500 to 5,000 rad to the midpelvis over a period of 6 to 7 weeks. Two large opposing portals or a 3-field technic are used in these cases. The 3-field method is chosen for cases in which the extent of the carcinoma is outlined in detail and thus a reduced dose can be given to the bladder, rectum and small bowel partly with the use of wedge-filters. The radiation is delivered through one large anterior and two lateral fields.

This radiation technic is applied *also in cases of true ovarian carcinoma in which the tumour was removed completely.* However, in such cases the dose from external radiation is decreased to about 3,000 to 4,000 rads.

The radiation therapy described has been used at the Radiumhemmet since 1964. At this time no conclusions can be drawn as far as results are concerned, but we do believe that they will be improved.

I have mentioned earlier that at the Radiumhemmet, radiotherapy was also given to *cases of true ovarian carcinoma with metastases above the pelvis.* Only two of 114 such patients with serous carcinoma are living symptom-free after 5 years. The corresponding number of endometrioid carcinoma is 4 of 24. Probably radiotherapy will be a palliative in advanced cases of true ovarian carcinomas, but it is questionable whether the 5-year survival in 6 of 138 cases can be attributed to the radiation, delivered in rather small doses. It is possible that the survival is due to a slow growth of the disease. However, we have tried recently to deliver dosages of 3,500 to 5,000 rads to the *total abdominal cavity* in selected cases of ovarian carcinoma with extensive metastases spread out over the entire peritoneal cavity. The radiation has been applied through six fields with central doses of 700 rads over a period of 5 days. Remarkably enough the patients have stood the radiation satisfactorily. Their general condition has improved, the ascites has disappeared and, sometimes, the tumour has decreased considerably in size. However, it is still doubtful whether the survival in cases of serous carcinoma has been prolonged. Such a radiation technic may be tried from a research point of view but should not be applied routinely.

Another attempt to increase the dose to the entire abdomen has been made at the M.D. Anderson Hospital. Megavoltage irradiation has been given through multiple narrow horizontal strips. Actually, this is a modification of the overlapping x-ray strip technic recommended by PATERSON for radiation of the trunk. This radiation technic is difficult to use in cases of carcinoma with ascites.

Chemotherapy. Great attention has been given to radiomimetic substances in the hope that they may delay the growth of the carcinoma. Experience has shown that the use of compounds similar to nitrogen mustard has been a success in causing regression of ovarian carcinoma. Since the publications by BATEMAN (1955) and others, Thio-TEPA has been reported to be useful in the management of ovarian carcinomas, but also Chlorambucil, E-39, Endoxan, Sarcolysin, Hemisulphur mustard etc. have yielded good palliation in many cases. At the Radiumhemmet we have chosen Thio-TEPA in the treatment of ovarian carcinoma and have used it exclusively or in combination with irradiation.

The intracavitary application of cytotoxic agents has also been used to a large extent at the Radiumhemmet. For years we hoped that intraperitoneal instillation of nitrogen mustard or similar drugs would lead to palliative results similar to those achieved by colloidal radioactive substances. Unfortunately, experience has shown that this does not hold valid for patients with ascites. Neither does prophylactic instillation of Thio-TEPA into the peritoneal cavity after laparotomy seem to be of real value, irrespective of whether the method used is continous application or a single injection.

In 1960 through 1962 an investigation was carried out to determine whether chemotherapy given in addition to radiation would improve survival rates. Thio-TEPA was given intravenously in moderate doses in 32 cases in which the ovarian carcinoma had been incompletely removed, but no extrapelvic metastases

ed only radiation (Fig. 3). The plan was to maintain combined therapy until depression of the bone marrow had appeared. In 42 of the 131 patients, therapy was given until the leucocytes and thrombo-

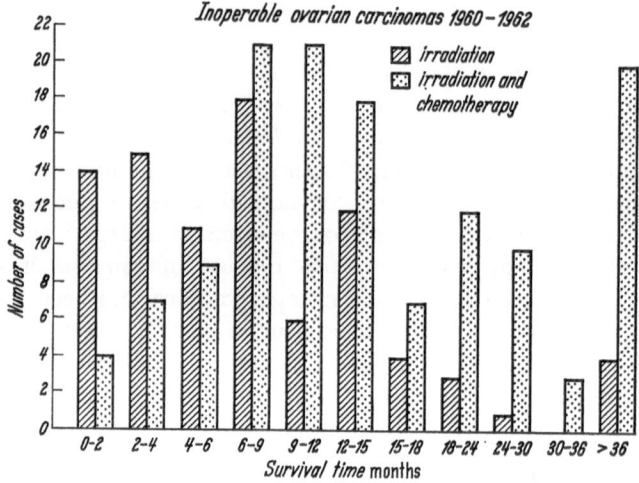

Fig. 3. Comparison of survival curves in patients who received X-ray and Thio-TEPA in any sequence and those who received Thio-TEPA only

Table II. *Distribution of 219 cases with inoperable ovarian carcinoma according to histopathological type*

Pathologic type	Treatment applied	
	Irradiation No. of cases	Irradiation/ chemotherapy No. of cases
Serous	33 (38%)	74 (56%)
Mucinous	2	1
Endometrioid	15 (17%)	18 (14%)
Unclassified	14 (16%)	22 (17%)
No microscopic examination	24 (27%)	16 (12%)
Total	88	131

were found. The follow-up of these cases has not revealed any benefit which can be attributed to chemotherapy.

To study the effect on cases of ovarian carcinoma that were either completely inoperable or had given rise to several unresectable metastases above the pelvis, Thio-TEPA was injected intravenously in 131 patients, while 88 patients receiv-

cytes were depressed to very low levels. Table II presents the distribution of the cases in regard to the histopathological type of the growth. The serous carcinomas constitute 38 per cent of the irradiated group and 56 per cent of those which had received combined therapy.

From the study it is obvious that combined treatment has proved to be

effective in producing a prolonged survival and a noticeable subjective improvement in many cases of extensive
ovarian carcinoma in which chemotherapy was given in large doses.

As a consequence of this trial we give
Thio-TEPA intravenously to patients
with extensive ovarian carcinoma, especially if the growth is of the serous type.
It is important to continue chemotherapy
until a depression of the bone marrow
has occurred. It is, therefore, not sufficient to keep the blood count under
close observation. Repeated bone marrow biopsies have to be made during
the course of therapy, especially as occasionally the blood count has not cor-
responded to the cellular pattern of the
bone marrow taken from the sternum.

Thio-TEPA is given intravenously
in a dose of 10 mg daily or every second
day. The initial dose varies considerably.
The patient is also kept under close observation for several weeks after the
completion of therapy, as a severe late
depression of the leucocytes and platelets
may sometimes occur two to four weeks
later. The patients have a decreased immunity to infections. The treatment involves a risk of aplastic bone marrow or
septicaemia. Five patients have died as
the result of therapy.

At present, we do not know whether
a combined treatment of irradiation and
chemotherapy is to be preferred to
chemotherapy alone in cases of true ovarian carcinoma with extension above the
pelvis. We suppose that a combined
treatment is appropriate in cases of endometrioid carcinoma. In our opinion,
therapy should begin with radiation and
chemotherapy should be given subsequently. Investigations have shown
that an apparent hyperplasia of the cellular pattern in the marrow from the sternum occurs during the first two weeks
of irradiation to the pelvis.

Table III. *Sustained palliation in 219 cases of inoperable carcinoma of the ovary*

Treatment applied		Effect
Irradiation No. of cases	Irradiation/ chemotherapy No. of cases	
47	17	None
41	116	Good

Recent observations support the opinion that chemotherapy alone is preferred
to combined treatment in cases of extensive serous and mucinous carcinomas.
Provided initial treatment has yielded a
good effect, further chemotherapy with
Thio-TEPA, Alkeran or Endoxan in
moderate doses should be given, under observation, though, of the blood count. In
our experience, however, the platelets will
never return to normal level. In addition
blood transfusions and testosterone in
large doses should be given.

Repeated Surgery. One important question remains: should surgery be carried
out in cases of extensive ovarian carcinoma which, on initial examination and/or
laparotomy, were considered completely
inoperable and which responded satisfactorily to treatment applied? The Radiumhemmet has advocated for years that, in
these cases, a laparotomy should be done
with removal of as much of the disease
as is possible. In the years 1958 through
1962 this was carried out in 45 cases of
serous carcinoma, in 8 cases of endometrioid carcinoma and in 10 cases of
unclassified true carcinoma. Six, 2 and
3 patients respectively have survived
three years after initial therapy. Five
patients are living at 5 years; only one
survived of the 45 patients with serous
carcinoma. However, it should also be
noticed that in 24 of the 63 patients operated upon, the disease "exploded" following surgery. As a consequence of
these poor results, we advocate surgery

only occasionally in cases of extensive ovarian carcinoma that from the beginning were considered completely inoperable. It may be that chemotherapy given in repeated series will widen the indications for repeated surgery.

Ovarian Carcinoma of Low Potential Malignancy. Our experience with the so-called questionable carcinomas includes 121 cases treated 5 years ago and 156 at least 3 years ago. In cases of unilateral growth a preservation of the normal ovary may be permissible. Radical excision is important especially in cases of mucinous tumours as fragments of neoplastic tissue left behind may lead to pseudomyxoma peritonaei. Radiotherapy with doses not exceeding 3,000 rads is useful when the tumour cannot be completely removed. Re-operation is indicated in cases initially considered as inoperable and which improved after radiation therapy. A 5-year survival rate of 79.6 per cent has been attained in 49 cases of low potential carcinomas with metastases. The corresponding 3-year survival rate in 67 cases is 85.1 per cent.

Summary

Principles for the treatment of ovarian carcinoma are outlined. Emphasis has been laid on histology and on anatomical extent of the growth. The extent of the tumour should be outlined in detail at clinical examination and at laparotomy. Excision of the carcinoma should be as complete as possible. Every effort should be made to keep the capsule intact. When serous and endometrioid carcinomas are fixed to surrounding tissue by firm adhesions it may be appropriate to restrict the operation to an explorative laparotomy and to re-operate upon the patient 10 to 14 days after completion of radiation.

Intraperitoneal application of colloidal radioactive sources following surgery seems to decrease the risk of peritoneal implants and is superior to radiomimetic substances in the palliation treatment of ascites. Removal of the primary cancer is occasionally followed by regression of disseminated metastases.

Radiotherapy, using adequate doses, should be administered to all cases of true ovarian carcinoma limited to the pelvis. Endometrioid carcinomas may respond better to radiation than serous tumours. In advanced cases of carcinoma, with unresectable metastases above the pelvis, chemotherapy should be administered either as the only treatment or in combination with radiation. Chemotherapy should be applied in doses that lead to depression of the bone marrow. Recent experience has shown that often the palliation effect from chemotherapy is superior to that from radiotherapy.

Discussion

RUTLEDGE asked for clarification of these points: 1. Did the recommendation that irradiation be used only in combination with chemotherapy for disease which has spread to the upper abdomen apply to all cell types, such as endometrioid carcinoma, for example? 2. What are the sources of treatment failure when the patient is not cured, although the disease is restricted to the pelvis and the maximum radiation dose has been given? Does this represent a lack of sensitivity of the tumour to irradiation, the ineffectiveness of the irradiation, even though it was in the range of 5,000 or 6,000 roentgens, or failure to detect subclinical evidence of spread of the disease to other parts of the abdomen? Could the disease possibly be multifocal in type? 3. Is it possible to identify endometrioid carcinoma as accurately as serous or mucinous carcinoma? Should some of the material from institutions that have had considerable experience in detecting endometrioid carcinoma be circulated among the cooperating institutions so that, in another five or ten years, results could be compared with accuracy? 4. Is x-ray therapy superior to chemotherapy in achieving regression of the ovarian cancer mass?

TEILUM recommended that, since in 1967 the cooperating centers are to meet and discuss with the international center the classification of ovarian tumours, practical measures should be taken to establish criteria for the identification of the unusual types of endometrioid cancer, the so-called unclassified adenocarcinoma and the so-called mesonephric tumours. In this latter group, there should also be a classification regarding the degree because many cases in this group are benign.

J. GRAHAM said that he appreciated the "blueprint" for management that KOTTMEIER outlined. He added that in his experience with Thiophosphoramide

(TSPA) used in conjunction with radiotherapy for advanced ovarian carcinoma, no advantage was obtained with the use of the larger doses of the drug.

KOTTMEIER, in closing, said that although irradiation had been used at the Radiumhemmet for advanced cancer for many years, it was regarded as a palliative procedure unless the disease was limited to the pelvis. LENZ's investigation also showed that radiation was of questionable value except as a palliative procedure. He added, however, that palliation was important in this disease. In recent years he had been more and more convinced that better palliation was achieved with satisfactorily applied chemotherapy than with radiation when upper abdominal disease is present. Furthermore, if radiation is used, even palliatively, large doses are necessary. The other questions he could not answer. KOTTMEIER expressed his sincere thanks to Dr TEILUM and hoped that a close collaboration would soon begin between the W.H.O., the UICC and the Figo as far as classification of ovarian neoplasms was concerned.

References

ABEL, S., Ovarian carcinoma: diagnosis and treatment. *Missouri Med.* **54**, 423 (1957).

ALLAN, M. S., and HERTIG, A. T., Carcinoma of ovary. *Amer. J. Obstet. Gynec.* **58**, 640—653 (1949).

BATEMAN, J. C., Chemotherapy of solid tumors with triethylene thiophosphoramide. *New Engl. J. Med.* **252**, 879—887 (1955).

—, and WINSHIP, T., Palliation of ovarian carcinoma with phosphoramide drugs. *Surg. Gynec. Obstet.* **102**, 347—354 (1956).

BRODY, S., Clinical aspects of dysgerminoma of the ovary. *Acta radiol. (Stockh.)* **56**, 209—230 (1961).

BRUNSCHWIG, A., Attempted palliation by radical surgery for pelvic and abdominal carcinomatosis primary in ovaries. *Cancer (Philad.)* **14**, 384—388 (1961).

CORSCADEN, J. A., *Gynecologic cancer* (ed. 3). Baltimore: William & Wilkins Co. 1962.

DAVIS, B. A., LATOUR, J. P. A., and PHILPOTT, N. W., Primari carcinoma of the ovary. *Surg. Gynec. Obstet.* **102**, 565—573 (1956).

DESAIVE, P. J. L., Chemotherapeutic and hormonal control of neoplasms of the female genital system. In: G. T. PACK and I. M. ARIEL (eds.), *Treatment of cancer and allied diseases,* vol. 6, p. 14. New York: Harper & Brothers 1962.

GEIST, S. H., *Ovarian tumors.* New York: Paul B. Hoeber 1942.

GRAHAM, J. B., GRAHAM, R. M., and SCHUELLER, E. F., Preclinical detection of ovarian cancer. *Cancer (Philad.)* **17**, 1414—1432 (1964).

GRAY, L. A., and BARNES, M. L., Carcinoma of the ovary. Report of 106 cases. *Ann. Surg.* **159**, 279—290 (1964).

GREEN jr., T. H., Hemisulphur mustard in the palliation of patients with metastatic ovarian carcinoma. *Obstet. and Gynec.* **13**, 383—393 (1959).

HERTIG, A. T., and GORE, H., *Tumors of the female sex organs*, sect. IX, fasc. 33, part 3. Armed Forces Institute of Pathology, Washington, D. C. 1961.

HRESHCHYSHYN, M. M., A critical review of chemotherapy in the treatment of ovarian carcinoma. *Clin. Obstet. Gynec.* **4**, 885 (1961).

KENT, S. W., and McKAY, D. G., Primary cancer of ovary. Analysis of 349 cases. *Amer. J. Obstet. Gynec.* **80**, 430—438 (1960).

KERR, H. D., and EINSTEIN, R. A. J., Results of irradiation of ovarian tumors. *Amer. J. Roentgenol.* **53**, 376—384 (1945).

—, and ELKINS, H. B., Carcinoma of the ovary. *Amer. J. Roentgenol.* **66**, 184—190 (1951).

KLIGERMAN, M. M., and HABIF, D. V., The use of radioactive gold in the treatment of effusion due to carcinomatosis of the pleura and peritoneum. *Amer. J. Roentgenol.* **74**, 651—656 (1955).

KOTTMEIER, H. L., Radiotherapy in the treatment of ovarian carcinoma. *Clin. Obstet. Gynec.* **4**, 865—874 (1961).

LATOUR, J. P. A., and DAVIS, B. A., Critical assessment of value of X-ray therapy in primary ovarian carcinoma. *Amer. J. Obstet. Gynec.* **74**, 968—981 (1957).

LONG, M. E., and TAYLOR jr., H. C., Endometrioid carcinoma of the ovary. *Amer. J. Obstet. Gynec.* **90**, 936—950 (1964).

MASTERSON, J. G., CALAME, R. J., and NELSON, J., A clinical study on the use of chlorambucil in the treatment of cancer of the ovary. *Amer. J. Obstet. Gynec.* **79**, 1002—1007 (1960).

MEIGS, J. V., The surgical treatment of cancer of the ovary. *Clin. Obstet. Gynec.* **4**, 846—854 (1961).

MONTGOMERY, J. B., and FARRELL jr., J. T., Value of postoperative irradiation in carcinoma of ovary. *Amer. J. Obstet. Gynec.* **28**, 365—377 (1934).

MORRIS, J. McL., and SCULLY, P. E., *Endocrine pathology of the ovary*. St. Louis: C. V. Mosby Co. 1958.

MULLER, J. H., First 5-year results of routine intracavitary administration of colloidal radioactive gold (Au 198) for the treatment of ovarian cancer. *Prog. nuclear Energy,* Series VII, 265 (1959).

PUROLA, E., Serous papillary ovarian tumors. A study of 233 cases with special reference to the histological type of tumour. *Acta obstet. gynec. scand.* **42**, Suppl. 3 (1963).

STANIČEK, J., ČERNOCH, A., u. ZAVŘEL, I., Die Grundsätze der chirurgischen Behandlung des Ovarialkarzinoms in der Kombination mit Radiogold 198 Au-Anwendung. *Neoplasma (Bratisl.)* **11**, 307 (1964).

TAYLOR jr., H. C., and MUNNELL, F. W., Treatment of tumors of the ovary. In: *Treatment of cancer and allied diseases.* (G. T. PACK and I. M. ARIEL, eds), vol. 6, p. 254. New York: Harper & Brothers 1962.

ULTMANN, J. E., HYMAN, G. A., CRANDALL, C., NAUJOKS, H., and GELLHORN, A., Triethylenethiophosphoramide (Thio-TEPA) in the treatment of neoplastic disease. *Cancer (Philad.)* **10**, 902 (1957).

WALTER, R. I., BACHMAN, A. L., and HARRIS, W., The treatment of carcinoma of the ovary. *Amer. J. Roentgenol.* **45**, 403—411 (1941).

WESTIN, B., Personal communication.

WINTZ, H., Die Röntgentherapie des Ovarialkarzinoms. *Strahlentherapie* **44**, 201 (1932).

WOODRUFF, J. D., and NOVAK, E. R., Papillary serous tumours of the ovary. *Amer. J. Obstet. Gynec.* **67**, 1112 (1954).

UICC Publications

Kaposi's Sarcoma. S. Karger AG., Basle (Switzerland) — New York (1963).

Cancer of the urinary bladder. S. Karger AG., Basle (Switzerland) — New York (1963).

Prognosis of malignant tumours of the breast. S. Karger AG., Basle (Switzerland) — New York (1963).

The lymphoreticular tumours in Africa. S. Karger AG., Basle (Switzerland) — New York (1964).

Cellular control mechanisms and cancer. Elsevier Publishing Company, Amsterdam — London — New York (1964).

Illustrated Tumor Nomenclature. Springer-Verlag Berlin — Heidelberg — New York (1965).

Structure and control of the melanocyte. Springer-Verlag Berlin — Heidelberg — New York (1966).

Public education about cancer; cancer education programmes in various countries. UICC, Geneva (1966).

Cancer incidence in five continents. Springer-Verlag Berlin — Heidelberg — New York (1966).

UICC Monograph Series

Vol. 1: Tumour specific antigens. Munksgaard, Copenhagen (1967).

Vol. 2: Cancer of the nasopharynx. Munksgaard, Copenhagen (1967).

Vol. 3: Choriocarcinoma. Springer-Verlag Berlin — Heidelberg — New York (1967).

Vol. 4: Cancer detection. Springer-Verlag Berlin — Heidelberg — New York (1967).

Vol. 5: Public education about cancer; research findings and theoretical concepts. Springer-Verlag Berlin — Heidelberg — New York (1967).

Vol. 6: Mechanisms of Invasion in Cancer. Springer-Verlag Berlin — Heidelberg — New York (1967).

Vol. 7: Potential Carcinogenic Hazard from Drugs. Springer-Verlag Berlin — Heidelberg — New York (1967).

Vol. 8: Treatment of Burkitt's Tumour. Springer-Verlag Berlin — Heidelberg — New York (1967).

Vol. 9: Proceedings of the Ninth International Cancer congress — Congress Lectures and Official Speeches. Springer-Verlag Berlin — Heidelberg — New York (1967).

Vol. 10: Proceedings of the Ninth International Cancer Congress — Panel discussions. Springer-Verlag Berlin — Heidelberg — New York (1967).